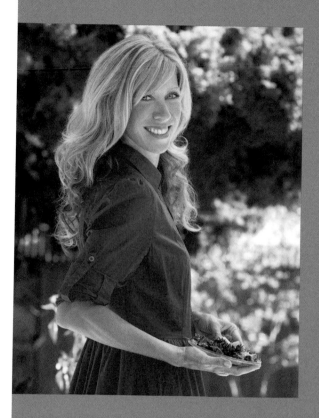

The 30-Day Vegan Challenge

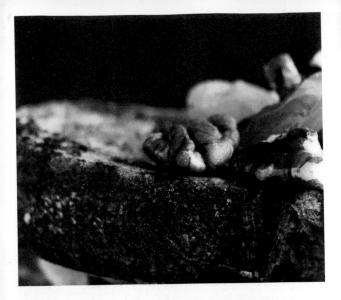
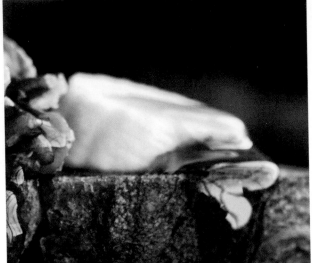

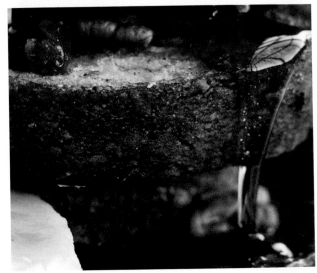

ALSO BY COLLEEN PATRICK-GOUDREAU

The Joy of Vegan Baking: The Compassionate Cooks' Traditional Treats and Sinful Sweets

The Vegan Table: 200 Unforgettable Recipes for Entertaining Every Guest at Every Occasion

Color Me Vegan: Maximize Your Nutrient Intake and Optimize Your Health by Eating Antioxidant-Rich, Fiber-Packed, Color-Intense Meals That Taste Great

Vegan's Daily Companion: 365 Days of Inspiration for Cooking, Eating, and Living Compassionately

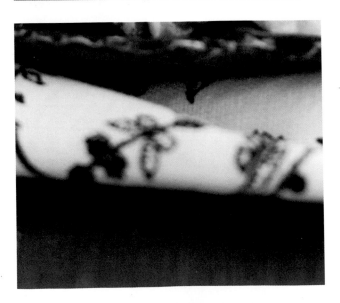
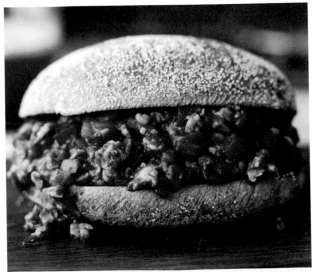

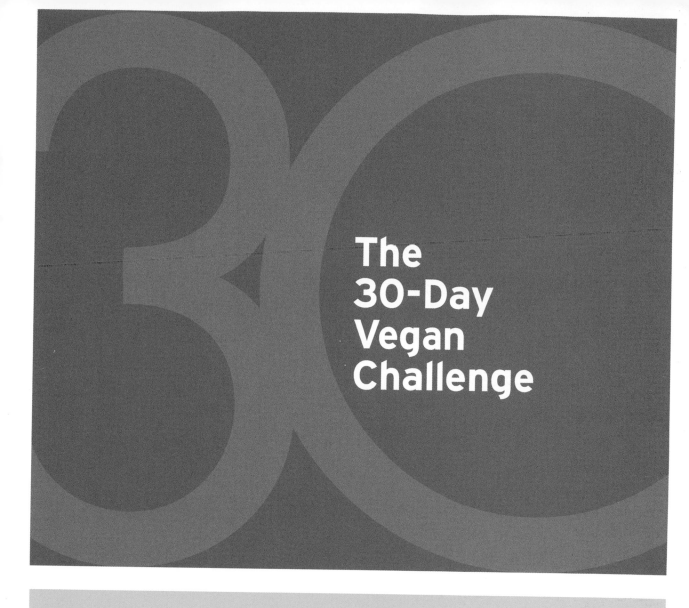

The
30-Day
Vegan
Challenge

THE ULTIMATE GUIDE TO EATING CLEANER, GETTING LEANER, AND LIVING COMPASSIONATELY

Colleen Patrick-Goudreau

BALLANTINE BOOKS   NEW YORK

No book can replace the diagnostic expertise and medical advice of a trusted physician. Please be certain to consult with your doctor before making any decisions that affect your health or extreme changes in your diet, particularly if you suffer from any medical condition or have any symptom that may require treatment.

A Ballantine Books Trade Paperback Original

Published in the United States by Ballantine Books,
an imprint of The Random House Publishing Group,
a division of Random House, Inc., New York.

BALLANTINE and colophon are registered trademarks of Random House, Inc.

LIBRARY OF CONGRESS CATALOGING-IN-PUBLICATION DATA
Patrick-Goudreau, Colleen.
The 30-day vegan challenge : the ultimate guide to eating cleaner,
getting leaner, and living compassionately / Colleen Patrick-Goudreau.
p. cm.
Includes bibliographical references and index.
ISBN 978-0-345-52617-5 (pbk. : alk. paper) − ISBN 978-0-440-42367-6 (ebook)
1. Vegetarianism. 2. Veganism. 3. Vegan cooking. 4. Diet therapy. 5. Nutrition.
6. Health. I. Title. II. Title: Thirty day vegan challenge.
TK392.P38 2011   613.2'622−dc23   2011017446

Printed in the United States of America

www.ballantinebooks.com

9 8 7 6 5 4 3 2 1

Katie Christ: food styling
Nissa Quanstrom: prop styling

Design by Debbie Glasserman

To my husband and fellow joyful vegan, David Goudreau,
whose unshakable support and unconditional love
are the foundation on which I stand

Foreword

In all likelihood, you have already made a spirited decision to accept the 30-Day Vegan Challenge and embark on what may very well be the journey of your life. While at this moment it may seem rather daunting, fear not; you could not have chosen a wiser way to begin.

The 30-Day Vegan Challenge is no ordinary book; it is an extraordinary vehicle of change that is beautifully crafted to offer every morsel of support imaginable as you venture through what may feel like unfamiliar territory. While your head may be spinning with questions, I can assure you that each and every one of those questions will be thoughtfully addressed in the pages that follow. Take a deep breath and know that you are in very capable hands.

My personal experience is as a registered dietitian. When I first decided to become vegan in the late 1980s, I was employed as a public health nutritionist. I was not sure if there was another vegan dietitian on the planet. I thought that once the truth was uncovered, I might very well be ousted from the profession. I wondered how I could remain in a career that had at its very foundation four food groups, two of which were animal-based. The only reference to vegan diets made during my entire university training was a stern warning that such extreme regimes were downright dangerous. After considerable soul-searching, I decided that I would stick with my chosen profession and make no apologies for my ethical choices. I decided that the balance of my career would be spent helping to ensure that those who had chosen a similar path would have the necessary nutrition information to succeed brilliantly.

With each passing year, the evidence in favor of plant-based diets grows stronger. Today, even the most conservative medical and dietetic organizations in the world acknowledge the safety, adequacy, and health benefits associated with vegan diets. This shift is solidly reflected in the marketplace, where mainstream manufacturers are increasingly using the word *vegan* on labels to sell their product. It is quite possible that these companies could find no single word that better captures the ideals consumers are seeking out—healthful, wholesome, responsible, ethical, and eco-friendly.

The evidence is quite clear that vegans have lower body mass indexes and are at reduced risk for most chronic diseases, including heart disease, hypertension, type 2 diabetes, and some forms of cancer. These are the very things that fill our doctors' offices, hospitals, and graveyards. We live in a food environment that is essentially toxic. The incontrovertible fact is that our food system is responsible for the vast majority of our health care expenditures. Well-planned vegan diets produce a dramatic shift in this paradigm. And while the personal health benefits of vegan diets are impressive, their consequences beyond personal health are perhaps even more compelling.

Adopting a vegan lifestyle is arguably the most powerful step any one individual can take toward the preservation of this planet. It takes about one-twentieth the resources to feed a vegan that it takes to feed a non-vegetarian. Intensive animal agriculture is simply not sustainable—it pollutes the air, the water, and the soil, and it is among our greatest contributors to deforestation, desertification, and species extinction. A 2008 award-winning study by researchers at Carnegie Mellon University found that our carbon footprint is more effectively reduced by eating 100 percent vegan one day a week than by eating 100 percent local seven days a week.

Perhaps the most gripping argument of all is that of ethics. Despite the fact that compassion is a guiding principle in all the world's religions and even in secular philosophies, the primary message we receive by the time we're adults is that compassion is acceptable as long as it is conditional and reserved only for certain groups—and species. One could argue that the process of turning innately compassionate children who identify deeply with animals into desensitized adults who participate directly and indirectly in violence against animals is what keeps us from being the fully enlightened, unconditionally compassionate human beings we are meant to be. Operating within the boundaries of selective compassion, we cannot but feel a weight on our minds and in our hearts.

Dr. Albert Schweitzer, one of the greatest humanitarians of all times, once predicted that "the time is coming when people will be amazed that the human race existed so long before it recognized that thoughtless injury to life is incompatible with real ethics. Ethics is in its unqualified form extended responsibility with regard to everything that has life."

Perhaps that time is here. Perhaps we need to put an end to viewing animals as resources to use as we please. The use of animals for human consumption is a cruel custom that is deeply entrenched in tradition and is both unnecessary and unjustifiable. Each and every one of us who dreams of a kinder, gentler world, who shares Schweitzer's vision of real ethics, has the capacity to turn thoughts into actions and to bring us a little closer to this reality. By picking up this book, you have taken the first courageous step toward this end.

When I had the privilege of reading *The 30-Day Vegan Challenge* in its entirety, I was touched by the compassion woven through each and every sentence. I was awed by the painstaking attention to detail and impressed by its reliability and readability. In a laudable effort to provide you with the most complete and practical guide possible, no stone was left unturned. Colleen Patrick-Goudreau is an outstanding writer and a remarkable human being. I cannot imagine finding a more capable and delightful partner in this journey. I am grateful that such a comprehensive resource exists and delighted that you have chosen to accept this challenge. May this journey be the journey of a lifetime. May it be a source of immeasurable rewards for you and for those with whom you are connected.

—Brenda Davis, R.D., author of *Becoming Vegan* and *Becoming Raw*

CONTENTS

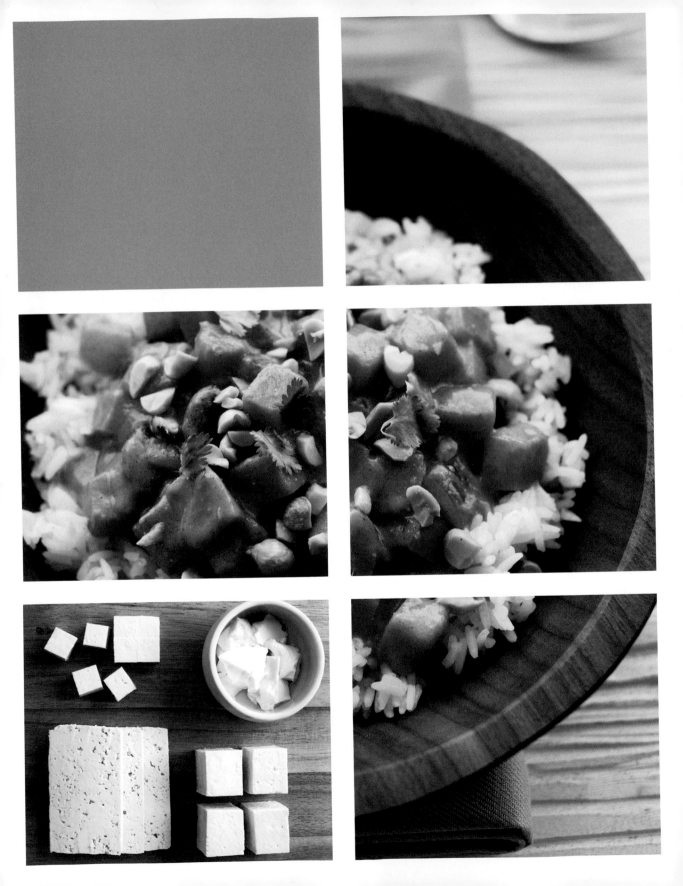

get ready!

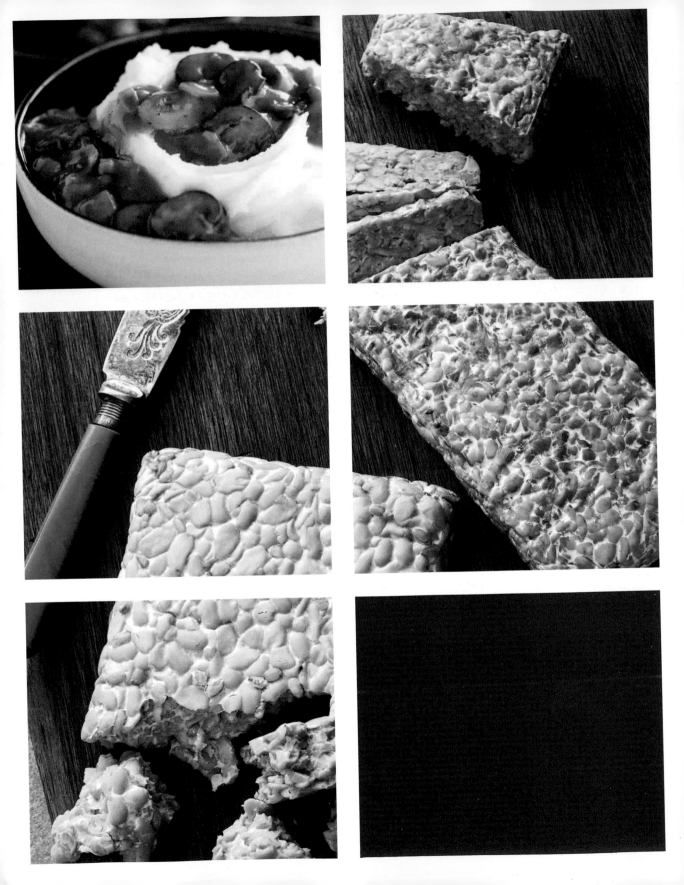

CHAPTER 1 Welcome to Positive Change

You may have come to the 30-Day Vegan Challenge motivated by a need to get healthier or lose weight, the desire to help decrease the use of the world's resources, or the compulsion to manifest your compassion for animals. Whatever your motivation, eliminating animal products from your diet—even for 30 days—will reap many benefits, some of which you may never have considered before.

Many of the changes people experience are immediate, some are noticeable by the end of 30 days, and all of them can be broken down into several categories of positive change in terms of nutrient consumption, disease prevention and reversal, physical changes, palate sensitivity, and a sense of ethical congruency.

NUTRIENT CONSUMPTION

Being vegan is as much about what you take in as it is about what you eliminate.

Expect More

As soon as you eliminate meat, dairy, and eggs from your diet and fill it instead with plant foods, I can absolutely guarantee you will be eating more fiber, more antioxidants, more folate, and more phytochemicals, because the source of these healthful substances is plants, not animals. You will also be taking in more essential vitamins and minerals, because—as you will discover on the following pages—the nutrients we need are *plant-based*, not animal-based.

Expect None

I can also guarantee that you will be consuming no dietary cholesterol, no lactose, no animal protein, no animal hormones, no animal fat, and no aberrant proteins that cause mad cow disease (bovine spongiform encephalopathy)—all of which originate in animal products and not in plants. Not only are these things unnecessary, they can all be harmful to the human body.

Expect Significantly Less

Making whole foods the foundation of your diet, which is what I recommend, means that you will be significantly reducing your consumption of many other disease-causing substances, including:

- **SATURATED FAT:** Though it exists mostly in animal flesh and secretions, saturated fat is also found in small amounts in plant foods, primarily from coconuts. However, plant-based saturated fat is chemically different from animal-based saturated fat and does not appear to have the same negative effect on our bodies. In other words, a little coconut butter or coconut milk in your diet is fine—possibly even beneficial.

- **HEAVY METALS:** Heavy metals such as mercury and other toxins settle in the fatty flesh of animals and are consumed by humans through their consumption of fish, dairy, and meat. The reason I didn't add this to the "Expect None" category is because even vegans consume low levels of heavy metals that end up on our food, but in significantly smaller quantities.

- **FOODBORNE ILLNESSES:** Although fruits and vegetables you buy in a store or restaurant can be contaminated by animal feces (and thus salmonella, campylobacter, E. coli, etc.), if you keep a vegan kitchen, the worst things you might find are aphids in your kale and a borer worm in your corn.

- **TRANS FATS:** By following my recommendations for eating whole foods, you take in far fewer trans fats, which are prevalent in processed foods via partially hydrogenated oils and which are also present in animal-based meat.

DISEASE PREVENTION AND REVERSAL

Decades of research have borne out the many benefits of a vegan diet in terms of disease prevention and reversal.

If your goal is prevention, treatment, or reversal of cardiovascular disease (particularly atherosclerosis, which causes heart attacks and strokes), you couldn't make a better dietary change than switching to a whole-foods, plant-based diet. And by the end of 30 days, you will see changes in the markers for these diseases.

Countless studies also point to the fact that a vegan diet contributes to reduced risk of type 2 diabetes, certain cancers—particularly prostate, colon, and breast—macular degeneration, cataracts, arthritis, and osteoporosis. See "Resources and Recommendations" for books and experts who specialize in these fields of research and treatment.

PHYSICAL CHANGES

Typically, the physical changes people detect have to do with what they tend to lose, but there are gains to be made, too.

Expect to Lose

People tend to lose weight when they remove fat- and calorie-dense meat, dairy, and eggs from their diet; they tend to notice a decrease in the severity of their allergies; and women tend to experience fewer PMS and menopausal symptoms.

Expect to Gain

Many people who switch to a vegan diet notice they have more energy, brighter skin with fewer blemishes, and an increase in the number of times they move their bowels, which is definitely beneficial for short- and long-term gastrointestinal health.

PALATE SENSITIVITY

Many people report that once their palate and body begin to know life without being coated by fat and salt, cravings for these things are greatly reduced or totally eliminated. As a result, your palate may become more sensitive, you may taste flavors you never noticed before, and you may even have a more acute sense of smell.

ETHICAL CONGRUENCY

The harder-to-measure goals are those that have to do with what it feels like to make choices that reflect our values. Prior to becoming vegan, I perceived myself as a conscious, compassionate person, yet I was supporting what is very likely the most violent industry on the planet. I was paying people to be desensitized and to do what I would never do myself: hurt and kill animals. I still consider myself a conscious, compassionate, nonviolent person, but now those values are authentically reflected in my everyday behavior. There is much joy and peace in living in alignment with my values.

GETTING STARTED

Since you're holding this book in your hands now, I'll assume that you know *why* you want to make some changes and that you're eager to reap one or more of the benefits I've identified above. Perhaps, though, you're unclear about *how* to make this transition—smoothly, joyfully, healthfully, and confidently. Let me assure you that whatever compels you to become vegan and however you identify yourself at this moment (carnivore, omnivore, pescetarian, flexitarian, vegetarian), the transition process is the same for everyone: it's a matter of undoing old habits and creating new ones.

In my experience, when most people contemplate becoming vegan, they feel utterly over-whelmed because it seems so unfamiliar and they don't know where to start. Many who try and fail conclude—mistakenly—that being vegan is an ideal that only a disciplined few can attain. They think being vegan requires willpower they don't have, so either they don't even try or they give up after a short time. Filled with questions and misconceptions, what they need is a personal guide to hold their hand through the transition period, debunking myths and demystifying what it means to "be vegan."

Enter *The 30-Day Vegan Challenge*—your very own personal guide.

I take the approach that it is not the fault of "being vegan" that people revert back to eat-ing meat and animal products or that they are unable to even go a month without them. Rather, I believe it's because core habits and perceptions remained unchanged, support during the transition process was nonexistent, and a dietary foundation was removed but not replaced with anything else to stand on. You won't have those issues. You will have my guidance and support the entire time.

Throughout the next 30 days, I will:

- Debunk myths using common sense so you will make informed decisions with confi-dence
- Get to the root of old perceptions and behaviors so that change is effortless
- Anticipate your challenges and provide validation and support
- Help you create a strong foundation of new habits
- Provide practical solutions for a variety of scenarios

You might choose to read only one chapter per day, or you may want to read well ahead. You may want to dive into the recipes dispersed throughout the book or use the weekly menu ideas on page 297 to plan your bountiful meals. Whichever way you choose to digest the information, you can be sure that along the way, some old thought patterns will be challenged and some new behaviors will be created.

If change is what you're looking for, then change is what you'll get, and I commend you for seeking it out. Change is often one of the most difficult things for humans to cope with—even when that change is positive. How many of us avoid making changes until we're absolutely forced to? How many of us engage in habits that make us sick rather than sim-ply change the way we eat? I've even heard doctors freely admit that they don't always give their patients the option of making true diet changes—beyond advising them to switch from "red meat" to "white meat"—because they believe people won't change.

Now, you can call me crazy, but I have more faith in people than that. I know people change. I see it every single day. When the bar is raised and people are given the tools and resources they need to feel empowered, they do change. The problem is, the more we keep telling people it's too hard to change, the more they just believe it.

The more we buy into the myths that there's something radical about eating fruits, vegetables, nuts, grains, seeds, beans, mushrooms, herbs, and spices and something extreme about *not* eating the bodies and secretions of nonhuman animals, the less we'll expect of ourselves and others. And nothing will change.

But by holding the bar high, we see radical changes take place in people—physically, emotionally, and spiritually.

All I ask is that you remain open. Never say never. Embrace the journey that encourages us to be humble, to learn new things, to become better people. That's what being human is all about, isn't it? We can continually make new choices, better choices, more compassionate choices—once we know better.

By virtue of your picking up this book and being willing to take the 30-Day Vegan Challenge, you've raised the bar. I thank you for letting me be part of your journey, and may you find joy and abundance in the changes you make.

CHAPTER 2 Defining "Vegan"

Because there are many misunderstandings and misconceptions about what being vegan means, let's start out defining what I mean when I say *vegan*. In the most literal sense:

- Being vegetarian means to eat everything but the flesh of animals, whether they are from the land or sea (including fish).

- To be vegan—pronounced VEE-gun—means to eat everything but the flesh *and* secretions of animals (including their milk and eggs).

In defining what it means to be vegan, it's important to talk about the history of the word *vegan*, which was coined in 1944 by British activist Donald Watson (1910-2005). Founder of the first vegan organization, Watson crafted the word *vegan* from the beginning and the end of the word *vegetarian*, because he was frustrated that being vegetarian had come to include eating dairy products and eggs.

Watson defined veganism as "a philosophy and way of living which seeks to exclude—as far as is possible and practical—all forms of exploitation of and cruelty to animals for food, clothing, or any other purpose."

And although being vegan—as Watson defined it—is about making conscious, compassionate choices, I think he would agree with my perception that it is not about trying to attain an impossible level of purity or striving to become a 100 percent certified vegan. There is no such thing—the world is just too imperfect for that. Even Watson acknowledges this in his definition when he uses this qualifier: "as far as is possible and practical."

Contrary to what many people believe, being vegan is not an end in itself. It is a *means* to an end. For me, that end is unconditional compassion: doing everything we can to make choices that cause the least amount of harm, both to ourselves and to others. And being vegan is an easy and effective step toward attaining that goal.

Though Watson coined the term *vegan* less than a century ago, the principle of compassion has been a guiding force in all the world's religions and secular philosophies for centuries. The idea of nonviolence, of *ahimsa*—causing no harm—is certainly not a new idea, and veganism is simply an extension of that principle. This is why I use the words *vegan* and *compassionate* interchangeably.

However, when people hear the word *vegan,* they tend to associate it with asceticism or martyrdom, deprivation or sacrifice. They often think being vegan is about rejecting things—about saying no. On one hand, this is true. Being vegan *is* about saying no. It's about saying no to suffering, exploitation, and violence. It's about saying no to unhealthful and unnecessary food. It's about saying no to the wasteful abuse of natural resources and the destruction of the remaining wild places in the world.

But at its core, being vegan is about saying yes. It's about saying yes to our values; after all, what's the use in having values if they don't manifest themselves in our behavior? It's nice to say that we're against violence and cruelty. Most of us are. But how many of us actually take these abstract values and put them into concrete action? For me, being vegan, which extends to every area of my life, is an opportunity to do just that: to put my abstract values into concrete action.

By choosing to look at what happens to other animals—human and nonhuman—on my behalf, for my convenience, I'm saying yes to my values of accountability, responsibility, and commitment to truth and knowledge.

By standing up for what I believe in and speaking on behalf of those who have no voice, I'm saying yes to my values of justice and of service to others.

By choosing to eat life-giving rather than life-taking foods, I'm saying yes to my values of peace, kindness, compassion, health, and simplicity.

The problem isn't that we wake up in the morning wanting to contribute to cruelty or violence. The problem is that we don't wake up in the morning wanting to create more compassion, peace, and nonviolence. If that were on our to-do list every day, imagine what we could accomplish. Imagine what our world would be like. Making choices that reflect nonviolence has an undeniable effect on our own psyches. That is to say, whereas violence creates more violence, nonviolence also creates more nonviolence, and I like being on that side of the equation.

TAKING VEGAN FOOD OUT OF THE BOX

In the many years I've been doing this work, what I know for sure is that people want to make healthful choices, but they also want these choices to be convenient and familiar, and they assume being vegan is neither.

This assumption has more to do with our perception than reality.

We tend to put "normal" or "regular" food in one box and "vegan" food in another, as if the latter were its own alien food group. The truth is, vegan food is food that we're all familiar with—it's vegetables, fruits, grains, legumes, nuts, seeds, mushrooms, herbs, and spices. In the case of baked goods, it's flour, sugar, cocoa, chocolate, vanilla, spices, baking soda, baking powder, cornstarch, and yeast.

When you get down to it, vegan food is food we already cook with and already love. You just might not call it vegan. If you've had an apple, you've had "vegan food." If you've ever eaten spaghetti with marinara sauce, you've had "vegan food." When we take it out of the box called "vegan," we recognize that it's not so unfamiliar after all.

It's no surprise we have these misconceptions about veganism. We are taught this early on in our culture: that meat, dairy, and eggs are "normal" food for regular folk and that vegan food is unsubstantial and lacking, reserved for "health freaks" or the allergy-prone. In fact, these misperceptions lead people to believe that many familiar favorites are not vegan, so let's set the record straight here and now.

- **BREAD IS VEGAN:** It's true that some brands and types of commercial breads have animal's milk added to them—but not all. Good bread—real bread—is naturally vegan. Just think of the definition of bread according to French law: it can contain nothing more than flour, salt, water, and yeast.

- **PASTA IS VEGAN:** Although some pastas (namely, egg noodles) have chicken's eggs added to them, by definition pasta is really just made from flour and water. In fact, the word originally meant "pastry dough sprinkled with salt."

- **COCOA BUTTER IS VEGAN:** We tend to associate the word *butter* with dairy, but it really has more to do with fat than with cow's milk. Peanut butter, cocoa butter, coconut butter, almond butter, and shea butter are all plant-based fats. Just because it says "butter" doesn't mean it's an animal product.

- **VEGANS EAT YEAST:** Considering the fact that yeasts are microorganisms classified as fungi, not animals, of course vegans eat yeast!

These and other myths will be debunked throughout *The 30-Day Vegan Challenge*. The good news is we can change our minds and change our behavior. After all, the foods we choose, the meals we plan, and the choices we make are all habits. They're deeply ingrained cultural, personal, familial, and social habits, but they're all habits.

I learned long ago that it's not that we *can* make a difference in the world and in our own lives; it's that we *do* make a difference—every day, with every choice we make. Every action we take, every product we buy, every dollar we spend, *everything* we do or eat has an effect on something or someone else. *There are no neutral actions.*

I think this idea is both empowering and frightening to many of us. It's empowering because it means *we're* responsible and have a tremendous amount of power. It's frightening because it means that *we're* responsible and have a tremendous amount of power. We get to choose not whether we want to make a difference but whether the difference we inevitably make is positive or negative. That's it. Those are our only two choices. There are no neutral actions.

My hope is that your daily choices become a reflection of your deepest values—for the next 30 days and the rest of your journey.

> **CHALLENGE YOUR THINKING:** We get to choose not whether we want to make a difference or not but whether the difference we inevitably make is positive or negative. Those are our only two choices. There are no neutral actions.

CHAPTER 3   Why 30 Days?

Most behavioral experts agree that it takes three weeks to change a habit, and that to do so successfully, the key is to replace old behaviors with new ones. The 30-Day Vegan Challenge is all about creating new habits and new perceptions, and I provide an extra week just to make sure we cover all of your questions and challenges. I also like the roundness of a 30-day cycle, giving your body enough time to respond in such a way that you will be able to measure improvement.

Most people find it remarkable that the body can change and heal so quickly with food and not pharmaceuticals, though it's been demonstrated again and again. We know this simply on an anecdotal level—feeling energized and clean after eating a healthful nutrient-dense meal or heavy and sick after a rich fat-laden meal—and this is validated on a clinical level by taking blood before and after a meal and noting differences in blood cholesterol, blood pressure, blood glucose, and the like. With our ability to measure such specifics, we know that after *one meal* our body chemistry changes negatively or positively depending on what we eat. After *one meal*.

The body is a complex organism, but in many ways its needs are simple. In fact, if we whittled it down, we can say that a healthy body is all about blood flow—keeping that blood flowing through our arteries to get to all the places it needs to go, easily and without hindrance.

Each time we eat, we have the choice to consume substances that hinder this blood flow or help it. After decades of research in the field of food and health, one thing is clear: animal products (meat, dairy, and eggs) hinder blood flow, and plant foods increase blood flow. This is why people see significant, tangible, measurable changes in their blood within 30 days of beginning to eat vegan. Like water that runs through an unblocked hose, the blood is able to run easily through the arteries—both because of the improved consistency of the blood and because of the openness of the arteries themselves.

To experience these changes, however, requires a little openness. It requires surrendering some old notions and being willing to have a new understanding. I've heard every excuse in the book and know how attached people are to their meat and animal products.

- **SOME PEOPLE ARE SKEPTICAL.** Having been utterly disempowered by the modern medical system, many people believe that their genes have already determined their fate. Rather than believe they have a part to play in their health, they have made scapegoats of their ancestors and thrown up their hands. To them I say, try it for 30 days. You have nothing to lose.

- **SOME PEOPLE SAY THEY "DON'T EAT A LOT OF MEAT AND DAIRY"** and so wouldn't benefit very much from taking this stuff out of their diets completely. In the many years I've been doing this work, I haven't met one person who doesn't have this perception of him- or herself. But I have to ask: compared to what? Compared to how much you *could* eat? Compared to how much they ate a hundred years ago? What barometer are we using when we say that? The truth is, you don't know how much of this stuff you're eating until you stop, and that's one of the benefits of the 30-Day Vegan Challenge. Your dietary habits become crystal clear.

  So to those who don't think you eat that much meat, dairy, and eggs, I say great. It just means it will be that much easier for you to stop completely for 30 days!

- **SOME PEOPLE THINK THEY'RE TOO OLD TO MAKE CHANGES.** Resigning themselves to the "inevitable" diseases and medications associated with "getting older," these folks insist you can't teach an old dog new tricks. I disagree. The reality is, it doesn't matter how old we are when we decide to make changes. Our food habits were ingrained in us by the time we were about 5 years old, and we carry these habits with us into adulthood. It doesn't matter if you're 30 or 40 or 18 or 80, a habit is a habit is a habit.

  The behaviorists who say it takes three weeks to change a habit don't make qualifications based on age. They don't say it takes three weeks to change a habit if you're 25 years old but three months to change a habit if you're 70. It's the same no matter how old you are. You just have to be willing to cast off some familiar behaviors and perceptions and try on some new ones.

Although they are deeply ingrained in us, our habits do not reflect who we really are. By definition, a habit is just a behavioral pattern we've created over time. In fact, the word *habit* originally referred to something that was worn (and is still used to refer to the garb of some religious persons, such as nuns), which means it can just as easily be put on as taken off.

That's the good news and that's the bad news. It's the bad news because we're tenacious creatures of habit, but it's the good news because habits are meant to be broken. And 30 days gives you plenty of time to take off the old and don the new.

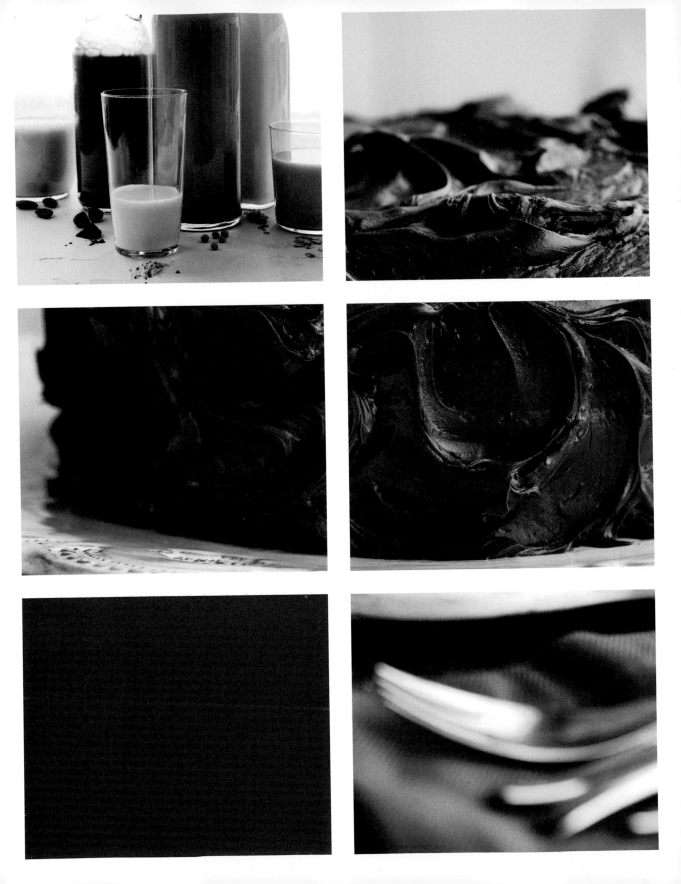

get set!

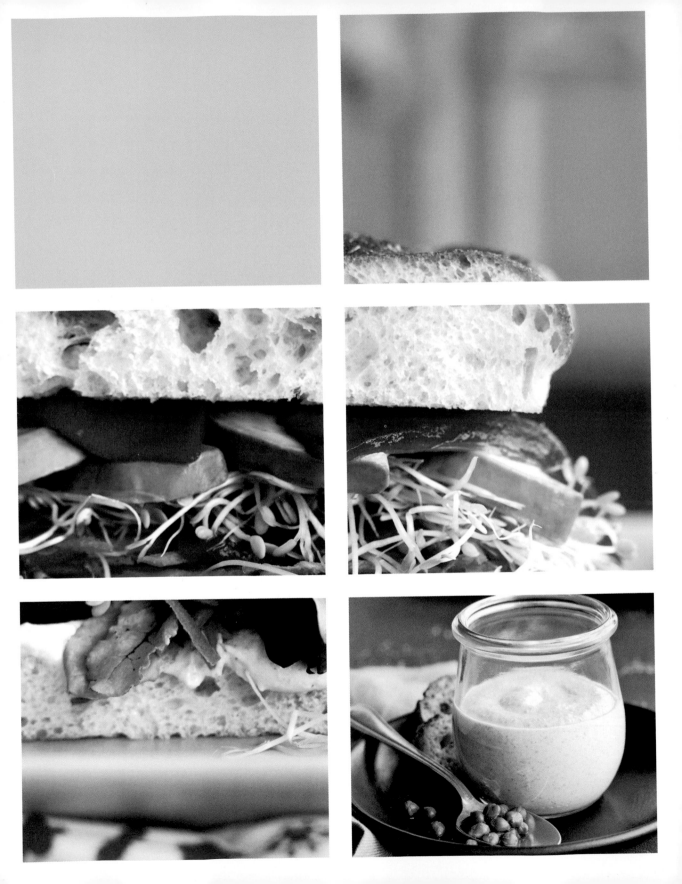

CHAPTER 4 Know Your Numbers

By the end of the 30 days, you will no doubt experience changes that are impossible to measure—changes in your outlook, energy level, perspective, and overall well-being—but you will also most likely experience physiological and biochemical changes that you can track and measure.

In order to see the tangible differences yourself, if would be helpful to visit your health professional before you start the 30-Day Vegan Challenge to get a health check as well as a full blood and urine panel. (To get an accurate B_{12} level, request a urine MMA test or get it online through www.b12.com.) Once you have the results back and understand what they mean, *let the 30-Day Vegan Challenge begin.*

You may be surprised to learn that measurable differences can be seen by eliminating meat, dairy, and eggs for just 30 days, but the more closely you follow my guidelines for eating a healthful, whole-foods, plant-based diet (including the recommendations for supplements), the greater the likelihood of noticeable improvements in your numbers.

The results of these laboratory tests are helpful tools for evaluating your health status, but keep in mind that there is the normal or standard value and then there is the optimal or therapeutic target, which are levels associated with the most minimal risk for developing diseases. For some of the tests I mention below, when these numbers differ, I provide both. Obviously, the numbers to shoot for are those that are optimal, not average; after all, do we want ideal health or just average health? Also, keep in mind that some recommendations for normal values are based on old research and may be influenced by biased sources. I note those below, too.

Common laboratory tests span a wide spectrum, so I'm including only a few. Your health professional can help you interpret others not listed here.

BODY WEIGHT

When it comes to evaluating weight and its impact on your health, it's not just a matter of what the scale says. Rather, your percentage of body fat, waist circumference, and body mass index (BMI) should all be considered.

In the last several decades, a number of different tables have been devised to help people determine their "ideal weight." The ones that were most widely used for decades were those created by the Metropolitan Life Insurance Company in 1942 and subsequently updated over the years. (You can find these tables with a quick search online.) Although on an individual basis, these height/weight tables provide very little information about an individual's health risk, they may be helpful when used in conjunction with other measurements to indicate whether or not you are within a healthy weight range.

BMI (BODY MASS INDEX)

One of the most accurate ways of assessing whether or not you are overweight or obese is to determine what percentage of your body weight is fat. However, getting accurate body fat measurements can be expensive and difficult, so the body mass index (BMI) was created in 1998 by the National Institutes of Health (NIH). This guide has essentially replaced the old life insurance tables as a method to gauge healthy weight and helps doctors, researchers, dietitians, and government agencies get on the same page regarding weight recommendations. The same scale is used for men and women.

Body mass index is a measure of body weight relative to height. Using the table opposite, find your height in the left-hand column, and move across the same row to the number closest to your weight. The number at the top of that column is your BMI.

According to NIH standards, you are considered overweight if you have a BMI between 25 and 29.9 and obese if you have a BMI of 30 or higher. You're at a healthy weight if your BMI is between 18.5 and 24.9.

One of the main problems with using body mass index *alone* is that it doesn't factor in muscle mass, so people such as body builders will have a high BMI but actually low body fat. Thus, it's useful to factor in waist circumference.

WAIST CIRCUMFERENCE

Waist circumference is a helpful measurement because your health is affected not only by excess body fat but also by where the fat is located. Some people gain weight in the abdominal area (the so-called apple shape), others around their hips and buttocks (pear-shaped bodies). People with the former are at higher risk for heart disease and type 2 diabetes.

COMPASSIONATE COOKS BMI INDEX CHART

HEIGHT WEIGHT (lbs / kgs)

		100	105	110	115	120	125	130	135	140	145	150	155	160	165	170	175	180	185	190	195	200	205	210	215	220	225	230	235	240	245	250
in	kgs	45.5	47.7	50.0	52.3	54.5	56.8	59.1	61.4	63.6	65.9	68.2	70.5	72.7	75.0	77.3	79.5	81.8	84.1	86.4	88.6	90.9	93.2	95.5	97.7	100	102.3	104.6	106.8	109.1	111.4	113.8
5'0"	152.4	19	20	21	22	23	24	25	26	27	28	29	30	31	32	33	34	35	36	37	38	39	40	41	42	43	44	45	46	47	48	49
5'1"	154.9	18	19	20	21	22	23	24	25	26	27	28	29	30	31	32	33	34	35	36	37	38	39	40	41	42	43	44	45	46	47	48
5'2"	157.4	18	19	20	21	22	22	23	24	25	26	27	28	29	30	31	32	33	34	35	36	37	38	39	40	41	42	43	44	45	46	47
5'3"	160.0	17	18	19	20	21	22	23	24	25	26	27	28	28	29	30	31	32	33	34	35	36	36	37	38	39	40	41	42	43	44	45
5'4"	162.5	17	18	19	20	21	21	22	23	24	25	26	27	28	29	29	30	31	32	33	34	34	35	36	37	38	39	40	40	41	42	43
5'5"	165.1	16	17	18	19	20	21	22	22	23	24	25	26	27	27	28	29	30	31	32	33	33	34	35	36	37	38	38	39	40	41	42
5'6"	167.6	16	17	18	19	19	20	21	22	23	23	24	25	26	27	27	28	29	30	31	31	32	33	34	35	36	36	37	38	39	40	40
5'7"	170.1	15	16	17	18	19	20	20	21	22	23	24	24	25	26	27	27	28	29	30	31	31	32	33	34	34	35	36	37	38	38	39
5'8"	172.7	15	16	17	17	18	19	20	21	21	22	23	24	25	25	26	27	28	28	29	30	30	31	32	33	33	34	35	36	36	37	38
5'9"	175.2	14	15	16	17	18	18	19	20	21	21	22	23	24	24	25	26	27	27	28	29	30	30	31	32	32	33	34	35	35	36	37
5'10"	177.8	14	15	16	16	17	18	19	19	20	21	22	22	23	24	24	25	26	27	27	28	29	29	30	31	31	32	33	34	34	35	36
5'11"	180.3	14	14	15	16	17	17	18	19	20	20	21	22	22	23	24	24	25	26	27	27	28	29	29	30	31	31	32	33	33	34	35
6'0"	182.8	13	14	15	16	16	17	18	18	19	20	20	21	22	22	23	24	24	25	26	26	27	28	28	29	30	30	31	32	33	33	34
6'1"	185.4	13	14	15	15	16	17	17	18	19	19	20	21	21	22	23	23	24	24	25	26	26	27	28	28	29	30	30	31	32	32	33
6'2"	187.9	12	13	14	14	15	16	16	17	18	18	19	20	20	21	22	22	23	24	24	25	25	26	27	27	28	29	29	30	31	31	32
6'3"	190.5	12	13	13	14	15	15	16	16	17	18	18	19	20	20	21	22	22	23	24	24	25	25	26	27	27	28	29	29	30	31	31
6'4"	193.0	12	12	13	14	14	15	15	16	17	17	18	18	19	20	20	21	22	22	23	24	24	25	25	26	27	27	28	29	29	30	30

Underweight
Healthy
Overweight
Obese
Extremely Obese

THE 30-DAY VEGAN CHALLENGE ■ 19

According to the NIH, a waist circumference greater than 40 inches for men and 35 inches for women is linked to a higher risk of type 2 diabetes, high blood pressure, high cholesterol levels, and heart disease.

To properly measure your waist, place a tape measure around your middle, just above your hipbones but below your rib cage. Breathe out, and measure.

PERCENTAGE OF BODY FAT

You can determine your body fat percentage by using one of those little devices called calipers, often available at your local gym or doctor's office. This is basically a skinfold test to determine the thickness of the subcutaneous fat layer at three or seven sites on the body, which is then converted to estimate fat percentage. A body fat level greater than 17 percent in men and 27 percent in women indicates you're overweight, while a body fat level of more than 25 percent in men and 31 percent in women indicates obesity.

BLOOD PRESSURE

Blood pressure is a measure of how hard blood is pressing against artery walls, like water running through a hose. Ideally, you want the top number to be under 120 and the bottom number under 80. The risk for strokes and heart attacks starts progressively climbing after 115/75 mm Hg. You can test your blood pressure using machines available in many pharmacies and doctors' offices, or buy a device to check at home. See "Resources and Recommendations."

BLOOD GLUCOSE

According to the American Diabetes Association, it is estimated that 18 million people in the United States have been diagnosed with diabetes, another 5.7 million are undiagnosed, and 57 million are prediabetic.

One to three different glucose tests are given by doctors to make a diagnosis.

- The first test checks the amount of glucose in your blood at any given time during the day, regardless of the last meal eaten. A glucose value of 200 mg/dl (plus diabetes symptoms) is a good indicator of diabetes.

- The second test is a fasting blood glucose, which is done after you have fasted for a minimum of eight hours. Fasting glucose should be in the range of 70 to 110 mg/dl; a fasting glucose level of 126 mg/dl or more indicates diabetes.

- The third test is an oral glucose tolerance test to see how well your body deals with sugar. Normally, blood sugar rises after you eat and then returns to normal levels (70 to 110 mg/dl) within an hour or two. Higher values mean your body has trouble moving glucose out of the blood and into the cells.

The 57 million people with prediabetes have a fasting blood glucose level of 110 to 125 mg/dl and a postmeal level of 140 to 200 mg/dl—not high enough to be considered diabetes but higher than what is considered normal.

CHOLESTEROL

We all throw around words such as *cholesterol,* and "good and bad cholesterol," though many of us don't really know what this stuff is or what it does. Made in the liver of animals, cholesterol is a fatlike substance we consume in our diets via meat, dairy, and eggs (there is no dietary cholesterol in plant foods). Though our bodies also produce cholesterol—we are, after all, animals—we have no requirement to *consume* dietary cholesterol. The cholesterol made by our bodies travels through the bloodstream in little packages called lipoproteins.

- Low-density lipoproteins (LDL or "bad" cholesterol) deliver cholesterol *to* the body.

- High-density lipoproteins (HDL or "good" cholesterol) take cholesterol *out* of the bloodstream.

When there is too much cholesterol in the bloodstream, it's a major risk factor for heart and blood vessel disease. To determine cardiovascular disease risk, doctors look at total cholesterol, LDL, HDL, and the ratio of the latter two.

Because the average cholesterol level in the United States is so high (around 235), recommendations indicate that total cholesterol should be reduced to below 200. Although it's true that people with a level of 200 are at lower risk than those at 235, they are still at significantly high risk. In fact, about 35 percent of those who have heart attacks have cholesterol levels between 160 and 200.

After decades of research, including longtime landmark studies such as the Framingham Heart Study and the China Diet Study, it is evident that the optimal level for total cholesterol is below 150. What's more, with a cholesterol level under 150, you don't really have to concern yourself with the further breakdown of "good" and "bad" cholesterol, outlined below.

LDL ("bad") cholesterol: less than 100 is optimal
HDL ("good") cholesterol: between 40 and 60 is optimal

Important note: A nutrient-dense plant-based diet makes the HDL portion of cholesterol *lower* because *all* portions of the total cholesterol number are reduced. In other words, don't be misguided into thinking something is wrong when your HDL level falls when you become vegan. On the other hand, a very high HDL level (60 or above) is not always a good sign, either. It means the HDL is working harder to get cholesterol out of the bloodstream. The more cholesterol, the more work it has to do.

TRIGLYCERIDES

Triglycerides are fatty substances that—like cholesterol—are made in the liver and circulate in the bloodstream. High levels indicate a risk of cardiovascular disease and are associated with pancreatitis.

Although medical establishments consider triglyceride levels of 100 to 150 mg/dl "normal" or "good," many experts feel that optimal fasting blood triglyceride levels should be 50 to 150 mg/dl. Levels of 200 to 500 mg/dl are considered high.

HOMOCYSTEINE

Homocysteine is an amino acid that is normally found in small amounts in the blood. Higher levels are associated with increased risk of cardiovascular disease, venous thrombosis, dementia, and Alzheimer's disease. The optimal range is between 6 and 8 μmol/l.

Note: Keeping homocysteine at levels associated with lower rates of disease requires adequate intake of both vitamin B_{12} (through supplements or fortified foods) and folate (through green leafy vegetables) or folic acid (through multivitamins).

VITAMINS

Because there are some vitamin deficiencies in the typical American diet, it is also worth looking at the following prior to and after the 30-Day Vegan Challenge.

- VITAMIN D. Americans are deficient in vitamin D more any other vitamin. Experts' opinions vary between shooting for 35 to 45 ng/ml and 50 to 70 ng/ml as the optimal range although some believe that levels as low as 20ng/ml may be sufficient.

- VITAMIN B_{12}. A level above 400 pg/ml is optimal.

See "Resources and Recommendations" for at-home testing kits for vitamin D levels.

Don't forget to return to your health professional to get another blood/urine panel taken at the end of the 30 days in order to note improvements.

CHAPTER 5

Complete Your 3-Day Food Diary

Though many people protest that they "don't eat a lot of meat, dairy, and eggs," the truth is you have no idea how much you're eating until you stop and examine your daily food choices more closely.

For this reason, I recommend keeping a food log for three days prior to starting the Challenge (including at least one weekend day, since we tend to eat differently and usually more decadently on Saturdays and Sundays) to help you see in black and white what your diet is like before you begin. You may be surprised.

For three days before beginning (perhaps while you're waiting for your blood test results), simply write down everything you eat and drink (except water). Be sure to include every last morsel: condiments, what you put in your coffee, the soda you order at lunch, a candy bar you get from the vending machine at work, and even the cheese you sprinkle on your pasta.

Carry a small notebook around with you to make it easier, and be as thorough as possible. This kind of food tracking will not be necessary once you begin the Challenge. It's simply to enable you to accurately assess your current diet as compared to how you'll be eating once the 30-Day Vegan Challenge begins. It will also help you identify your favorite and most regularly eaten foods so you can easily veganize them, as suggested in subsequent chapters.

CHAPTER 6 Find a Buddy

Whether you're taking the 30-Day Vegan Challenge on a whim or want to make long-lasting changes in your life, this process will be a lot more enjoyable if you do it with someone else—perhaps a friend or coworker. Together you can exchange ideas, compare notes, provide support, and cook with and for each other.

In addition, I encourage you to ask your family members or anyone with whom you live to join you in the Challenge. Because you share meals and values, it will make the process less stressful if everyone is on the same page and eating the same foods at home.

Any kind of change is hard, and the more support you can get from your loved ones, the more successful you will be. However, when the changes we make affect the people closest to us or reflect back to them something they're not comfortable seeing in themselves, it can create tidal waves in an otherwise calm sea—especially when food is a factor.

I hear from so many people whose otherwise loving and supportive family members become irate at the idea that their spouse or sibling or adult child has become vegan. Keep in mind that because they have not experienced the same desire to eschew animal products, they may not understand why their loved one has, and they may feel threatened by any change in their normal routine. Even if you've said nothing to make them feel this way, they might feel judged or guilty for wanting to continue to eat meat, dairy, and eggs.

Taking the 30-Day Vegan Challenge—and reading this book—*together* will potentially lessen the tension that mixed households experience, particularly in the first few weeks when everyone is struggling with new habits, new routines, and new ways of seeing the world.

If they protest, remind them that it's only 30 days!

Also, if you do find resistance or hostility as you continue on this path, please take comfort in the fact that given time, that initial reaction usually subsides. Over and over, I've seen loved ones come around after they've had time to adjust to the changes.

CHAPTER 7

Create Your Goals and Intentions

Because our motivations tend to determine our experience, I think it's important to be clear about why you want to do this Challenge and what you hope to get out of it. In other words, I recommend creating some intentions and goals, and there is indeed a difference between the two.

The best way to differentiate between the two is to say that goals tend to be tangible and potentially measureable; intentions are more about having a particular mind-set. A goal is about the *end,* and an intention is having the proper mind-set to achieve that end.

For example, your intentions for this 30-Day Vegan Challenge might be:

- To be open-minded
- To be willing to confront information or images that may be difficult or painful
- To be joyful and enthusiastic
- To not let fear (of the unknown, of something new, of something painful) guide me

Your goals might be:

- To learn three new recipes
- To lose 5 pounds
- To lower your cholesterol
- To get a better understanding of nutrition and animal issues

Intentions create a framework of consciousness, a motivation for *why* and *how* you want to approach something. They're more about the process than the end result. Goals, on the other hand, are about results, and there's nothing more satisfying than returning to a list of goals and crossing off the things you set out to accomplish.

However, I do encourage you to keep your goals realistic. While it is perfectly reasonable to set a goal to lose some weight, you will want to be realistic about your expectations. For example, experts recommend losing no more than 2 pounds a week, for reasons of safety. And although some people may lose more than 8 pounds in 30 days depending on what their starting weight is, I *do not recommend* making your goal "lose 30 pounds in 30 days." If you want to keep it less specific, just make "lose weight" a goal; even if you lose 1 pound by the end of the 30 days, you'll have accomplished your goal!

That goes for any number you may be measuring, including how many points your cholesterol and blood pressure drop. The idea is to create goals that are realistic so that you can feel proud of yourself by the end of 30 days. Perhaps just going 30 days without meat, dairy, and eggs is enough of an accomplishment for you; if that's the case, just make *that* your goal and then be pleasantly surprised by anything you may experience.

I also recommend writing your intentions and goals down on paper (or on your computer). Seeing them in black and white makes them more concrete and more satisfying to look at when the 30 days are over.

The following questions provide a guide to help you create your goals and intentions and to help you assess them once the 30 days are over.

- **HOW DO I FEEL NOW?**
  Physically?
  Emotionally?
  Spiritually?

- **WHAT ARE MY INTENTIONS FOR DOING THE 30-DAY VEGAN CHALLENGE?**

- **WHAT GOALS DO I WANT TO ATTAIN BY THE END OF THE 30 DAYS?**

- **WHAT AM I MOST AFRAID OF OR ANXIOUS ABOUT?**

- **WHAT AM I ANTICIPATING BEING THE MOST CHALLENGING ASPECTS OF THESE 30 DAYS?**

- **WHAT AM I ANTICIPATING BEING THE MOST EXCITING ASPECTS OF THESE 30 DAYS?**

At the end of the 30 days, write down your answers to these questions:

- **HOW DO I FEEL NOW?**
  Physically?
  Emotionally?
  Spiritually?

- HAVE I LEARNED ANYTHING ABOUT MYSELF DURING THESE 30 DAYS?

- HAVE I LEARNED ANYTHING ABOUT MY FRIENDS? FAMILY MEMBERS?

- DID I STAY CLEAR ABOUT MY INTENTIONS THROUGHOUT THE 30-DAY PROCESS?

- DID I MEET ANY OF MY GOALS?

- IF NOT, HOW DO I FEEL ABOUT THAT? ARE THESE GOALS I CAN RETURN TO NOW AND AGAIN?

- DID THE FEARS I HAD COME TO FRUITION? HOW DID I HANDLE THESE SITUATIONS? HOW WOULD I WANT TO HANDLE THEM IN THE FUTURE?

- WHAT DID I FIND CHALLENGING ABOUT THE 30 DAYS? IS THERE ANYTHING I CAN DO TO MAKE IT EASIER MOVING FORWARD?

May you approach these next 30 days with an open mind and an open heart and find much joy along the way. Where you find discomfort, may it make you stronger, enhancing the person you are and strengthening the values you hold.

That is my hope for you.

With the intention of providing the best recipes to guide you on your journey, I have included my favorites, honed and perfected over many years and only slightly adapted—if at all—from my existing three cookbooks (see "Resources and Recommendations"), where you'll also find nutrition information for each recipe. The recipes run the gamut of breakfast dishes, lunch options, dinner mains and sides, and desserts, and many of them can be used for special occasions and holidays. Reluctant to simply stick them at the back of the book, I've placed them within the various chapters so you can recognize them within the context that made sense for each one. In addition to the formal recipes, there are dozens of suggestions for ingredients you can throw together to create quick and easy dishes in a jiffy, as well as weekly menu ideas that begin on page 297.

Always striking a balance between providing easy-to-prepare recipes and encouraging people to get into the kitchen to cook, my recipes are meant to be accessible, familiar, healthful, and delicious. Having written three cookbooks, taught cooking classes for eleven years, and heard directly from many of my students and readers, I've had the privilege of learning exactly which of my recipes have been the most celebrated. I'm so honored that many of them have become part of people's repertoire, helping them to transition to veganism and to impress skeptics along the way, and I hope they will do the same for you.

I always say that once my recipes are in the reader's hands, they're not mine anymore. Short of adding animal products, please feel free to modify the following recipes in order to customize them to your palate. For instance,

- If the baked goods are too sweet, add less sugar.
- If you need more salt in any of the recipes, then add a little more.
- If you like to reduce the little oil I recommend, then use water to sauté vegetables instead.
- If you like spicier flavors, just increase the heat.
- If your oven temperature is different from mine and requires that something cook a little longer than I've indicated, then follow your oven and not my instructions.

Most of all, enjoy the process of resensitizing your palate to all the flavors in plant foods. One final note: because wheat and soy are common allergens for people, you'll notice that each recipe indicates whether it is wheat-free and/or soy-free.

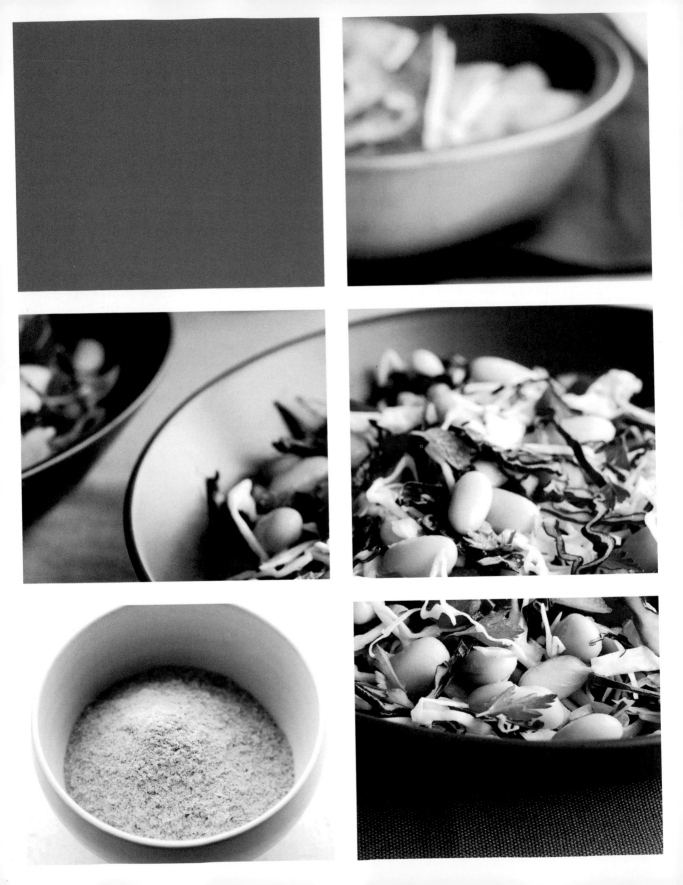

go!

The 30-Day Vegan Challenge

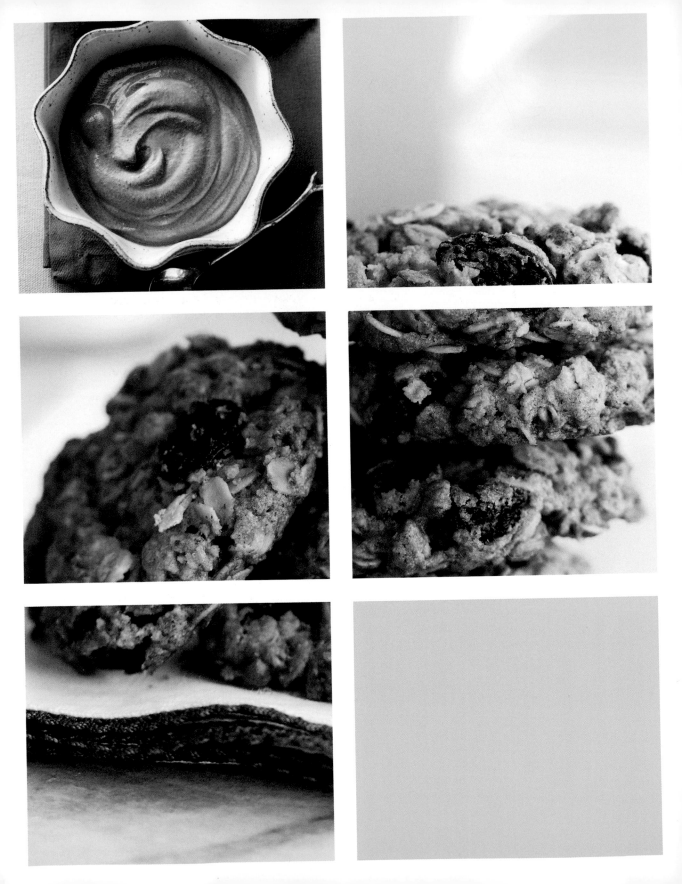

Stocking a Healthful Vegan Kitchen

Today being your first day, no doubt you will want to know what to eat! Before I send you to the grocery store, I encourage you to take a look in your cupboards, refrigerator, or freezer and note what you already have that is vegan. You will most likely find pasta, marinara sauce, peanut butter, jelly, rice, canned beans, and frozen and fresh vegetables and fruits. You're certainly welcome to grab a few staples from the store based on the lists below (such as nondairy milk for your cereal or coffee), but my hope is that you will see that you already have some vegan food in your house.

At the same time, just as when you wrote your 3-Day Food Diary you noticed how many animal-based foods you may have been eating prior to starting the Challenge, so too may you notice all the non-vegan food in your kitchen, whether they are such obvious things as the meat in your freezer; animal-based milk, dairy-based cheeses, and eggs in the fridge; or the processed and packaged foods with animal-derived ingredients in your cabinets, such as macaroni and cheese and Jell-O.

Having familiar animal products in the kitchen makes it too convenient to reach for them when you're ravenous or in a rush. Best to make a clean break. Some people will discard all the animal products immediately, some will decide to eat them up, and still others may decide to donate them to a local animal shelter/wildlife center or feed it to their cats or dogs.

However, one mistake people make when getting rid of what is undesirable and unhealthful is not replacing them with healthful versions. Having a variety of nutritious ingredients on hand—particularly fresh fruits and veggies—is key to ensuring that you can whip up delicious, compassionate meals anytime. Though a lot of junk food is technically vegan (Cocoa Puffs, Oreo cookies, and Skittles, for example), my intention is to guide you toward *healthful* plant-based foods, and I'm always walking the line of making suggestions that allow for fast, easy cooking, while recommending foods that are as unprocessed as possible.

There are many vegan-friendly brands in addition to the ones I name below; once you know what to look for on the label, which we go over on Day 3, you'll find options everywhere you look.

CANNED GOODS

- **CANNED BEANS:** Some people mistakenly believe that canned beans are lower in nutrition, but that's not true; in fact, many people digest canned beans much better than they do beans made from scratch because canned beans have been extensively soaked and cooked, which removes the sugars that people have a hard time digesting. The only thing you sacrifice with canned beans is money, because you pay extra for convenience. You can decide which means more to you.

Varieties to stock: Chickpeas (garbanzo beans), kidney, black, cannellini, navy, great northern, black-eyed peas, pinto, soybeans, vegetarian refried.

Favorite brands: Eden Foods, Whole Foods 365, Westbrae, Trader Joe's.

Tip: Always rinse and drain canned beans to get rid of the liquid they've been sitting in. This also rinses away some excess sodium.

- **CANNED TOMATOES:** When fresh tomatoes are out of season, canned tomatoes save the day.

Varieties to stock: In order to always have a variety for different dishes, buy cans of diced tomatoes, whole peeled, stewed, crushed, and fire-roasted tomatoes. Also stock up on tomato paste, since it adds so much depth of flavor to sauces, stews, stir-fries, pasta, and chili.

Favorite brands: Muir Glen, Whole Foods 365, Trader Joe's.

Tip: As you look over these categories, you may want to begin writing out your shopping list in preparation for going to the grocery store.

- **CANNED SOUPS:** Though it's infinitely less expensive (and yummier) to make your own soups from scratch, canned soups are great when you're in a pinch.

Varieties to stock: Split pea, lentil, minestrone, carrot, tomato, bean, and chili are typical choices across all brands, though the more natural brands tend to be made from vegetable stock rather than animal-based stock.

Vegan-friendly brands: Amy's, Health Valley Foods, Muir Glen, Simply Organic, Trader Joe's, Walnut Acres, Whole Foods 365, Westbrae. Instant soups, such as Dr. McDougall's, are also available. Some brands of soup, such as Imagine Foods and Pacific Foods of Oregon, are packaged in aseptic (cardboard) boxes that don't need to be refrigerated until opened.

Tip: Many brands carry fat-free, low-fat, and low-sodium versions of their soups, and many are also organic.

SAUCES AND DRESSINGS

- PASTA, MARINARA, AND PIZZA SAUCES: Some brands add cheese or chicken broth, so just check the label. Choose sauces that have the fewest and most recognizable ingredients. (Sometimes sugar is added—even in homemade sauces—though better brands will use sugar and not corn syrup.)

Vegan-friendly brands: Muir Glen, Whole Foods 365, Trader Joe's, Newman's Own.

- SALAD DRESSINGS: Some commercial dressings are made with eggs, honey, cow's milk, or cow's milk derivatives; just check the labels and look for more healthful brands, which also tend to be free of corn syrup or hydrogenated oil.

Vegan-friendly brands: Annie's Naturals, Whole Foods 365, Spectrum Organics, Newman's Own, Organicville, Trader Joe's.

- CURRY PASTES: Having curry pastes on hand allows you to whip up fast, flavorful meals simply by combining them with coconut milk and adding to sautéed vegetables. The best stuff can be found in Asian markets or large natural food stores, but wherever you're shopping, look for versions without fish sauce or fish paste. Green, red, yellow, or Massaman, and Panang are common varieties.

- STIR-FRY SAUCES: Although you can always opt for making your own stir-fry sauce, bottled varieties provide convenience. Many are vegan and can be added while vegetables are sautéing for instant flavor.

- SALSA AND HUMMUS: Kept in the fridge, these are two essential foods that add instant flavor and nutrients to many dishes. Choose fresh salsa in the refrigerated section over salsa in jars.

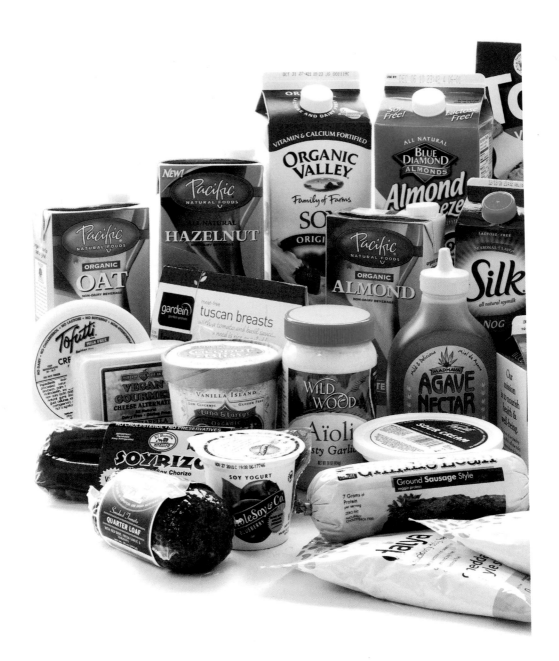

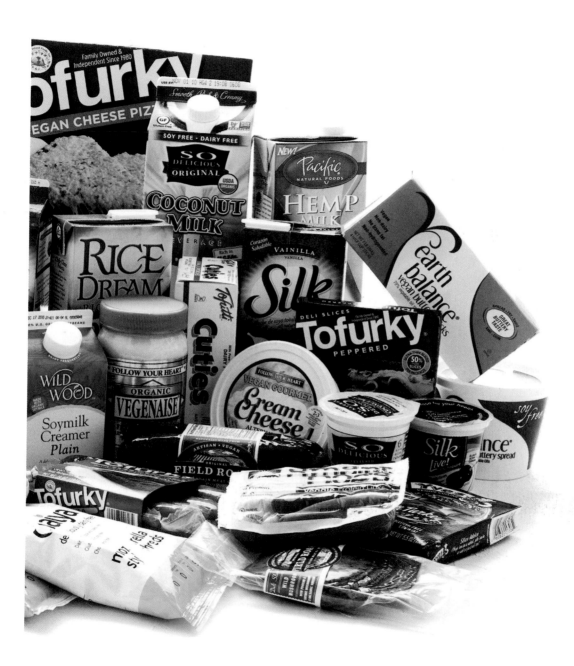

CONDIMENTS

If you take a closer look at all of your condiments, you'll realize that most of them are naturally vegan. In fact, most of the things we flavor meat with are plant-based, as illustrated by all the condiments listed below and by the ones you most likely have in your pantry already, such as ketchup, mustard, relish, and chili sauce.

- **TAMARI SOY SAUCE:** Brewed longer than Chinese soy sauce, Japanese tamari is much fuller-bodied and just tastes better. Try Shoyu or Bragg's Liquid Amino Acids for a similar flavor. Most tamari brands are also wheat-free.

- **TAHINI:** Essentially sesame paste (like peanut butter, only using ground sesame seeds instead of peanuts), tahini is used to make hummus, salad dressings, and sauces.

- **EGGLESS MAYONNAISE:** You'll soon be enjoying Better-Than-Chicken, Better-Than-Tuna, and Better-Than-Egg Salads (see pages 97, 162, and 97), for which you'll need this essential ingredient. Use in all the same ways you'd think to use egg-based mayonnaise; vegan mayo just relies on the fat from plant oils rather than fat from eggs. The best vegan brands are Vegenaise (by Follow Your Heart), Nayonaise, and Wildwood's Garlic Aioli, although Spectrum Organics and Trader Joe's have eggless versions, too.

- **BARBECUE SAUCE:** Many people have half-consumed bottles of BBQ sauce in their fridge. Now's the time to start fresh! Look for flavors and brands without honey.

- **WORCESTERSHIRE SAUCE:** Considered essential for Bloody Mary cocktails, or even added to Caesar salad (feel free to add it to the recipe on page 133), vegan Worcestershire sauce contains no anchovies. Look for such brands as Annie's Naturals, Edward & Sons, and The Wizard's.

SPREADS AND SYRUPS

Most jams, jellies, relishes, nut butters, and syrups are naturally vegan, but while you're in cleanout mode, take a look at the labels and get rid of those spreads and syrups that contain unhealthful corn syrup and hydrogenated oils.

- **LIQUID SWEETENERS:** Agave nectar, maple syrup, and brown rice syrup can generally be used interchangeably.

- **JAMS, JELLIES, PRESERVES:** Look for those sweetened with fruit concentrate.

- **NUT AND SEED BUTTERS:** Almond, peanut, cashew, macadamia, sunflower seed, and hemp seed butters are all fabulous. Look for those without added oil and sugar.

VINEGARS

I have an entire cupboard shelf dedicated to vinegars, since they lend so much flavor and depth to a variety of dishes and dressings. Now is the opportunity to experiment with new tastes and infusions.

- SEASONED RICE: "Seasoned" means a little sugar is added, taking the edge off the vinegar and making it a little sweeter. If you can't find seasoned, just buy plain rice vinegar and add a little of your own sugar.

- BALSAMIC: Use the cheap stuff for cooking and the good stuff for dressings. (Hint: if the label says "Modena," it's cheap.) Try different varieties, such as balsamic cherry vinegar or white balsamic vinegar. Each is as special as the next and makes a great base for salad dressings.

- APPLE CIDER: Good for salad dressings and baked goods (see "Day 16: Better Baking Without Eggs").

OILS

All cooking oils are vegan, but not all are created equal. Choose olive, sesame, canola, and coconut for cooking (the latter two for baking), and avoid those high in polyunsaturated fats, such as vegetable, corn, safflower, and sunflower. Regardless, I recommend that you use oils sparingly just for a little added flavor or to keep food from sticking to pots and pans.

Tip: Buy an oil mister at a kitchen supply store in order to spray pans with oil while still using very little.

HERBS, SPICES, AND VEGETABLE STOCKS

- DRIED HERBS AND SPICES: Because herbs and spices tend to intimidate people, they sit on the spice rack for years until they're stale and flavorless. Use them!

Tip: If you consider that the shelf life of dried herbs is about six months and that for spices is twelve months, perhaps that will inspire you to take inventory. If yours are past their prime (or if you can't remember when you bought them), replace them. It's my hope that over the course of this Challenge, you'll gain more confidence using herbs and spices in your cooking.

VEGETABLE STOCK: A wonderful ingredient that adds depth to so many dishes, vegetable stock is an easy switcheroo from chicken or beef stock. Prepared broths and stocks (also in low-sodium versions), such as No-Chicken, No-Beef, Vegetable, and

Mushroom, are available in aseptic boxes, but I prefer veggie bouillon cubes for their convenience.

Vegan-friendly brands: Prepared—Imagine Foods, Health Valley, Pacific Foods of Oregon. *Bouillon cubes/powder*—Rapunzel, Edward & Sons, Better Than Bouillon, Herb-Ox.

■ NUTRITIONAL YEAST FLAKES: Although it suffers from what I think is a terribly un-appetizing name, nutritional yeast is found in the bulk section of natural food stores and adds cheesy flavor to sauces, pasta dishes, and popcorn. (And I know from experience that cats and dogs also love it sprinkled on their food!)

BAKING ITEMS

Along with various flours (all-purpose, whole-wheat, pastry, bread), you most likely already keep yeast packets (for making leavened breads), baking soda, baking powder, vanilla extract, and unsweetened cocoa powder in your pantry. Great. You might want to have muffin, scone, and cake mixes on hand in your kitchen as well. They're more expensive than when you bake from scratch, but sometimes the convenience is worth the extra expense. If the mix you buy calls for eggs or dairy-based milk, just follow the guidelines in "Day 16: Better Baking Without Eggs" to make them vegan.

CHALLENGE YOUR THINKING:
By definition, chocolate is vegan. Only when cow's milk is added is it not vegan anymore.

CHANGE YOUR BEHAVIOR:
Look at labels for milk fat, milk powder, whey, and casein as indications of non-vegan ingredients in chocolate bars and chips.

Favorite brands of prepared mixes: Simply Organic, Oetker Organics, Bob's Red Mill, Arrowhead Mills, Hodgson Mills.

Chocolate

Chocolate is an essential in baking (at least in my house it is). One of the biggest misconceptions about being vegan is that you have to forgo chocolate. Not true. By its very nature, chocolate is vegan; it comes from the cacao tree. Cocoa butter, cocoa powder, bittersweet chocolate, semisweet chocolate, dark chocolate, and white chocolate are all vegan by nature. Only when you add cow's milk is chocolate not vegan. Some companies (such as Hershey's and Nestlé) play with definitions by adding cow's milk to what they call semisweet and dark chocolate bars and chips. Just take a quick peek at the ingredients to make sure there is no added milk fat, milk powder, or casein. See page 96 for specific brands of vegan chocolate bars.

DRIED BEANS AND LENTILS

Cooking beans from scratch is a breeze. Lentils are even easier, since they don't have to be soaked first. Keep red lentils, brown or green lentils, and yellow or green split peas on hand for quick soups, stews, salads, pâtés, and loaves.

WHOLE GRAINS

Acting as a base or complement to many of the dishes you'll be preparing, whole grains are also simply delicious. Stock up on a variety, from amaranth to quinoa, so that you have options aplenty. Most whole grains have cooking instructions on the packaging, but if you're buying in bulk, see page 52 for a cooking chart.

PASTA AND NOODLES

Most commercial pastas (penne, angel hair, spaghetti, fettuccine, linguine) and noodles (soba, udon, and rice) are vegan, made with flour (semolina, buckwheat, or rice), water, and salt. (Gluten-free pastas are also available.) A few brands may add eggs, so just check the label.

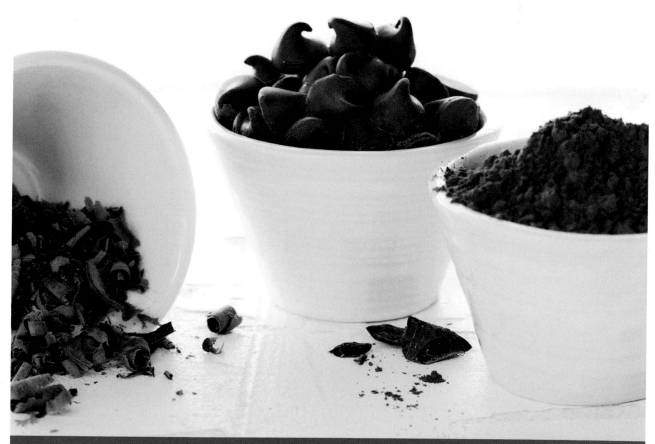

(FROM LEFT TO RIGHT): SHAVED DARK CHOCOLATE, SEMISWEET CHOCOLATE CHIPS, BITTERSWEET CHOCOLATE CHUNKS, COCOA POWDER

NONDAIRY FOODS

Nondairy versions of familiar foods abound in the dairy section of the grocery store. No deprivation here.

- YOGURT: Cultured with all the "good bacteria" such as *L. acidophilus* and *B. bifidum* that people look for in dairy-based yogurts, there are soy-milk-based (Silk, Wildwood, Trader Joe's, Whole Soy & Co.), coconut-milk-based (Turtle Mountain/So Delicious), rice-milk-based (Ricera), and even almond-milk-based (Amande) yogurts available.

- BUTTER: Earth Balance is my favorite; it's free of hydrogenated oils and trans fats, it's made from non-genetically-modified ingredients, and it comes in soy-free, organic, whipped, and stick versions. Use it just the way you would use dairy-based butter. It's the same measure for measure.

- MILK: Most plant-based milks come in aseptic boxes you can keep in the cupboard until they're ready to open. (Then they get stored in the fridge.) Soy, rice, oat, almond, hemp, hazelnut, and coconut milks are available in a number of brands and flavors. (See "Day 14: Choosing Plant-Based Milks.")

- CHEESE: You can find vegan cheeses in all shapes and sizes these days, and more will continue to flood the market. Larger health-oriented grocery stores will have the widest selection, but vegan grocery stores online and off (see the sidebar on page 60) will most definitely carry them. (See "Day 12: Discovering That There *Is* Life After Cheese")

VEGETARIAN MEATS

There are a variety of veggie meats that provide the salt, fat, texture, and familiarity that you crave in your animal-based versions. Though they're certainly healthier than the animal-based versions, some of these lil' buggers are definitely processed and should be treated as convenience or transition foods—not daily health food.

- DELI SLICES: Soy-based Yves and Tofurky brands carry vegetarian turkey, ham, bologna, salami, and pepperoni, and wheat-based (soy-free) Field Roast's deli slices come in Lentil Sage, Wild Mushroom, and Smoked Tomato flavors.

- CUTLETS: Field Roast makes delicious wheat-based (soy-free) nut-breaded cutlets, and Gardein specializes in soy-based versions.

- MEATLESS MEATBALLS, GROUND VEGGIE MEAT, AND MEAT LOAF: Nate's, Trader Joe's, Match Meat, Gardein, and Yves are all vegan-friendly brands. Field Roast makes a fantastic meat loaf.

- **SAUSAGES:** My favorite brands are Field Roast (wheat-based and soy-free) and Tofurky (tofu-based) for dinner-type sausages; Lightlife makes a gluten-based version called Gimme Lean that is ideal as a breakfast sausage.

- **VEGGIE DOGS:** Yves (Tofu Dogs and Veggie Dogs) and Lightlife (Smart Dogs and Tofu Pups) will be in the refrigerated section; Loma Linda's Little Links are sold in a can.

- **CHICKEN-FREE NUGGETS:** A great transition food for kids because of their crispy coating. Just pop them in the oven and serve with ketchup or BBQ sauce.

Vegan-friendly brands: Gardein, Health Is Wealth, Lightlife, Boca—found in both the refrigerated and freezer sections.

- **VEGGIE BURGERS:** Whether you're looking for tofu-based, veggie-based, or wheat-based, meatless burgers abound. Some are more processed than others; some are vegetarian (not vegan) and contain chicken's eggs, so check the label.

Vegan-friendly brands: Dr. Praeger's, Amy's, and Gardenburger are found in the freezer section. Wildwood Foods and Soy Deli brands make tofu burgers found in the refrigerated section.

Tip: Even within the category of vegan meats, there is a spectrum in terms of how processed they are. Those made from tofu or wheat gluten are definitely less processed than those made from soy isolate protein or soy protein concentrate.

FREEZER ITEMS

Frozen food tends to get a bad rap, but lots of healthful foods are found in the freezer section. Fruits and veggies are flash frozen before being sold and retain all their nutrition.

- **FRUIT:** Keep a combination of frozen fruits on hand for delicious smoothies.

Tip: When bananas are at their ripest, peel them, break the bananas into chunks, place in a freezer bag, and store in the freezer for instant, thick smoothies any time of the day. Check out the recipes for Blueberry, Mango, and Green Smoothies on page 83.

- **BREAD:** Some brands of sliced whole-grain sandwich breads contain honey, while others contain cow's milk derivatives, such as whey or casein. However, pita bread, lavash, sandwich rolls, French baguettes, and nice Italian rolls in the bakery section are more often vegan than the sliced breads meant to have a long shelf life.

Vegan-friendly brands: Sliced bread–Ezekiel (often in the freezer case), Rudi's Organic Bakery, Arnold's, Alvarado Street Bakery, Garden of Eatin'; *hot dog and hamburger buns*–Alvarado Street Bakery, Rudi's Organic Bakery; *English muffins*–Rudi's Organic Bakery.

- **FROZEN PIZZA:** Varying in the type of crust and nondairy cheese they use, the most popular brands are Tofutti, Amy's, and Tofurky.

Tip: Prepared pizza crust, cornmeal crust, and phyllo dough found in the freezer are typically vegan.

- **ICE CREAM AND SORBET:** I grew up with a father who owned ice cream stores, so I'm a tough critic. Once you get dairy out of your palate, though, you stop comparing what you knew with what's new. There are more options than I name here. Check the freezer section.

Vegan-friendly brands: Turtle Mountain/So Delicious, Whole Soy, Temptation, Soy Dream, Double Rainbow, Trader Joe's, and Tofutti are popular soy milk ice creams with lots of flavors and frozen treats. Coconut Bliss is a delicious coconut milk ice cream. Rice Dream is made from rice milk, and Almond Dream is made from almond milk.

Tip: Though sherbet and frozen yogurt are dairy-based, sorbet is vegan by definition, and many gelato shops have vegan options, made with fruit or soy milk. Choose brands that use cane sugar as a sweetener, not corn syrup.

That should be enough to get you started. Many more brands and products are mentioned throughout the book in various sections, so feel free to read ahead.

Eating Healthfully Affordably

When people make the transition to a whole-foods, plant-based diet, one of the things they notice is how much less money they spend on food. I've seen it time and again. Now, I realize you may be saying, "But wait! I just spent a lot of money restocking my kitchen!" I understand you may have had to replace some animal-based products with plant-based ingredients, but I imagine we're talking mainly about condiments and the like. Because these items will last you a long time, keep in mind that you won't be buying these staples week after week. I think once you get beyond the initial 30 days, you'll be better able to more accurately calculate what you're spending on your weekly groceries.

My hope here is to debunk the myth that eating a vegan diet is more expensive than eating an animal-based diet, and guide you to eating healthfully affordably.

COST COMPARISON

Animal proteins are generally more expensive than plant proteins. The cheapest cuts of beef, such as ground round, average $3.00 per pound in the United States; boneless chicken breasts average $3.40 a pound, and canned tuna is about $2.00 per pound. Contrast that with dried beans and lentils at less than $1.00 a pound and rice well below $1.00 per pound. Tofu is also usually under $2.00 a pound. The cost of nuts and seeds varies, and although pine nuts tend to be expensive, you can always choose sunflower seeds, which contain nearly the same amount of protein at a fraction of the price.

If you price out vegetarian meats, such as veggie dogs, they do tend to cost about $5.00 a pound, so this is just another reason I emphasize basing your diet on whole foods. If you want to indulge in these convenience foods once in a while, that's fine, but keep in mind that even when you buy non-vegan convenience foods, you're paying more than if you bought whole foods. Ulti-

> **CHALLENGE YOUR THINKING:** Convenience foods—vegan or non-vegan—simply cost more than whole foods.
>
> **CHANGE YOUR BEHAVIOR:** In order to make the most healthful and affordable choices, make whole plant foods the foundation of your diet.

mately, in terms of the most healthful and most affordable food, whole plant foods win every time—over processed foods *and* over animal products.

COSTS BEYOND DOLLARS

Notice I'm using the word *affordable*—not the word *cheap*. There's a big difference between eating affordably and eating cheaply. I'm not talking about eating cheap food, which is what we've all become accustomed to, primarily due to government subsidies and buy-backs for meat, dairy, and eggs. Because of these artificially cheap products, we tend to complain when we have to pay the true cost of whole, organic, nonsubsidized foods. The problem isn't that healthful plant foods are expensive; the problem is that unhealthful animal products are priced artificially low.

Aside from changing our buying habits, we need to change our *thinking* when it comes to the money we spend on what we eat. Traditionally, people have praised "cheap" animal products because it means more people can buy what are in reality very expensive things to produce, ignoring the fact that there are costs to consider other than the actual dollars we spend—costs to our health, costs to the Earth, costs to the people who produce our food, costs to the animals—and there are many ways to reduce these costs, to the benefit of everyone involved.

CHOOSING SIMPLICITY

I admit I tend to romanticize the stories my parents tell me about their families during the Depression. They were very poor and literally counted every penny. They tell me how excited they and their siblings were when they had enough money to buy half a loaf of bread or a lollipop. I'm certainly not trivializing the difficulties they experienced; rather, I appreciate the simplicity of how they lived and the gratitude they felt being able to afford what they could. We all know how much we appreciate something we have to fight for. And in our days of plenty, we don't have to fight for much, and so I think we tend to appreciate less.

Admittedly, I'm overwhelmed when I go into a grocery store, because the choices we have are frankly ridiculous—almost embarrassing. So although I'm grateful for the privilege of having so many options, they actually just make me more inclined toward simplicity—the simplicity we're often forced into when we're in a recession, when income is low, or when we need to get a better handle on our budget. This simplicity has so many benefits, including:

- Appreciating what we have
- Saving up for what we really want

- Using up what we have in our cupboards before going shopping
- Choosing healthful whole foods rather than expensive packaged products

EATING AT HOME

Cooking at home is one of the best ways to eat affordably. Today, almost 50 percent of Americans and 30 percent of U.K. residents eat their meals outside of the home. Eating out that much takes a toll on our wallets, on our bodies, and even on our taste buds. Restaurant chefs are trained to maximize the use of oil and salt, so their calorie-dense dishes contribute not only to weight gain and health problems but also to our palates lacking sensitivity, coated as they are with fat and sodium. Eating out should be regarded more as a treat than as a daily rite.

I say this aware that people working in offices are often bound by lunchtime meetings and people who travel extensively for work have little choice but to eat in restaurants. What I'm suggesting is that *when we are able,* we choose home-cooked meals over restaurant fare. Although this may not be as possible for the lunchtime meal (although you can pack sandwiches and salads—see "Day 9: Packing Lunches for School and Work"), I do recommend that you at least strive to eat breakfast and dinner at home. You will notice a huge difference in how you feel and how much money you save.

CHALLENGE YOUR THINKING: Because restaurant chefs are trained to maximize the use of oil and salt, their calorie-dense dishes contribute to weight gain, health problems, and dulled palates.

CHANGE YOUR BEHAVIOR: Make eating at home the norm and eating out a treat.

BUYING IN BULK

When I suggest buying in bulk, I'm not referring to going to those large warehouse stores and buying fifty packages of paper towels. I'm talking about shopping in the bulk section of grocery stores and natural food stores, where you can buy dried foods, such as pasta, grains, flour, oatmeal, lentils, beans, and even herbs and spices, from bins, choosing exactly how much you want and paying for the weight of that food rather than for the brand name or packaging. Not only is buying in bulk less expensive, it is also much more Earth-friendly, especially if you bring your own bags or containers.

Keep in mind that if you want to be a savvy shopper, it's best to look at the cost per unit to determine the true cost of an item. The unit price tells you the cost per pound, quart, or other unit of weight or volume of a food package, and it's usually posted on the shelf below the food. You save money when you compare the cost of the same food in different-sized containers or different brands. For example, if you want to buy frozen orange juice, you may find a 6-ounce can that cost 64¢. The unit price for this small can is $3.42 per quart.

A 12-ounce can of frozen orange juice in another brand may cost 89¢, and the unit price is $2.38 per quart. Here, the larger container is less expensive.

COOKING FROM SCRATCH

Perhaps it takes more effort than calling the pizza guy (see "Day 6: Making the Time to Cook"), but cooking from scratch is healthier and more affordable, including when it comes to baking.

It's true there are vegan cake, brownie, and biscuit mixes out there, but if you're looking to save money, those are unnecessary expenses. Let's take a look at the cost of my Drop Biscuits (page 259). Parsing out and pricing all of the ingredients called for, it works out to $1.15 to make 12 biscuits; that's a little more than 10¢ per biscuit.

Look at the Chocolate Cake recipe (page 179). Depending on the type of cocoa you use (organic, fair-trade will be more expensive), the cost for the entire cake is $3.46 if using more expensive cocoa and $2.75 if using less expensive cocoa. This is less than any cake mix you'll buy in the store, especially when you consider that when you use those cake mixes, you still have to add your own oil, so you're paying a lot of money for just flour, sugar, and cocoa. And it costs substantially less than buying a pre-made cake in your grocery store or bakery. That goes for the frosting, too. It's true a lot of frostings sold in grocery stores are vegan, but they're usually loaded with corn syrup and artificial preservatives. Making your own frosting is not only less expensive but also healthier.

CHOOSING NUTRIENT-DENSE FOODS

Cost considerations go well beyond dollars and cents. We want to get the best monetary bang for our caloric buck, but ideally, we want to get the most nutritional bang for our caloric buck as well. Physiologically, we need calories (i.e., food) in order to give us the energy to function properly. Just as we need to fill a car with high-quality fluids in order for it to run well, so too do we need high-quality fuel in order for our own bodies to run well. When we fill our cars or bodies with junk, they'll run all right, but not at their optimal level, and that should be our goal.

This is the principle behind avoiding eating empty calories. They may fill you up, but they don't provide you with the nutrients you need to function well. It's like filling up a gas tank with water. The tank might be filled, but it's not filled with a substance that allows it to run, and in a short period of time the car will break down. Processed and refined foods are basically empty calories, because though they have the same energy content of any other calorie, they lack vitamins, minerals, antioxidants, phytochemicals, and fiber. The same can be said of meat, dairy, and eggs—they provide a lot of calories but very little nutrient value in return. No fiber. No antioxidants. No phytochemicals.

You want to make the most of the calories you take in—and make these calories nutrient-dense. Think of how much money we spend in the form of empty calories, including beverages, sodas, juices, and fancy coffee drinks. A lot of calories are spent with very little return in terms of nutrition.

Based on their nutrient-per-calorie density, the winners are:

- **FIRST PLACE:** dark green leafies such as kale, collard greens, chard, mustard greens, and turnip greens.

- **SECOND PLACE:** other green vegetables, such as Brussels sprouts, broccoli, artichokes, asparagus, celery, cucumbers, peas, green peppers, snow peas, snap peas, string beans, and zucchini.

- **THIRD PLACE (BUT STILL COMPLETE WINNERS):** non-green veggies like beets, tomatoes, carrots, squash, bell peppers, and cauliflower and fresh fruits.

Make no mistake about it: eating nutrient-dense foods also has very tangible cost benefits in terms of the medical bills you won't be paying in the long term. Coronary bypass surgery and cholesterol-lowering drugs, diabetes drugs, and dialysis—all correlated with animal-based diets—are incredibly expensive; a bypass surgery or angioplasty procedure can cost nearly $60,000. Some 16 million people are living with some form of coronary heart disease, and 1.2 million people suffer a heart attack every year. As a result, there are more than 425,000 coronary artery bypass graft surgeries performed in the United States each year, making it one of the most commonly performed major operations. All this pain, misery, expense, and death for a preventable disease.

As one of my favorite vegan doctors, Dr. Caldwell Esselstyn, always says: "Coronary artery disease is a toothless paper tiger that need never ever exist, and if it does exist, it need never ever progress. When people learn to eat plant-based to eliminate heart disease, it could inaugurate a seismic revolution in health."

BECOME A SAVVY SHOPPER

Don't fall into the traps of overspending and making unhealthful food choices at the grocery store. To avoid this:

CHALLENGE YOUR THINKING: Processed and refined foods as well as animal products may fill you up, but they don't provide much nutrient value in return.

CHANGE YOUR BEHAVIOR: Get the most nutritional bang for your caloric buck: choose nutrient-dense foods.

GET COOKIN': Take advantage of some of these nutrient-dense foods by making the Garlic and Greens Soup on page 231, Roasted Brussels Sprouts with Caramelized Onions and Toasted Pistachios on page 255, and Muhammara (Roasted Red Pepper and Walnut Spread) on page 227.

- **MAKE A LIST:** Having a list and sticking to it is vital to saving money. This is where planning your meals ahead comes in handy (see "Day 6: Making the Time to Cook"). Knowing what you want to eat for the week enables you to look through your recipes carefully enough to create your shopping list and prevents you from having to run out to the store for one item, which always winds up turning into several by the time you leave the store. According to studies, 70 percent of shoppers enter the grocery store with a shopping list but only 10 percent adhere to it. Commit to buying only what you need and resist temptations along the way.

- **LOOK DOWN:** Items on the lower shelves tend to be less flashy, less processed, less intensively packaged—and thus less expensive.

- **EAT BEFORE YOU SHOP:** Old but helpful advice. We never make the best choices when we're ravenously hungry.

- **CHOOSE LOCAL:** Because most supermarket produce travels thousands of miles before arriving, it's bred for longevity, not flavor. To experience maximum flavor and freshness while supporting your own local farms, choose locally grown fruits and veggies as much as possible, either by buying them at farmer's markets or by shopping in grocery stores that adhere to the law that requires them to notify customers where certain foods were grown.

- **KNOW WHEN TO CHOOSE ORGANIC:** Because organic produce is priced according to its true cost, it feels more expensive than subsidized, artificially cheap conventionally grown produce. To help you make the best decisions about when to buy organic, it's helpful to know which fruits and veggies have more pesticide residue than others so you can make informed choices. Check out the Environmental Working Group's "Shopper's Guide to Pesticides" at foodnews.org.

  At a glance, the following produce tends to be so heavily sprayed with toxic chemicals that many experts recommend eating them only when they're organic: apples, bell peppers, celery, cherries, imported grapes, kale, nectarines, peaches, pears, potatoes, raspberries, and strawberries. These are called the Dirty Dozen. Those least sprayed are called the Clean Fifteen and include asparagus, avocado, cabbage, cantaloupe, eggplant, grapefruit, honeydew melon, kiwi, mangos, onions, pineapple, sweet corn, sweet peas, sweet potato, and watermelon.

- **DON'T BROWSE:** Think of the different departments as separate stores within the supermarket. Just as you wouldn't shop at every store at the mall, think of the grocery store this way. Just target the sections that provide the healthiest fare and avoid altogether those that are filled with empty-calorie products.

- PUT OFF GOING TO THE GROCERY STORE: When you "haven't a thing to eat," take a long hard look at your newly veganized cupboards, freezer, and refrigerator. Most likely you have enough to make a few more meals before heading to the store. Make a stew with those canned beans; make a pilaf with that brown rice. Spoiled as we are, we think we have to run to the store every time we're low in the staples. Be creative and stretch out the time between your visits a little longer. You'll save a little money and perhaps enjoy seeing what you can come up with.

Applying these principles, you'll save loads of money and prevent costly and life-threatening diseases.

COOKING GRAINS

Grains are one of the easiest things to cook, as long as you know how to boil water. Cooking times and grain: liquid ratios vary. Here is a helpful guide.

GRAIN TYPE	GRAIN : LIQUID	COOKING TIME
Brown rice (short or long grain)*	1 cup : 2 or 2½ cups	Simmer 45 minutes.
Basmati rice* (white)	1 cup : 1¾ cups	Simmer 20 minutes.
Basmati rice* (brown)	1 cup : 2 cups	Simmer 40 to 45 minutes.
Bulgur wheat	1 cup : 2½ cups	Simmer 25 minutes, fluff, let sit for 10 minutes. Or boil the water, pour over bulgur, cover and let sit for 1 hour.
Quinoa* (pronounced KEEN-wah)	1 cup : 2 to 3 cups	Rinse quinoa in a strainer, and add to pot along with water. Cover, and bring to boil for 10 minutes or until water is absorbed. Fluff, and cover until time to serve.
Couscous (pronounced KOOS-koos)	1 cup : 1½ cups	Bring water to boil. Add couscous, 1 tablespoon Earth Balance or olive oil, and ½ teaspoon salt. Remove from heat, stir, cover and let stand for 10 minutes. Fluff with fork.
Amaranth*	1 cup : 3 cups	Mix with corn, scallions, and cooked beans. Simmer 25 to 30 minutes. Do not salt until thoroughly cooked.
Pearled barley	1 cup : 4 cups	Simmer 60 to 70 minutes.
Millet*	1 cup : 2½ cups	Simmer 15 minutes, remove from heat, fluff, and let sit uncovered for 20 minutes.
Wild and brown rice mix*	1 cup : 3 cups	Simmer 35 minutes.
Polenta* (cornmeal)	1 cup : 4 cups	Bring water to a boil, add 1 teaspoon salt, and slowly add polenta, stirring constantly. Reduce heat to gentle simmer, stirring for 2 more minutes. Cover and cook for 40 to 45 minutes, stirring every 10 minutes.

* Gluten-free

DAY 3   Reading Labels

With a good idea of what to fill your cupboards with, and in preparation for going to the grocery store to stock up *and* save money, let's take a look at how to read labels so you can identify the most prevalent animal products that appear in various items.

Contrary to what many people think, vegans do not spend all their time deciphering labels. The truth is that once you know what to look for, one quick glance at the label will tell you if it has an animal product in it. Having said that, if you have to weed through a long list of ingredients to determine if it's vegan or not, you probably shouldn't be eating that product anyway. Why would you want to put into your mouth something that resembles a chemistry experiment rather than actual food? You shouldn't feel like you're in science class when you read a label.

The best way to avoid labels altogether is to eat whole foods as much as possible. The more you eat whole foods, the less you have to worry about animal products or unnecessary and potentially harmful ingredients in your food.

Having said that, I realize that we eat things other than just whole fruits and vegetables, so when we buy such things as canned beans, pre-made soups, store-bought tortillas, and other processed foods, I recommend we try to choose those with

- The fewest ingredients possible
- Ingredients whose names we can recognize
- Ingredients that are animal-free

Now, some people argue that once you eliminate the most obvious animal products from your diet (meat, animal's milk, and eggs), you can relax a bit when it comes to the animal products hidden in commercial foods. Although I agree that being vegan is not about obsessing over being perfect, the fact is I simply don't want to consume the blood, bones, or fat of animals, even when they're hidden among other ingredients. I would never buy any of these things if they were sold individually, and I don't want to eat them shoved into my food as filler or fat. In fact, many of these animal products are given names other than what they really are because even the manufacturers know that people wouldn't buy them if they knew exactly what they were.

Gelatin: Made by boiling the slaughterhouse remains of bones, skin, and connective tissues of animals—most often cattle, pigs, horses, and fishes—gelatin is the by-product of the meat and leather industries. If it says "gelatin" on the label, it is animal-derived. Though there are vegetable-derived gelatinlike products available, such as agar, guar gum, carrageenan, and pectin, they would *not* be the source if a label simply says "gelatin."

- **PRODUCTS MOST ASSOCIATED WITH GELATIN** are Jell-O, marshmallows, vitamin capsules, gummy candies, and ice cream. Vegan versions of each are available. For marshmallows, check out Dandies made by Chicago Soy Dairy (chicagosoydairy.com) and those made by Sweet and Sara (sweetandsara.com).

- **ETHICAL CONSIDERATION:** Though gelatin is made from the by-products of slaughterhouse waste, it is misguided to think that using the remains of the animals is a noble use of what would "go to waste," as many people assert. We unnecessarily kill 10 billion land animals and countless marine animals every year, and the industries that profit off these animals have come up with sundry ways to make even more money by selling their by-products. These very profitable by-product industries simply wouldn't exist if we didn't kill animals in the first place. By purchasing animal by-products, we are supporting the primary industries we ethically oppose.

Whey and casein: Both are derived from animal's milk. When you curdle dairy-based milk (to make cheese), you are essentially separating the milk solids (casein) from the milk liquid (whey). If the label says "casein," "caseinate," "milk protein," "sodium caseinate," or "whey," they are most definitely animal-derived. Some soy- and rice-based cheeses have casein added to them. Although a similar process takes place to make tofu (see "Day 21: Demystifying Tofu: It's Just a Bean!"), no plant-based milk naturally contains casein or whey.

- **PRODUCTS MOST ASSOCIATED WITH CASEIN AND WHEY:** Some—but not all—brands of protein powders, boxed cereals, cereal bars, processed sandwich breads, prepared bread crumbs, and crackers contain these cow's milk derivatives. Vegan versions of these foods are definitely available, so just check the label.

- **HEALTH CONSIDERATION:** When you separate the curds from the whey to make cheese, you're tangling up all the milk proteins (the casein) into solid masses or curds. What remains contains only whey proteins. In cow's milk, 80 to 87 percent of the proteins are caseins, which is not a good thing. According to renowned researcher and professor emeritus of nutritional biochemistry at Cornell University T. Colin Campbell, casein is the "number one carcinogen [cancer-causing substance] that people come in contact with on a daily basis." In dairy-based cheeses, the casein is even more concentrated, and in low-fat dairy milks, there tends to be more casein to make up for the fat that has been removed.

Lactose: The sugar in all mammalian milk (including that of humans), lactose appears on labels as such. However, "lactate" or "lactic acid" is not animal-derived.

■ HEALTH CONSIDERATION: There seems to be a misunderstanding about the components that make up mammalian milk, since I often hear people mistakenly assert that they're "allergic to milk" and thus drink lactose-free cow's milk. Casein is the *milk protein* to which people can become allergic; lactose is the *milk sugar* that gives many people gas, bloating, and cramps. Since so many people are suffering from "lactose intolerance," which is our body's natural revulsion to a sugar we're not equipped to digest after we're weaned, the dairy industry came up with a profitable solution: lactose-free milk. Though the milk may not contain lactose, it still contains saturated fat, dietary cholesterol, and casein. If you want truly lactose-free milk, drink those derived from plants.

Lanolin: A fat derived from sheep's wool, lanolin is a by-product of the wool industry, and it is most commonly found in cosmetics, lotions, moisturizers, and lip balms. The product Oil of Olay is derived from the word *lanolin,* which is a primary ingredient. Plenty of beauty products are made without lanolin.

Stearate or stearic acid: A fat derived from either plant or animal sources, it's used for making candles, soaps, and plastics; it's sometimes used in chewing gum and candy. The best way to know its source is to read the label. If it's plant-derived, it will most likely say so.

Carmine or cochineal: Both of these terms refer to the ground-up bodies of beetles that are then used as a coloring in red-colored juices, dairy-based yogurt and ice cream, and cosmetics. The word *carmine* is derived from a word that means "crimson," so essentially you'll find it in products that are some shade of red, pink, or purple. It also appears on labels as "carminic acid."

Bonito: These are dried fish flakes and are frequently seen in Japanese foods.

Lard: The fat taken from pigs' stomachs.

Lipoids or lipids: The fat and fatlike substances found in animals and plants. When they're from plants, they usually say so.

Rennet or rennin: An enzyme taken from the fourth stomach of young ruminants to make dairy-based cheese. Each ruminant produces the special kind of rennet needed to digest his or her mother's milk. There's kid-goat rennet especially for goat's-milk cheese, lamb rennet for sheep's-milk cheese, and calf rennet for cow's-milk cheese. In the case of the latter, most of the stomachs are from the discarded males of the dairy industry who are sold to the veal industry.

Urea or uric acid: Excreted in urine and other bodily fluids, it's used to give a brown color to baked goods, such as pretzels. It will appear on the label as such.

Isinglass: This is derived from the swim bladders of sturgeon fish and is used as a clarifying agent in some wines and beers. It won't appear on the label, but any beer or wine labeled "vegan" means that it wasn't clarified with isinglass. The isinglass is typically not present in the finished beer or wine.

INTENTION, NOT PERFECTION

These days we also see a lot of warnings on labels that say the food was manufactured in plants and on equipment that have also been used to handle cow's milk and other allergens. This is more about liability protection than anything else. The Food Allergy Labeling and Consumer Protection Act now requires labeling of any food that contains or was in contact with machinery that processed one or more of the following allergens: peanuts, soybeans, cow's milk, eggs, fish, crustacean shellfish, tree nuts, and wheat.

CHALLENGE YOUR THINKING:
Being vegan is not about striving for an unattainable level of purity. Being vegan is about intention—not perfection.

CHANGE YOUR BEHAVIOR:
Do the best you can to make compassionate, healthful choices that cause the least amount of harm to others.

People have asked me if I—from a vegan perspective—buy or eat products that may be processed using machinery that also has non-vegan products processed on it. My answer is yes, I do. That kind of low-level concern about purity is not why I'm vegan, and it doesn't mean I'm less vegan if I eat chocolate chips that were processed on machinery that *may* also process non-vegan chips.

Being vegan is about doing the best we can in this imperfect world. It's not about being perfect or pure. If we lose sight of that, if we treat veganism as the end rather than the means, not only will we drive ourselves crazy, we'll also forget what being vegan is all about. Though there are some things we have no control over, I think it makes more sense to focus on what we can do rather than on what we can't. And there's so much we *can* do.

DAY 4 Getting to Know the Grocery Store

You've cleaned out your cupboards, made your shopping list, and learned how to identify animal-based ingredients at a glance. It's time to go shopping and perhaps visit aisles you've never ventured down before!

Habituated to choosing the same items again and again, we're not even aware of how unconscious our choices are when we shop. But make no mistake about it. Though it appears you're exercising personal choice and freedom when you choose one product over another, massive efforts and huge amounts of money go into influencing—that is, manipulating—your decisions. Careers are built on the study of consumer behavior, and each and every item sold in the grocery store—the average supermarket sells 40,000 edible products—is methodically shelved, priced, and advertised based on the results of these studies.

At a time when cardiovascular disease, diabetes, and obesity are at an all-time high, food companies famously shirk responsibility and deny their own influence, claiming that individuals have the freedom to make their own personal choices and are clearly choosing the foods that they want.

You often hear this type of reasoning in the attempt to justify people's consumption of meat, dairy, and eggs: "If people didn't want these things, they wouldn't buy them. The animal products industries are just filling a consumer demand." Never mind that the demand is created and shaped by the very companies that have the most to gain. Every day, every moment—whether it's through radio and television commercials; magazine, newspaper, and Internet advertisements; supermarket product placement; billboards; or celebrity endorsements—*we are told what to eat,* especially when it comes to animal products. We're told that "real men eat beef," that humans are *supposed to* consume

> **CHALLENGE YOUR THINKING:** Though it appears you're exercising personal choice and freedom when you choose one product over another, massive efforts and huge amounts of money go into influencing— that is, manipulating—your decisions.
>
> **CHANGE YOUR BEHAVIOR:** Make informed food choices by becoming a conscious, informed, savvy shopper.

the milk of another animal, that chicken's eggs are "nature's perfect food." Unless you live in a hole in the ground, you're not immune to these messages, which are so powerful, so prevalent, and so effective that any recommendation against consuming meat, dairy, and eggs appears *biased*.

This plays out in the number of times I've heard people declare that vegans have an "agenda": "It's fine if they want to eat that way, but they shouldn't tell other people how to eat. They shouldn't impose their opinions on others." Yet the companies that have the most to gain are telling us how to eat *all the time*. We've been conditioned to believe that to consume meat, dairy, and eggs is to take a neutral position but to be vegan is to have an agenda. Just one critically minded walk through a typical grocery store is enough to demonstrate that we choose—almost hypnotically—what the food companies want us to choose—primarily in the form of unhealthful animal products and processed junk.

> **CHALLENGE YOUR THINKING:**
> To eat and promote meat and other animal-derived products is to take a position; meat is not neutral.

So how do you take this inevitable weekly or biweekly trek through the supermarket and make the most healthful, conscious, compassionate choices possible? Consider the next 30 days an exercise in looking through a vegan lens. As you begin to look at the world this way, you see options you never noticed before. It's just a matter of opening your eyes and venturing down some new aisles.

- **LEARN THE LAYOUT:** Once you begin seeking it out, you'll find vegan food all over the place, everywhere you look. Here are some tips for finding vegan items that may be new to you. Placement may vary from store to store, but in general:

  - Nondairy milks are next to dairy-based milks in the refrigerated section, but aseptically packaged milks are on the shelves where similarly packaged juice boxes are kept.
  - Nondairy butters, yogurts, and cheeses are next to dairy-based butters, yogurts, and cheeses.
  - Vegetarian meats, tempeh, and tofu tend to be shelved together in the dairy section. Some grocery stores shelve them in the freezer. Silken tofu, however, in cardboard aseptic packages, tends to be shelved either with baking ingredients or in the Asian section of a grocery store.
  - Some brands of eggless mayonnaise are in the condiment section, but some are refrigerated in the dairy section.
  - Commercial egg replacer powder tends to be with baking ingredients. Don't be led astray by a grocery clerk who brings you to the refrigerated section to show you Egg Beaters in the little carton. They're still eggs—they're just egg *whites*.
  - Nondairy ice creams are in the freezer with dairy-based ice creams.

- Veggie burgers are often in the frozen section, though tofu-based burgers tend to be in the refrigerated section next to the tofu. Burger mixes, such as those by Fantastic Foods, would most likely be in the aisle with similar types of prepared boxed foods that just call for adding hot water.

- **PICK UP A NEW FOOD:** The most familiar vegan foods for you will be vegetables, fruits, nuts, seeds, legumes, grains, mushrooms, herbs, and spices, but just because you know what a vegetable is doesn't mean you've tried them all. Pick up a new plant food today in any of the aforementioned categories and give it a try.

- **GO INTERNATIONAL:** Check out the shelves reserved for Asian, Middle Eastern, Mexican, and Indian food items. You'll find sauces, condiments, prepared meals, spices—most of which happen to be vegan.

- **ASK FOR WHAT YOU WANT:** If your store doesn't carry a vegan item you're looking for, ask them to stock it. If their distributors carry it, the store will more than likely be happy to sell it—especially if they know at least one person will buy it. (Most likely, more people will buy it once it's stocked, and the store will continue selling it.)

- **SHOP ON THE PERIMETER:** The outside aisles are where you'll find the fresh, whole foods, such as produce and bulk items such as grains and nuts. More processed products are in the center aisles.

- **SHOP BY COLOR:** This is easy to do when you're centering your diets on whole foods (not colorfully packaged items). When in the produce section, fill your cart with as much color variety as possible.

In addition to health food stores and vegan stores (see the box on page 60), don't forget to check out those little neighborhood markets that cater to specific cuisines. You can find an array of tantalizing plant-based condiments, spices, and herbs in Indian, Middle Eastern, Asian, or Mexican markets.

VEGAN GROCERY STORES

Although you can find almost any of the vegan food items I recommend in natural food stores, online and bricks-and-mortar vegan grocery stores are popping up all over the world. The following vegan-owned companies specialize in food but also carry an array of compassionate products such as clothing, shoes, and toiletries.

- **FOOD FIGHT VEGAN GROCERY** in Portland, Oregon. Online and retail store (foodfightgrocery.com).

- **COSMOS VEGAN** in Marietta, Georgia. Shop via the online store, and have items shipped or pick up your order at their showroom during visiting hours (cosmosveganshoppe.com).

- **PARK + VINE** in Cincinnati, Ohio. Retail storefront (parkandvine.com).

- **SIDECAR PIGS FOR PEACE** in Seattle, Washington. Shop online or in person (sidecarforpigspeace.com).

- **VEGAN ESSENTIALS** in Wisconsin. Online shopping; no in-person shopping, but they welcome you to pick up orders that are placed online, or visit to try on footwear (veganessentials.com).

- **VEGAN STORE** in Rockville, Maryland. Online store, open for walk-in customers during select hours (veganstore.com).

DAY 5   Trying New Foods and Creating New Habits

I've heard every excuse in the book for not going vegan, and I'm certain that each one stems from fear-based perceptions rather than experiential reality. This is evident in some of these common excuses:

- *Preparing and cooking vegetables is very different and much harder than cooking meat and animal products.*

- *I tried being vegan, but I got bored with eating the same foods over and over again. I wanted more options.*

- *If I become vegan, I'll experience restriction, limitation, and deprivation.*

The problem is that our perception of ourselves and our habits isn't always aligned with reality. As William Shakespeare wrote in *Hamlet,* "There is nothing either good or bad, but thinking makes it so." We need to take veganism out of the box and recognize that it's not as unfamiliar as we think.

If you've been looking in one direction your whole life, choosing the same foods over and over, and not leaving your comfort zone, you're most likely stuck in habits and routines that compel you to make snap judgments against vegan food, placing it in an ugly box marked "other" and allowing yourself to remain unchanged.

The truth is that when you become vegan, you become aware of the fact that you have more food choices than ever before. It's not that those choices weren't available to you when you were eating meat, dairy, and eggs; it's just that you weren't looking outside of your comfort zone. When you shift your gaze from one direction to another, an entire world opens up—of new cuisines, new flavors, new textures, new aromas, new experiences. And how exciting is that? Think about the process of going from eating Italian cuisine your whole life to learning how to prepare Indian cuisine. You're intuitively aware that

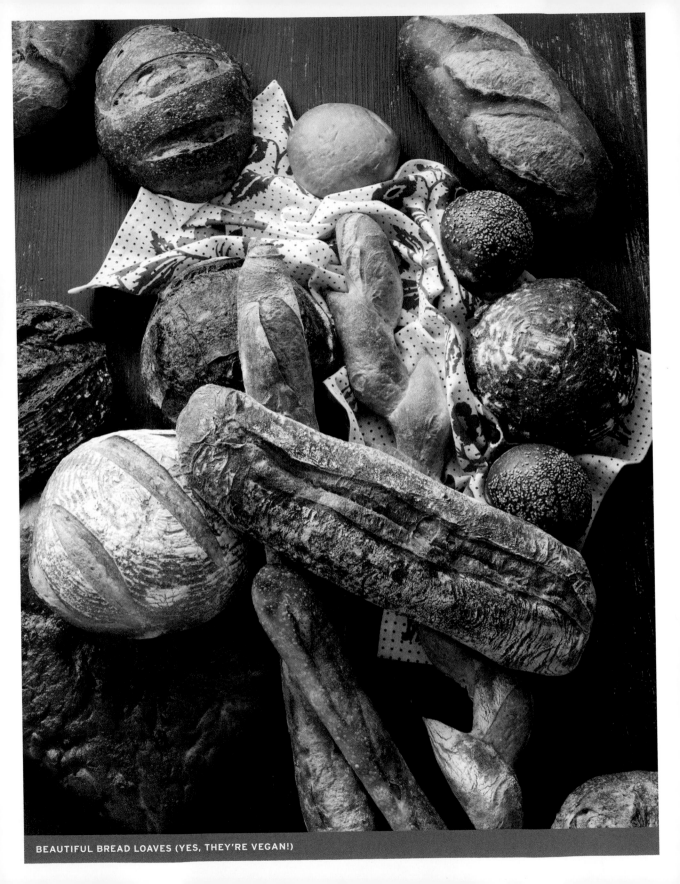

BEAUTIFUL BREAD LOAVES (YES, THEY'RE VEGAN!)

you need to learn some new techniques and explore some new ingredients, but you don't judge Indian cuisine as being inferior to Italian cuisine. You just recognize that it's different and unfamiliar to *you*.

Some of our blocks about veganism aren't simply about the food itself but are also about how we plate our food. In our meat-centric culture, we're accustomed to having a piece of meat at the center of our plate, surrounded by some token vegetables (most likely covered in dairy-based butter and cream sauces). Many people perceive a vegan meal as lacking because they imagine that piece of meat being removed, leaving the plate with only side dishes. I think this is one of the reasons people think vegans eat "only sides" or "only salads."

But the way we plate our food is a cultural construct—what we've been taught in our families and in our society. If you think about cuisines all around the world and how the food is plated, you'll remember that it can look very different from a Western meal. Think of Indian, Mexican, Thai, Chinese, Vietnamese, Italian, or Ethiopian cuisines. The plates are made up of what we in the West would call "side dishes." And yet these are the most healthful and flavorful dishes, based on vegetables, grains, lentils, beans, and greens. So we need to rethink what a plate of food "should" actually look like as well as embrace the notion of having a plate of what we would call "side dishes."

Perception also plays a huge role when we say "I don't eat a lot of meat/fish/cheese/eggs/fill-in-the-blank." Frankly, I don't know one person who hasn't said this. Everyone seems to have this perception of themselves, and yet 45 billion land and sea animals are killed every year in the United States for human consumption. Someone is eating the animals and their secretions!

The truth is, you really don't know how much you're eating until you stop. When you stop, you realize how many of the things you automatically reached for before were meat-, dairy-, or egg-based. We become acutely more aware of our habits once we make an effort to change them.

- The first step is eliminating meat, dairy, and eggs—which you're doing on the 30-Day Vegan Challenge.

CHALLENGE YOUR THINKING: If you've been cooking Italian food your whole life and decide to master Indian cuisine, you realize there are things you don't know and need to learn. You don't judge Indian cuisine as being *inferior* to Italian cuisine; you just recognize that it's *different* and *unfamiliar* to *you*.

CHANGE YOUR BEHAVIOR: Embrace whatever new "vegan foods" you discover on your journey, resisting the temptation to judge them as *inferior* to the animal-based foods with which you're familiar.

CHALLENGE YOUR THINKING: The way we plate our food is a cultural construct.

CHANGE YOUR BEHAVIOR: Rethink what a plate of food "should" look like, using cuisines from around the world as inspiration, and give yourself permission to create a plate of what we typically call "side dishes."

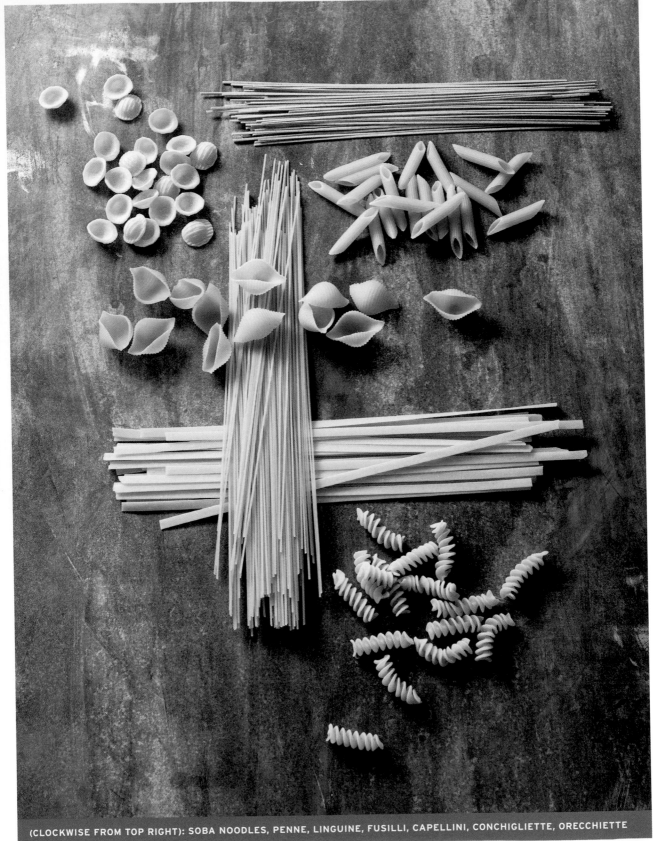

(CLOCKWISE FROM TOP RIGHT): SOBA NOODLES, PENNE, LINGUINE, FUSILLI, CAPELLINI, CONCHIGLIETTE, ORECCHIETTE

- The second step is recognizing your patterns.

- The third step is replacing these habits with new ones.

This last step is often what trips people up, but it need not. You don't have to create an entirely new repertoire of foods unless you want to. If you're like most people, vegan or not, you're most likely rotating the same dishes again and again. You make the same favorite meals, go to the same restaurants, and order the same items each time. We're such creatures of habit that experts estimate that we rotate the same seven or eight meals each month. This is one of the reasons I find it so ironic that people say *vegans* don't eat a variety of food. I have found it to be quite the opposite.

To create your new repertoire rotation, consult the 3-Day Food Diary you created before you started the Challenge, and do the following:

1. Write down or note what you already eat that's vegan. Common examples include:
   a. pasta with marinara sauce
   b. peanut butter and jelly sandwiches
   c. chips and salsa
   d. corn or flour tortillas with rice, beans, and guacamole
   e. vegetable stir-fry
   f. tossed green salad with raw veggies
   g. bean chili (see recipe on page 158)
   h. minestrone (vegetable soup)
   i. hummus (see recipe on page 159)

You'll most likely find that at least three dishes in your current repertoire are already vegan. Highlight those.

2. Next, take a look at your diary and pick out three of your favorite meat-, dairy-, or egg-based dishes. Now think of ways to easily "veganize" them. For instance, you can:
   a. use vegetable stock in place of chicken stock in your favorite soup
   b. add a few drops of liquid smoke or a chopped chipotle pepper to your favorite split pea soup (see page 233) instead of ham to get that smoky, salty flavor
   c. sprinkle toasted salted pine nuts on your favorite pasta dish instead of Parmesan cheese
   d. replace dairy-based sour cream with nondairy sour cream or guacamole
   e. add vegetarian meat crumbles or crumbled thawed tofu to marinara sauce and serve over pasta
   f. use mushrooms, tofu, or tempeh in place of meat in a stir-fry
   g. make pesto without the Parmesan cheese, enjoying the rich flavors of the pine nuts, basil, garlic, and olive oil with a little salt

Now you've got six vegan recipes—and they're all familiar favorites!

3. Finally, learn three new recipes. Consult the recipes throughout this book for a number of breakfast, lunch, dinner, dessert, and snack ideas.

Without making much effort, you've just discovered nine vegan recipes for your rotation, and only three of them are new. This enables you to still enjoy your favorites while discovering new dishes. One of the most gratifying comments I hear from people is that in becoming vegan they find a love of cooking. They find themselves excited to try new recipes and cuisines, and they gain a confidence in the kitchen they never had before. Even if you don't wind up loving cooking, just being willing to try new flavors is an improvement.

As time goes on, I encourage you to continue to rotate these nine dishes. I'm always struck by people who say they tried being vegan but became bored eating the same foods over and over again. The fact that we get stuck in ruts is not the fault of being vegan. It's because we became lazy and didn't rotate or expand our repertoire. Rotating the same meals is fine for a while, but be sure to explore the thousands of plant foods and flavors out there to keep things exciting and new.

CHALLENGE YOUR THINKING: The fact that we get stuck in cooking and eating ruts isn't the fault of being vegan. It's because we become lazy and don't rotate or expand our repertoire.

CHANGE YOUR BEHAVIOR: Periodically rotate your favorite dishes; even changing one meal every couple of months keeps things dynamic rather than static.

DAY 6 Making the Time to Cook

Let's assess things thus far. You've been to the grocery store, learned to recognize animal-derived ingredients on labels, restocked your kitchen with healthful foods, and realized that many of the things you were already eating were vegan. Now it's time to demystify cooking. Although I expect you will have prepared some vegan meals before today—perhaps some from your old repertoire—this chapter is about helping you lay a strong foundation that will empower you to feel confident in the kitchen. It's also an opportunity to start trying some of the recipes featured throughout the book.

One of the most common excuses for not eating a healthful, plant-based diet is "I just don't have time to cook." We've become so dependent on processed, packaged, frozen, and fast food that our barometer for how much time we should spend on preparing our meals has become completely skewed. Our idea of how long we should spend on cooking (and eating!) has become completely distorted. Our threshold for chopping vegetables is about zero.

We need a new measuring stick. It's true that cooking requires a little extra time, but compared to what? Compared to throwing a package of processed foodlike substances into the microwave? Sure, I'll concede. Cooking requires more time than that, but is that really the measuring stick we want to use?

Even if you think you're eating well but basing your diet on animal-based products, complaining that you have to chop vegetables is still not a viable excuse. *Everyone*, not just vegans, should be eating vegetables.

CHALLENGE YOUR THINKING: Our threshold for chopping vegetables has become completely distorted.

CHANGE YOUR BEHAVIOR: Create a new measuring stick. Decide what is a reasonable amount of time to spend on chopping vegetables each day, with 15 minutes being the minimum.

Fifteen to thirty minutes is a reasonable amount of time to spend making food for ourselves and our families, and it's not only possible, it's imperative. Taking fifteen to thirty minutes a day to nurture ourselves, to nourish our bodies, and to feed our families is really no time at all. In fact, whatever we're doing that we think is so much more important than taking care of ourselves and our loved ones will mean nothing when we're not well enough or not here to enjoy it. If we think we can't find a few minutes a day to take care of ourselves and those who depend on us, then perhaps we need to reexamine our priorities.

The bottom line is this: if we don't have time to be sick, then we have to make time to be healthy.

WE HAVE THE TIME; WE DON'T MAKE THE EFFORT

But if you want to know the truth, I think we *do* have the time. Although everyone complains about busy schedules, if we were really honest with ourselves, we'd admit that we *do* have the time to cook; we just don't *use* our time to make the effort.

If we have the time to pack the family into the car, drive to a restaurant, find a parking spot, stand in line to wait for a table, decide what to order, wait for the food, eat the food, wait for the bill, pay the bill, and drive back home, then we have time to chop some vegetables.

The goal is to make healthful, delicious, plant-based meals in a reasonable amount of time—not spend countless hours in the kitchen. With that in mind, let's look at a number of ways to make this a reality.

CHOP VEGETABLES IN ADVANCE

Most of us can identify with this scenario: You go to the grocery store and stock up on vegetables, then come home and store the vegetables in the refrigerator. When it's time to eat, you return to the fridge, stare into its great abyss, and declare, "There's not a thing to eat." You lament that it would take too long to cut up the veggies in time for dinner, so instead you call the pizza guy or heat up a frozen dinner, while said vegetables begin to break down without being eaten, eventually ending up in the trash can instead of in your belly.

Now picture this: You come home from the grocery store and instead of shoving all the vegetables in the fridge, you take 15 minutes to chop them—at least some of them. You store the chopped veggies in bags and containers and *then* place them in the fridge. Hours later, you return. Looking at the chopped peppers, sliced onion, and minced garlic, you're inspired to make a stir-fry. The sliced carrots serve as a snack while you put it all together, and the cooking process itself is enjoyable and stress-free.

For some reason, if the tops are still on the carrots, the broccoli is still joined at the stem, or the cauliflower is still in its head, we have a mental block. We complain that it will take us *forever* to chop them up, and so we leave them to compost in the refrigerator and wonder why we're always throwing vegetables away.

"If we chop them, we will eat them," say I. We know this works with kids, and it works with adults, too.

Once the vegetables are stored, how long will they keep in the fridge before they start to lose their freshness? The answer is about five days or so, but here's a secret: *don't let them sit in the fridge*. Eat them! The idea is to get them into your belly, not see how long they keep before they start to break down.

Store these veggies in water: If cut-up root vegetables and tubers, such as potatoes, yams, beets, sweet potatoes, and winter squash (butternut, acorn, Kabocha), are not kept in water, they'll turn brown.

Store these veggies in sealed containers: Cut-up carrots, celery, bell peppers, broccoli, cauliflower, and onions stay fresh in a well-sealed container or bag.

Store these veggies wrapped in a towel: Green leafy vegetables, including kale, collard greens, chard, beet greens, and lettuce, can be chopped in advance, but they need to be wrapped in a dish towel or paper towels and then stored in an airtight plastic bag. Their fridge life is a little shorter, particularly the more delicate lettuce, which will start to oxidize (turn brown) after two days.

Store these veggies in jars: Garlic, ginger, and shallots are perfect for mincing up in the food processor and storing (separately) in glass jars.

Many grocery stores sell cut-up vegetables, which is also an option. I'm always amused when people, especially those who aren't eating a lot of vegetables, become suddenly concerned that vegetables lose their nutrients once they're cut up and stored. It's an unfounded concern. You may be sacrificing a little flavor and freshness, but you're not sacrificing nutrition. Let's keep things in perspective: vegetables cut in advance are better than no vegetables at all.

> **CHALLENGE YOUR THINKING:**
> *If we chop them, we will eat them!* For all intents and purposes, vegetables chopped in advance are more nutritious than no vegetables at all.

DON'T WAIT UNTIL DINNERTIME TO DECIDE WHAT TO HAVE FOR DINNER

Because I argue that our blocks to eating healthfully and compassionately are all in our mind, I'm absolutely convinced that the secret to eating well and consuming more vegetables has more to do with planning in advance than anything else.

Giving our meals just a little forethought can make all the difference, and that doesn't require anything more than thinking. You don't have to *do* anything. Most people decide what they're going to eat once they're already hungry, and at that stage we don't make decisions based on nutrition; we make decisions based on speed or cravings. It might be another story if we follow my first piece of advice and have chopped-up vegetables in the refrigerator, but that only strengthens my point: *plan in advance*.

Though we can be a little more flexible with breakfast (since it tends to be the simplest meal of the day), when it comes to dinner in particular, we should know the *night before* what we're going to have for dinner the following night. Stretch it to the next morning at the very latest, but we should absolutely know what we're eating for dinner long before that time arrives.

Here's how it plays out:

- As you lie in bed tonight, think about what you have in the refrigerator. Decide to wake up 10 minutes earlier than usual, and take that time to chop a few veggies: a bunch of carrots, two potatoes, and an onion for a soup; bell peppers for chili; or lettuce, cauliflower, and celery for a salad.

- If you decide you want a grain dish tomorrow night, throw some rice or quinoa or barley into a saucepan tonight, along with water and a vegetable bouillon cube. Turn on the heat and before you know it, half of tomorrow night's dinner is already prepared.

- When you're preparing dinner tonight and your recipe calls for one chopped onion, chop *two* onions. Use one for your recipe, and store one in a container. You already have the cutting board and knife out, so take advantage of that.

- Before you leave for work in the morning, toss your favorite vegetables or tofu into a marinade and leave them all day. When you come home, roast or grill them.

- While you're getting ready in the morning, throw lentils, spices, chopped onion, and garlic into a slow cooker and turn the heat to low. Come home to a dinner ready to eat.

COOK MORE THAN YOU NEED

Though I stand by my recommendation for taking fifteen to thirty minutes a day to cook, if you're always planning ahead, you may not even need that much time each day. One night you might eat out, one night you may have leftovers, and another night you may have food you prepared in advance and froze, in which case all you need to do is thaw and reheat.

I've often heard single people lament that most recipes tend to be created for two or four people and that they're forever searching for recipes for one. *Au contraire! I encourage* people to cook for two if they're just one person or for four if they're just a couple. The idea is to always make more than you need so you have leftovers to eat the next day or to freeze for the coming week.

With that in mind, you can see how you won't necessarily have to prepare meals every day. Sure, you may have to reheat them or throw together a quick side salad, but the bulk of the meal is already made.

CREATE A MEAL SCHEDULE

We humans are fierce creatures of habit, which can work in our favor or against us. Habit connects us with what is familiar, making us feel comfortable and safe. We appreciate the predictable. We crave routine. Our food rituals and traditions bear this out, as do our meal rotations.

A memory I cherish from my childhood is pizza night. Every Friday night was pizza night—and not pizza we ordered from a pizzeria. I mean pizza we made ourselves, using our favorite base: English muffins. I could count on these nights like clockwork, and each member of the family made his or her own variations: sauce on top of the cheese, sauce under the cheese, shredded cheese, sliced cheese, chunky sauce, pureed sauce. It was serious work, and it always preceded our weekly jaunt to the movie theater.

A meal schedule doesn't have to be rigid, and it may not work for everyone, but having a general guide might be helpful. You might decide that:

- Monday nights are for soups or stews
- Tuesday nights are dedicated to stir-fries
- Wednesday nights are for Mexican cuisine
- Thursday nights are sandwich nights
- Friday nights are for pasta or pizza

The options are endless, and once you know how you want to break things down, you can create a list of favorite recipes or dishes you already have that fit into these categories. Hang these lists on the refrigerator door.

Knowing exactly what you plan to eat for the week enables you to go to the store with a game plan instead of wandering aimlessly around, spending more money than you want to or planned on. Shopping with a list means you're more likely to stick to it and not buy unnecessary ingredients for dishes you're not even planning on cooking.

With a game plan, you've already tackled the hardest part of cooking: deciding what to make!

Starting Off the Day Right: Breakfast Ideas

With six days of breakfast behind you, I imagine you're recognizing how familiar vegan food actually is. But in order to show you how many options you have, I'm providing a huge range of breakfast ideas here. As with all of our food choices, there is a spectrum in terms of nutrient density; though vegan breakfasts are more healthful than any animal-based version, the best thing we can do is choose the most nutrient-rich foods that are high in fiber and low in calories.

Assuming they're even making time for breakfast in the first place, most people—vegan or not—tend to rotate the same things every day. It's not that we don't have a bevy of options to choose from, but our desire for routine and familiarity tends to trump anything else. That's fine if that works for you. In fact, even within our regular repertoires, we can find a lot of variety, depending on the type of milk we use or what kind of bread we choose. You might also find that you change your breakfast depending on the season—if it's warm or cold—and according to the day of the week. Most of us eat lighter during the week than we do on the weekends.

CHALLENGE YOUR THINKING: Though plant-based breakfasts are more healthful than any animal-based version, the best thing we can do is choose the most nutrient-rich foods that are high in fiber and low in calories.

All of the suggestions below can be applied to kids or adults.

COLD BREAKFASTS

- FRUIT SMOOTHIES: Incredibly nutritious, very filling, and super-versatile, homemade smoothies provide the best bang for your calorie and monetary buck, whether you drink them at home or take them on the road. (See page 83 for recipes for a variety of smoothies.)

- NONDAIRY YOGURT WITH FRESH FRUIT, NUTS, AND GRANOLA: Options abound depending on the yogurt you use (soy, rice, and coconut milk yogurts are in many large food stores), and the type of fruit, cereal, granola, nuts, or seeds you add.

- CEREAL: Skip the sugary brands and choose those that are made with whole grains. Pour on your favorite nondairy milk (almond, oat, soy, rice, hazelnut, or hemp), and mix in some fresh fruit.

- MUESLI: This is a general term for a combination of uncooked rolled oats, fruit (dried and/or fresh), and nuts. Add ground flaxseeds or hulled hemp seeds and your favorite nondairy milk for a hearty, healthful breakfast.

- GRANOLA: Typically added to yogurts, cereal, muesli, or fresh fruit, some commercial granolas are heavily sugar-laden. Check out the bulk section of a large natural food store for more healthful varieties.

- FRESH FRUIT: There is nothing more beautiful and nutrient-dense than a plate of fresh fruit, which can vary according to the season. If it's not enough to fill you up, add nuts, rolled oats, or peanut butter for more sustenance.

- SLICED BANANAS WITH PEANUT OR ALMOND BUTTER: Fast and easy.

- BANANA WITH A HANDFUL OF NUTS: Quick and transportable for one of those on-the-run breakfasts.

- PEANUT BUTTER AND JAM SANDWICH: With banana slices tucked in, this standby is actually a very healthful meal any time of the day.

- LEFTOVERS: Some dishes are even better the next day—cold, right out of the fridge. If you're in a hurry and have the choice between grabbing a container of leftovers and eating nothing at all, choose the former.

- ENERGY BARS: When you're desperate, these are an option. Though most are vegan, some are more healthful than others. (See "Day 9: Packing Lunches for School and Work" for favorite brand names.)

HOT BREAKFASTS

Not all hot breakfasts are meant for the weekends or special occasions; hot porridges such as oatmeal can be whipped up in a jiffy and are perfect in the colder months.

- PORRIDGES: Whether you make them from oats, cornmeal, grits, quinoa, barley, rice, or cream of wheat, the components are the same: nondairy milk, cinnamon, sweetener (dry, such as cane sugar, or liquid, such as maple syrup or agave nectar), dried fruit (such as raisins or dried cranberries), and additional fresh fruit.

- **FRENCH TOAST AND BLUEBERRY PANCAKES:** See pages 79 and 82 for recipes for these incredibly simple breakfast staples. Crepes, which are just thin pancakes, are also an option, and yes, *all* of these can be made delicious and fluffy without eggs!

- **TOFU SCRAMBLE:** Choosing a firm tofu is the secret to the perfect scramble. A little turmeric turns the tofu a beautiful yellow color, leading many people to never notice that they're eating tofu and not scrambled eggs. See page 80 for recipe.

- **TEMPEH SCRAMBLE:** Replace tofu with steamed and crumbled tempeh, and proceed with the Tofu Scramble recipe on page 80.

- **MUSHROOM SCRAMBLE:** Chop up several different types of mushrooms, sauté them in just a little olive oil, season with salt and fresh herbs, and you've got a low-calorie breakfast that can be served with toast or atop polenta.

- **BREAKFAST BURRITO:** Either make it bean-based, just like a typical lunchtime burrito, or roll up your tofu scramble in a flour or corn tortilla along with salsa, chopped avocado, and lettuce.

- **BAKED BEANS:** A typical British breakfast item; you can also include tomato slices and toast with Marmite.

- **VEGAN SAUSAGE:** Gimme Lean and Yves breakfast links provide the fat, salt, and mouthfeel people identify with animal-based sausage.

- **HASH BROWNS:** Make from scratch using shredded potatoes, or buy frozen hash browns (natural brands will contain only potatoes and sometimes oil).

- **HOME FRIES:** Dice (but don't peel) a few potatoes, steam them, and then fry (or roast) them with diced onions in a little oil. Serve with ketchup or nondairy sour cream.

BREAD-BASED BREAKFASTS

- Enjoy whole-wheat toast with your favorite spreads: nondairy butter, peanut butter, almond butter, fruit preserves, Vegemite, or Marmite. For more nutrients, add banana or apple slices. For additional flavor, sprinkle cinnamon on top.

- Smear a bagel with nondairy cream cheese or peanut butter. Top with a sliced banana or strawberries.

- Biscuits and gravy make a heavier meal perhaps more conducive to a special occasion; use the recipe for Drop Biscuits on page 259.

- English muffins with a favorite spread and fruit slices bring me right back to my childhood. Some commercial brands contain whey, but vegan English muffins, such as those made by Rudi's Organic, are available.

PASTRIES

Vegan muffins, donuts, and other pastries can be homemade or found online and in many large natural food stores. You'd be surprised what you can find when you ask.

BREAKFAST BEVERAGES

In terms of vegan options, beverages abound; in terms of nutrient density, be aware that some fruit juices, aside from those you make yourself with a juicer, may be laden with sugar and preservatives, and vegetable juices such as tomato may exceed the recommended allowance for sodium. Coffee—especially as a replacement for breakfast—is not health food, and exotic coffee drinks and even what may appear to be healthful fruit shakes sold in specialty cafes and restaurants may be incredibly calorie-dense. Better to spend your calories on more healthful options.

Of course, fortified nondairy milks can be drunk as beverages, and other hot beverages such as tea, hot cocoa, and tisanes (herbal infusions) are delightful ways to start the day.

Hot Cocoa: Some (not all) commercial hot cocoa powder mixes include cow's milk, but many do not. Such brands include Dagoba (organic and fair trade), which makes Authentic Hot Cocoa as well as Xocolatl Drinking Chocolate; Ah!Laska's Organic Cocoa; Ghirardelli's Sweet Ground Chocolate and Cocoa; and Trader Joe's Natural Mint Cocoa.

You can easily make your own hot cocoa by combining unsweetened cocoa powder with sugar, nondairy milk, and a little vanilla extract. It's inexpensive, and you can determine exactly how sweet to make it. Hot chocolate can be made by melting dark chocolate into nondairy milk, along with a little vanilla extract. Whisk, and serve. Make a Mexican variation by adding cinnamon and chili powder.

While we're talking about chocolate beverages, though I'm not pretending it's health food, many chocolate syrups—for making chocolate milk or ice cream sundaes—are also vegan, including Ah!Laska and Hershey's, though the latter is made with corn syrup.

WHATEVER YOU EAT, DON'T SKIP BREAKFAST!

If you've heard it once, you've heard it a million times: don't skip breakfast—it's the most important meal of the day.

A quick glance at the word itself should tell you why this is so: it's a blend of the words *break* and *fast,* and that's quite literally what you're doing. After having gone without food for ten to fifteen hours, depending on when you ate dinner and how long you've slept, your body awakens in low gear and needs fuel to help you start your day. Your blood sugar has dropped, your metabolism has slowed, and your pistons aren't exactly firing at their optimal level. By eating nutrient-dense food, you create a foundation from which the rest of your day can be built.

CHALLENGE YOUR THINKING:
People who skip breakfast tend to have a higher body mass index than those who eat it. If weight loss is a goal, skipping breakfast is counterproductive.

CHANGE YOUR BEHAVIOR:
Eat breakfast!

CHANGE YOUR BEHAVIOR:
If we don't have time to be sick, we have to make time to be healthy.

Numerous studies strongly link skipping breakfast with being overweight and lacking the ability to concentrate, and this applies to children, adolescents, and adults. In fact, if weight loss is a goal of yours, skipping breakfast is counterproductive. When your body fasts, it goes into conservation mode, which means your metabolism slows down and remains slow until you give your body a message that it can stop conserving energy. That message is food. Calories. Energy. The other reason people who skip breakfast tend to be overweight is because they make up for it later and eat more throughout the day.

Whether they're vegan or not, most people complain that they don't have time to eat breakfast. Balderdash. Remember, *if we don't have time to be sick, we have to make time to be healthy.* If we have the time and forethought to make sure our coffee is ready when we wake up, we have what it takes to make sure we start our day on the right foot.

Tempeh Bacon

YIELD: 10 TO 14 SLICES

Let's face it: bacon is all about the fat, the salt, and the smoky flavor. This recipe provides these three components—and lots of flavor and nutty texture—without the saturated fat, dietary cholesterol, and all the other ickiness that characterizes animal-based bacon.

One 8-ounce package tempeh
¼ cup tamari soy sauce
2 teaspoons liquid smoke

3 tablespoons real maple syrup
¼ cup water
Canola oil for frying

Add the block of tempeh to a 3-quart pot fitted with a steamer basket, and steam for about 10 minutes. (Cut in half if it doesn't fit in your pot.)

Meanwhile, in a large bowl, combine the marinade ingredients: the tamari, liquid smoke, maple syrup, and water. Mix well.

Let the tempeh cool before slicing it into thin bacon-size strips. Place the slices in the marinade, and marinate for as long as you like. The longer you marinate, the stronger the flavor will be, but I often marinate for just less than a half hour. Toss now and then to make sure all the tempeh slices are coated.

Add some canola oil to a sauté pan and fry the tempeh strips over medium-high heat until crisp on one side. Turn, and fry again until crisp on the other. Sprinkle a little extra tamari and maple syrup (or remaining marinade) on the tempeh while it's on the heat, essentially caramelizing the tempeh. After a little time, the tempeh will turn brown, caramelize, and get crispier and chewier. (About 5 minutes on each side is a reasonable estimate.)

Remove from the heat, set on plate with a paper towel to absorb any excess oil.

Variations
- Use tofu in place of tempeh. Cut tofu into strips, marinate, and sauté. I suggest, however, that you use tofu that has been frozen and thawed. (See "Day 21: Demystifying Tofu")
- If you have extra marinade, simply prepare a second package of tempeh or tofu, or use it in a stir-fry.

Wheat-free

DID YOU KNOW?

Liquid smoke is produced by burning hardwood chips (hickory, mesquite, etc.) and condensing the smoke into a liquid form. The liquid is then scrubbed and filtered to remove all impurities. A little goes a long way, and it's a great flavoring for many dishes where you want a smoky flavor, such as Split Pea Soup (page 233).

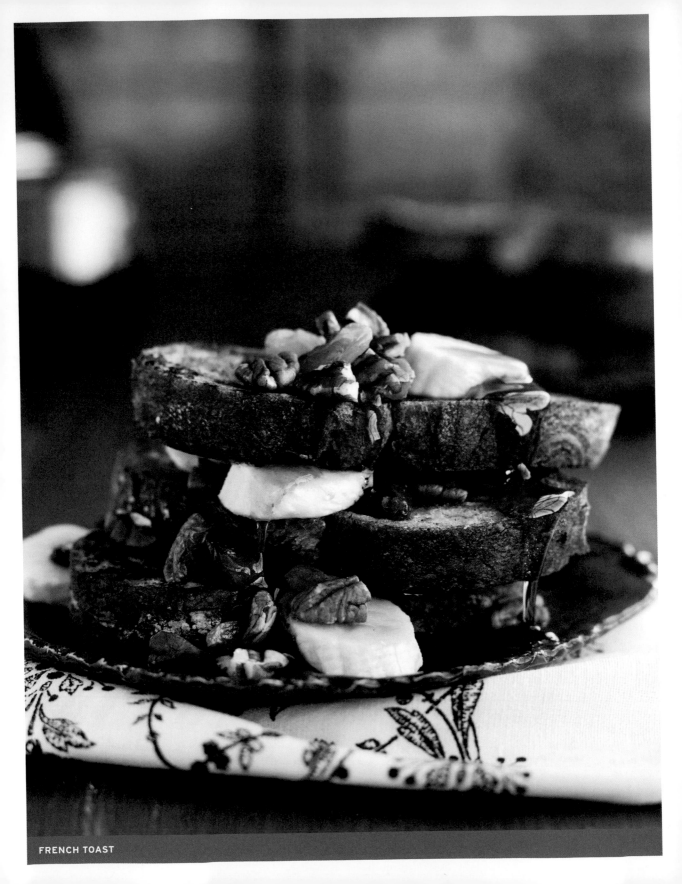

FRENCH TOAST

French Toast

YIELD: 8 TO 9 SERVINGS

First mentioned during the reign of Henry V in England when it was called *pain perdu* or "lost bread," French toast was originally devised as a way to use stale bread. Whether you use fresh or stale, once you try this incredibly easy and delicious dish, you'll ask yourself why we ever use eggs for this quintessential breakfast treat at all.

1 loaf thick Italian or sourdough bread
1 cup nondairy milk (soy, rice, almond, hazelnut, hemp, oat)
1 teaspoon ground cinnamon
¼ teaspoon ground nutmeg

1 teaspoon vanilla extract
4 tablespoons nonhydrogenated, nondairy butter (Earth Balance is best)
Maple syrup for drizzling
Powdered sugar for dusting, optional

Cut the bread into ½-inch slices.

In a shallow bowl, whisk together the milk, cinnamon, nutmeg, and vanilla. Set aside.

Melt the butter in a large skillet over medium heat. Dip each slice of bread into the milk mixture, then place in the hot skillet. Cook until each side is golden brown. You may need to add more butter, especially as you finish cooking the first batch and before you begin to add the second batch of bread.

Remove from heat and transfer to serving plates. Drizzle with maple syrup or dust with sifted confectioners' sugar just before serving.

Variations and Suggestions

- Mix together the maple syrup with raisins and/or ground-up toasted pecans or walnuts.
- Top with fresh berries.
- Use a loaf of cinnamon raisin bread.
- Add banana slices.

Soy-free, if using soy-free Earth Balance

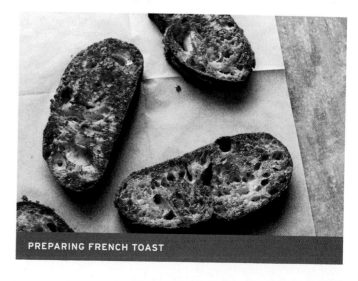

PREPARING FRENCH TOAST

Tofu Scramble

YIELD: 2 TO 4 SERVINGS

The secret to making the perfect Tofu Scramble is using just the right textured tofu. Use an extra firm, and squeeze out some of the water.

1 tablespoon olive oil for sautéing
1 medium yellow onion or 3 scallions (green onions), finely chopped
1 teaspoon minced garlic
1 bell pepper (red, yellow, orange, or green), finely diced
One 16-ounce package extra-firm tofu, drained and rinsed

1 cup loosely packed spinach leaves, rinsed and patted dry
½ teaspoon turmeric
1 teaspoon cumin
½ teaspoon paprika
2 tablespoons nutritional yeast
¼ teaspoon salt, or to taste
Freshly ground pepper to taste

Heat the oil in a sauté pan over medium heat. Add the onion, garlic, and bell pepper and sauté for about 5 minutes, until the onion and peppers are tender and turning a little brown.

Meanwhile, using your hands, crumble the tofu into a bowl to create the consistency of coarse bread crumbs. Add to the sauté pan and stir to combine.

Add the spinach, turmeric, cumin, paprika, and nutritional yeast, and sauté for about 5-8 minutes, stirring occasionally until the tofu is a bright yellow color (from the turmeric) and thoroughly heated.

Add salt and pepper to taste, and serve with toast or Tempeh Bacon (page 77).

Variations

- Sauté sliced cremini mushrooms along with the onions and peppers.
- For a Mexican scramble, add 1 cup of your favorite salsa after the tofu is cooked, and allow it to heat through. Make a Breakfast Burrito by wrapping the scramble in a tortilla and serving with tortilla chips, avocado, and nondairy, nonhydrogenated sour cream.
- For an Italian twist, add fresh herbs such as basil, oregano, rosemary, and/or parsley, and some finely chopped Kalamata olives.
- Keep it simple by eliminating the veggies, aside from the garlic and onion.

Wheat-free

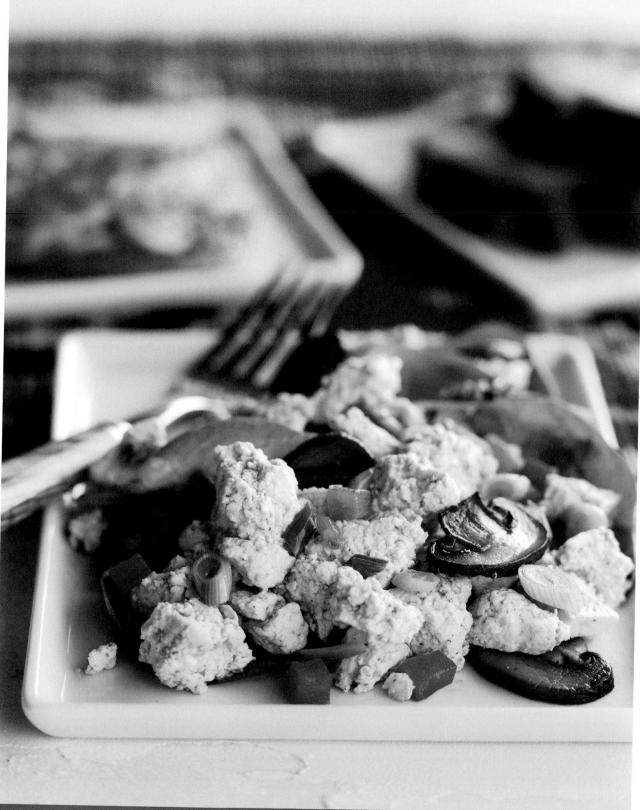

TOFU SCRAMBLE

Blueberry Pancakes

YIELD: 8 TO 10 PANCAKES

These fluffy pancakes are incredibly easy to make.

1 cup unbleached all-purpose or
    whole-wheat pastry flour
1 tablespoon baking powder
1/4 teaspoon salt
1/4 teaspoon cinnamon (optional)
1 cup nondairy milk (soy, rice, almond,
    hazelnut, hemp, oat)
2 tablespoons canola oil or
    nonhydrogenated, nondairy
    butter, melted (Earth Balance is
    my favorite)

3 tablespoons liquid sweetener, such as
    maple syrup, apple juice concentrate,
    or orange juice
1/2 cup blueberries
Additional oil or butter for cooking
    (optional)

Combine the flour, baking powder, salt, and cinnamon in a bowl. In a separate bowl, combine the milk, oil, and sweetener.

Add the milk mixture to the flour mixture and mix just until moistened; a few lumps are okay. Fold in the blueberries but don't overstir.

Heat a nonstick griddle or sauté pan over medium high heat. (You may add some oil or nondairy butter to the griddle or sauté pan and heat until hot, but with a nonstick pan, you don't even need it.)

Pour batter onto the griddle to form circles about 4 inches in diameter. Cook the pancakes for a couple minutes on one side until bubbles appear on the surface. Slide a spatula under the pancake and flip it over. Cook the pancakes on the other side for another 2 minutes or so. Continue until golden brown on each side, about 4 minutes in all.

Soy-free

Fruit Smoothie Trio: Blueberry, Mango, and Green

It's very difficult to create a "recipe" for smoothies, because there are so many options and variations depending on the season and your likes and dislikes. Here are three of my favorites; customize them to your taste as you please. Although fresh (unfrozen) bananas work perfectly fine, using frozen bananas adds a wonderful thickness to the smoothies.

Blueberry Smoothie

YIELD: ONE 16-OUNCE GLASS

1 or 2 ripe bananas, preferably frozen chunks from the freezer
½ cup or more frozen blueberries
¼ cup frozen strawberries
¼ cup fresh orange juice

½ cup nondairy milk (soy, rice, almond, oat, hemp, or hazelnut)
1 tablespoon almond butter or other nut butter
1 tablespoon ground flaxseeds

Mango Smoothie

YIELD: ONE 16-OUNCE GLASS

1 or 2 ripe bananas, preferably frozen chunks from the freezer
½ cup or more frozen mango
¼ cup frozen pineapple chunks
¼ cup fresh orange juice

½ cup nondairy milk (soy, rice, almond, oat, hemp, or hazelnut)
1 tablespoon peanut butter
1 tablespoon ground flaxseeds
¼ cup nondairy yogurt (optional)

Green Smoothie

YIELD: TWO 16-OUNCE GLASSES

1 or 2 ripe bananas, preferably frozen chunks from the freezer
1 or 2 apples, quartered (not peeled)
1 cup pineapple chunks
2 loosely packed cups spinach (or kale, chard, or other greens)

½-inch piece ginger, peeled
2 or 3 pitted dates
1½ cups cold water
¼ cup juice (apple, pineapple, orange)
1 tablespoon ground flaxseeds

For each smoothie, add all the ingredients to a blender and mix until thoroughly blended. You can make it thinner or thicker depending on your preference. Just vary the juice and milk for the consistency you prefer. Any blender will work, though a high-powered one, such as a Vitamix, creates the smoothest, creamiest consistency.

Wheat-free, soy-free if using soy-free milk

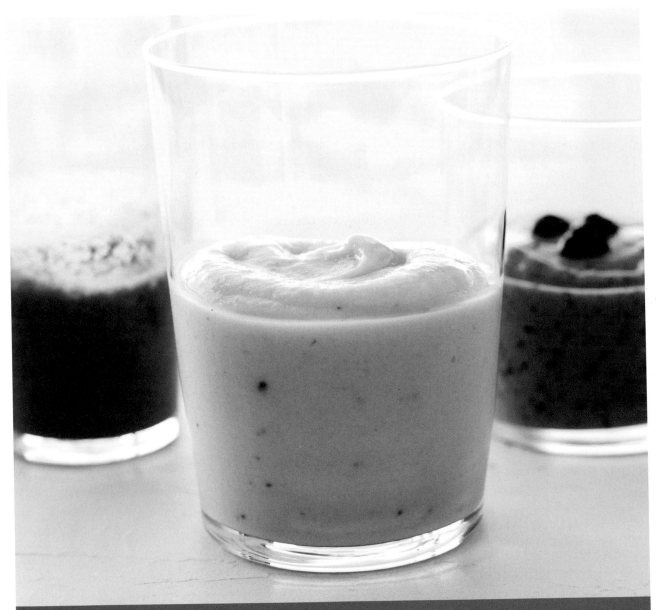

(FROM LEFT TO RIGHT): GREEN SMOOTHIE, MANGO SMOOTHIE, BLUEBERRY SMOOTHIE

DAY 8   Eating Out and Speaking Up

Having harnessed in the first week the tools and resources you need to eat vegan at home, let's address what many people anticipate being challenging about being vegan: eating in restaurants. You may be surprised at how easy it is.

Some people are afraid that their social lives will suffer when they eliminate meat and dairy from their diet, since social occasions and food tend to go hand in hand. For anyone who has ever thought it difficult as a vegan to dine out, to eat at the home of a non-vegan friend, or to find food to eat at parties, I can assure you it's just a matter of changing your perception. If you look for lack, that's what you will find; alternatively, if you look for abundance, that is what you will discover. Once you look at the world through a vegan lens, you realize how effortless it is to find an abundance of options in restaurants of all types; you just may have never noticed before because you weren't looking for it. Friends and family members most likely already have vegan recipes in their repertoire—they just may not call them "vegan."

> **CHALLENGE YOUR THINKING:**
> If you look for lack, that's what you'll find. If you look for abundance, that's what you'll discover.
>
> **CHANGE YOUR BEHAVIOR:**
> Take vegan food out of the box, and ask for what you want.

FINDING WHAT YOU WANT IN NON-VEGAN RESTAURANTS

Though you can find something to eat in every restaurant (see tips below), the most vegan-friendly restaurants are those that feature non-American fare. That leaves countless options—no matter what town you're in.

- Chinese restaurants offer many vegan dishes, and Buddhist Chinese restaurants serve vegetarian-only fare. Just be sure to tell them to leave out the eggs.

- Thai, Vietnamese, and Burmese restaurants are very vegan-friendly, featuring vegetable, noodle, and tofu dishes. Just ask for no fish sauce.

- Japanese restaurants feature edamame, vegetable nori/sushi rolls, tempura, salads made of lettuce or sea vegetables with house dressing, vegetable dumplings, and miso soup. Specify no fish sauce.

- Middle Eastern restaurants offer a smorgasbord of delights: baba ghanouj, hummus, dolmas, olives, tapenade, falafel, and pita bread.

- Any pizza place will make a cheese-free pizza for you. Request veggies for added flavor and nutrition. (Hint: If you bring in your own favorite nondairy cheese, they will most likely use it to make your pizza, and you can encourage them to carry it and offer it as an option on their menu.)

- Indian and Sri Lankan restaurants have a bevy of vegan options. South Indian restaurants tend to be vegetarian-only. Be sure to ask them to leave out the ghee (clarified butter).

- Italian restaurants offer lots of pasta (primavera, arrabbiata, puttanesca), vegetable dishes, salads, and starters such as bruschetta and antipasti. Just specify vegetable broth and no cheese.

- Ethiopian restaurant menus always have a huge array of vegan selections, including lentils, split peas, greens, and potatoes.

- Mexican restaurants always have rice, beans, tortillas, salsa, and guacamole. Specify to leave off cheese, and ask if refried beans are cooked in lard or vegetable oil. If they're cooked in lard, whole beans are the way to go.

- Sub shops can make a vegetable-only sandwich for you and flavor it with oil, vinegar, mustard, salt, and pepper. (To avoid potential contamination by foodborne pathogens, don't hesitate to ask employees to change their gloves before handling your veggies.)

- Look for all-you-can-eat buffets and salad bars. A good buffet can offer a wide range of healthful options such as salad greens, cooked and raw veggies, beans, fresh fruit—even baked potatoes and pasta.

- Many cafes sell chai tea and hot cocoa, using mixes that tend to be vegan. Also, authentic chocolate cafes tend to sell European-style hot cocoa, which by definition is vegan. Just ask.

- Ice cream stores often have sorbets, which are by definition dairy-free, unlike sherbet (which always has dairy). I've also been in many gelato shops that offer soy- and fruit-based versions of their gelati. Just ask to be sure.

- Even baseball stadiums, ballparks, and arenas have changed with the times, and many offer vegan fare from veggie hot dogs and burritos to french fries and pretzels. Check out soyhappy.org for a vegan's guide to ballparks.

Of course, vegetarian- and vegan-only restaurants are your best bets for those lucky enough to live near them. (See "Restaurant and Travel Resources" sidebar on page 114.)

ASKING FOR WHAT YOU WANT WITH CONFIDENCE

Eating outside of your home is not just a matter of choosing the restaurant, it's also a matter of communicating your food ethics in a confident, positive, effective way.

1. BE SPECIFIC: Though not everyone may know how to pronounce it, the word *vegan* (*VEE-gun*) is more familiar than ever. What it *means*, however, is still a mystery to some, so it's important to be specific about what your needs are. Plenty of people think chicken broth is acceptable for vegans simply because there aren't chicken parts floating around, and some people erroneously think vegans don't eat pasta, bread, or yeast. Give the server the benefit of the doubt, be clear, and ask for exactly what you want. And don't hesitate to send something back if they missed the mark; you're paying for the food and should get exactly what you ask for.

   SCENARIO SUGGESTION: When eating out, or when invited over to a friend's for dinner, it's helpful to state specific foods. You can say to your server, "This dish/menu sounds wonderful. Just to be clear, I'm vegan, so please tell me if I order something with eggs, meat broth, or animal-based cheese, milk, or cream."

2. BE POSITIVE: Most likely, you made the choice to leave animals and their secretions off your plate because it makes you feel good—physically, mentally, emotionally, and spiritually. If that's your truth, then that's exactly what you should express to those around you. Your attitude will influence the perception and attitude of others about what it means to be vegan.

   SCENARIO SUGGESTION: When ordering in a restaurant, of course it's appropriate to thank the server for accommodating you, but don't apologize to the point of being self-effacing. Politely thank the staff for their flexibility, and then just move on.

3. BE CONFIDENT: Food is a personal as well as political subject that has been known to bring up people's defenses, and vegans may find themselves on the receiving end of ridicule, criticism, interrogations, jokes, and plain old rudeness. Remaining confident that the attack has nothing to do with you personally will help you take the encounter in stride. Also, don't feel you need to carry the weight of defending all the benefits of

veganism. If asked why you make the choices you do, speak from your heart and tell your truth.

SCENARIO SUGGESTION: You're at a party, and someone hears that you've recently become vegan and feels the need to confront you about it. He says to you, "I just finished a book by a prominent anthropologist, and he provides a lot of evidence that humans were never pure vegetarians at any point in our evolution." Many might be tempted to respond with an assertion that the anthropologist is wrong, that humans gathered more than they hunted, that we're physically designed to eat plant-based diets, and so on, and if your goal is to win an argument, then argue away. But consider an alternative response that defuses the attack, speaks to the real issue, and enables you to remain true to yourself. You could say something like: "I don't know much about anthropology and I haven't read that book, but I do know that I feel really good about eating this way. It's better for my health and certainly better for the animals. And besides, isn't being human about doing things better than we did in the past, especially as we gain the benefit of more knowledge and more choices?"

4. BE PROACTIVE: For those times when you don't have a say in choosing the restaurant—at an employee lunch or office party, for example—it's worth calling in advance to find out which menu items can be made meat- and dairy-free. You'd be surprised how happy chefs are to create something new—and everyone will covet your special dish!

5. BE TECHIE: Many restaurants have websites with their menus online. Why not check out their options in advance? You'll know right away how friendly they are to vegan customers.

6. BE PREPARED: There may be times when a work or family event centers around meat (like a barbecue) or takes place in a restaurant that is unfavorable to vegans (such as a steakhouse). At such times, consider eating something before you go and/ or bringing your own food to eat when you get there. This may seem inconvenient, but it's better than not eating at all, and the food you bring will most likely inspire others to try something new.

7. BE HUMOROUS: Non-vegans as well as vegans can get a little uptight around such a sensitive subject, and humor has a way of defusing tension. Always keep in mind that whatever jokes non-vegans might make at your expense, it really has nothing to do with you. Passive-aggressive though these people are, it will help if you respond with humor and levity.

SCENARIO SUGGESTION: I try to keep things light while at the same time telling the truth. So, for instance, if I'm eating at a table with non-vegetarians, invariably someone will apologize for eating the chicken's leg they're about to bite into. Instead of lying and saying "It's okay" or reacting indignantly, I usually say—with a smile—something like, "Look, don't apologize to me. Apologize to the chickens." It's a good way to get people thinking without being judgmental.

8. BE CREATIVE: Wanna know a secret? You can ask for whatever you want—even in a restaurant. You don't have to order what's on the menu; you can modify whatever they already have and ask them to make it differently.

9. BE VOCAL: When in a group situation, speak up and ask your friends, family, or coworkers to dine at a local vegetarian restaurant. Not only will you have more than just a few menu options to choose from, but *everyone* can eat and experience the abundance and joy of a plant-based menu.

10. BE GENEROUS: Bring muffins in for your morning office meeting, leave cookies on your neighbor's porch, make a cake for a special occasion and share it with colleagues. See my recipes for such goodies on pages 173-182. Coworkers, neighbors, clients, friends, and family all appreciate the gift of homemade goodies, and sharing delicious food can sometimes be more powerful than anything you might say. Anytime non-vegetarians try your famous meatless chili or your decadent dairy-free cookies, they are exposed to dishes they might have never chosen on their own, and often they'll walk away with a new perception of "vegan food."

DAY 9 · Packing Lunches for School and Work

With more than a week behind you (bravo!), it's time to focus on food for the road, whether you're packing lunches for your children for school, packing a daily work lunch for your partner or yourself, or working outside in a garden or on a construction site. If you're traveling (see more about travel in "Day 10: Finding Abundant Food Options While Traveling"), you may need to prepare food for the car or the plane. You may want to go on a picnic, or you may be a college student in need of quick and easy on-the-go meals. Certain types of food are easier to transport than others, such as sandwiches, wraps, and all sorts of salads, whether they're based on pasta, greens, noodles, lentils, beans, or grains.

CHALLENGE YOUR THINKING:
If it tastes good, they will eat it.

CHANGE YOUR BEHAVIOR:
Make fabulous, familiar, filling sandwiches for your loved ones. Even the pickiest eaters will embrace them.

10 SANDWICHES AND WRAPS

If it tastes good, they will eat it. That's my motto. What it really comes down to is that people want their food to be satisfying, filling, and familiar. Sandwiches meet all three criteria, plus they're quick, they're easy, they're compact, and they travel well. Aside from the Better-Than-Egg Salad (page 97), Better-Than-Tuna Salad (page 162), and Better-Than Chicken Salad (page 97), all of which can be used as sandwich fillings, here are a number of other ideas.

1. NUT BUTTER AND JELLY: I don't care how old you are; this is a great sandwich to include in your rotation. The old standby of peanut butter with jelly/jam/preserves will be the least expensive, but try almond or cashew butter, too. Here are a few variations:

- Add a few apple or banana slices, grated carrots, or cucumber slices.

- Spread peanut butter on a tortilla or collard green leaf, top with banana slices and raisins, and roll it up.

- Try almond butter with agave syrup.

Tips

- Make the sandwiches the night before, and place a piece of waxed paper between the jam and the top slice of bread to prevent sogginess. Just remove the waxed paper before eating.
- Choose high-fiber whole-grain bread.
- Choose natural peanut butter that contains peanuts and possibly some salt—but no sugar or added oils. When you open the jar, just stir in the oil that has naturally separated.
- Choose all-fruit jams and jellies that are sweetened with fruit, not added sugars.

2. MEATLESS "LUNCH MEATS": There are a number of vegan lunch meats available, some less processed than others. Spread on some eggless mayonnaise such as Nayonnaise, Vegenaise, or Wildwood's Garlic Aioli; or add mustard, relish, ketchup, lettuce, pickles, and tomatoes. Veggie hot dogs on a bun are also very transportable.

3. VEGGIE SUBS: Onto thick slices of Italian bread or sandwich rolls, spread some hummus and/or some avocado. Add roasted red peppers, artichoke slices, alfalfa sprouts, arugula or any lettuce you prefer, shredded carrots, and shredded beets. (For variety, add your favorite meatless lunch meats.)

4. BURRITOS: Before leaving the house, just roll up your favorite beans (black, pinto, vegetarian refried) in a tortilla with rice, salsa, avocado, some shredded lettuce, and nondairy sour cream. Or make a Tofu Scramble (see page 80) the basis for your wrap. Roll it up, wrap it up, and carry it out. Burritos actually hold up for a few hours, so don't worry about their getting soggy.

5. PORTOBELLO MUSHROOM SANDWICH: Make the Marinated Portobello Mushroom Steaks on page 99. Add to a hearty roll, along with eggless mayonnaise and lettuce.

6. BACON, LETTUCE, AND TOMATO: Lightlife makes a veggie bacon, though my preference is for a more wholesome option, such as my Tempeh Bacon on page 77. With some tomato slices, lettuce, and eggless mayonnaise, you're good to go.

7. BURGERS: Stick your favorite veggie burger in a bun, and top with your favorite fixings. Don't forget about Field Roast's cutlets and meatless meat loaf—also great options for a bun.

8. SLOPPY JOES: See page 100 for a delicious meatless version of this hearty meal. Put on a hearty roll or fill a pita pocket, and wrap it up for the road.

9. PITA POCKETS: Add any of your favorite fillings, such as the ones I named above. A favorite light sandwich of mine is shredded lettuce, chopped apple, and chopped celery in a pita pocket with oil and vinegar dressing.

10. FALAFEL: Make your own falafel balls or chickpea burgers (see page 164), and add to a pita pocket or hearty roll, along with shredded lettuce, tomato slices, hummus, and sliced pickles.

Tip: Sandwich spreads abound, whether they're homemade or store-bought: mashed avocado, hummus, mashed banana (goes great with nut butters), nondairy cream cheese, baba ghanouj, agave nectar, fruit spreads, ketchup, eggless mayonnaise, mustard, pesto, tomato sauce (for an impromptu pita pizza), or Muhammara (see page 227).

10 ONE-DISH SALADS

Whether they're based on pasta, greens, veggies, beans, or lentils, healthful salads are so easy to prepare in advance and take from one location to the next.

1. CORN SALAD: Mix corn (fresh or frozen and thawed), chopped red onion, bell pepper, and sundried tomatoes, with a little olive oil, some balsamic vinegar, and salt and pepper. (Trader Joe's has delicious frozen *roasted* corn kernels.)

2. BEAN SALAD: Use a combination of different canned beans, and combine with fresh herbs, lemon juice, chopped bell pepper, some seasoned rice vinegar, and a few tablespoons of your favorite salsa. Make it heartier by including a cup of cooked brown rice and some chopped avocado. Check out the Cannellini Bean Salad with Fresh Herbs on page 107.

3. PASTA SALAD: There are so many different types of pasta out there, so even if you're not eating wheat or gluten, you can find rice pasta or quinoa pasta, particularly at large natural food stores. The options for pasta salads are endless; here are a few ideas:

   - Prepare penne, bow tie, wagon wheel, or whatever kind of small pasta you like. Add a chopped tomato, ½ cup chopped or sliced black or kalamata olives, ½ cup corn, ¼ cup chopped fresh basil, a few cloves of finely chopped garlic, a tablespoon or two of olive oil, a tablespoon or two of fresh lemon juice, a teaspoon or two of red wine vinegar, and salt and pepper to taste.

   - Prepare elbow pasta, let cool, and mix with finely chopped bell peppers, carrots, celery, and eggless mayonnaise.

4. **TACO SALAD:** You can use beans, vegetarian chicken, chopped tofu, or crumbled tempeh as your base. Whatever you choose, sauté it in a little oil, and add a packet of taco seasoning (such as a Bearitos packet) or your own combination of chili powder, cumin, and salt, along with ¾ cup water. Cook until mixture becomes thick and heated through, and you've got a hearty, flavorful mixture. Pack up with some tortilla chips or wheat or corn tortillas, along with some shredded lettuce and tomatoes.

5. **GREEN SALAD:** Choose your favorite leafy green, pile on the chopped veggies, avocado, some sunflower seeds, tofu, or a can of beans (rinsed and drained), and your favorite dressing (keeping the dressing separate until you're ready to assemble the salad), and you've got a great meal for the road.

6. **BREAD SALAD:** Great for a hearty Italian loaf that's going a little stale. Chop the bread into bite-size pieces. In a bowl, combine it with 1 cup chopped tomatoes, 1 cup chopped cucumbers (peeled and seeded), 1 cup chopped red onion, 1 clove garlic minced, 1 bunch basil, chopped, and 1 tablespoon fresh thyme. Add a few tablespoons olive oil and some balsamic vinegar to lightly coat, and toss.

7. **NOODLE SALAD:** My favorite noodle salad is made with soba noodles (see page 104), though there are many options for cold noodle salads, such as linguine or rice noodles with peanut sauce, sliced bell peppers, and sesame seeds.

8. **BETTER-THAN SALADS:** See page 97 for Better-Than-Egg Salad (mashed tofu), page 162 for Better-Than-Tuna Salad (mashed chickpeas), and page 97 for Better-Than-Chicken Salad (steamed tempeh), and add potato salad to the list. The ingredients for each vary somewhat, but they all rely on the eggless mayonnaise and some finely chopped veggies.

9. **FRUIT SALAD:** Chop up your favorite seasonal (unpeeled) fruits, and sprinkle on some cinnamon, a drizzle of agave nectar, and a squeeze of lemon juice. Add some chopped dates or raisins.

10. **LENTIL SALAD:** While brown lentils are cooking, sauté finely chopped garlic, carrots, onions, and celery. Add some dried thyme and lemon juice, and cook until veggies are soft. When lentils are done, add the veggie mixture, along with a little Dijon mustard and salt. Stir in some chopped fresh parsley, let cool, and pack up.

Or create your own using the table on page 94.

MIX-AND-MATCH GRAIN SALADS
Pick your favorite things from each column to design your grain-based salads.

GRAIN Select 1 from this column	RAW VEGGIES Select 1	FRUIT, NUTS, SEEDS Select 1 or 2	HERBS AND SPICES Select 1 or 2	DRESSINGS Select 1 or 2 or more
Quinoa, Couscous, Brown rice, Millet, Bulgur, Barley, Wild rice	Carrots, bell peppers, tomatoes, scallions/green onions, red onion, corn, snow peas, chopped broccoli, or chopped cauliflower	Raisins, currants, dried cranberries, dried apricots (finely chopped), chopped apple, chopped fresh oranges, chopped nuts such as almonds, walnuts, or peanuts (and toast them first if you prefer), pine nuts, sunflower seeds, sesame seeds, poppy seeds	Dried ginger, curry powder, turmeric, cardamom, coriander, cumin (and toast them first if you prefer), or fresh basil, fresh parsley, fresh cilantro	Salsa, combination of sesame oil and rice vinegar, an Italian salad dressing, a favorite creamy salad dressing from the bottle, a combination of garlic, lemon juice, and olive oil

OTHER SUGGESTIONS FOR PACKING LUNCHES

Leftovers: Whatever you had for dinner the night before will most likely transport well, including soups, stews, or chili. Buy an awesome thermos that will keep them hot, or if you work in an office, just heat them up in the kitchen. However, if you're like me, you'll enjoy leftovers at room temperature.

Storing and heating: Invest in some insulated containers and thermoses that will keep food and beverages hot.

BEVERAGES AND SNACKS TO PACK

Fresh fruit: The obvious and most healthful and transportable snacks are fresh fruit (apples, apricots, Asian pears, bananas, blueberries, cherries, figs, grapefruit, grapes, kiwi, mango, melon, nectarines, orange sections, papaya, peaches, pears, pineapple, plums, raspberries, and strawberries). In a separate container, bring peanut, almond, apple, or pumpkin butter for dipping the fruit.

Raw veggies with dip: Carrot, celery, or bell pepper slices pair well with hummus or peanut butter.

Dried fruit: Dried dates, prunes, raisins, mangoes, and apricots are road foods by definition.

Nuts, seeds, and trail mix: Toasted or raw nuts and seeds mixed with dried fruit are great to snack on. Buy pre-made (Trader Joe's specializes in these mixes) or make them yourself.

Popcorn: Make your own and divide the batch up into little bags or containers. I make popcorn with an air popper, spritz on a little oil from a sprayer, and toss with salt, cumin, chili powder, and nutritional yeast. If it's for the little ones, skip the chili powder. Otherwise, most already-popped bagged popcorn tends to be vegan, unless it's a variety that features cheese.

Tip: Feel free to bring your own homemade popcorn with you to the movies, but keep in mind that most movie theaters' popcorn is made with oil, not dairy-based butter. Just ask for no butter added.

Pita bread with hummus or tabouli: Make your own or buy pre-made hummus or tabouli.

Crackers with peanut butter: I keep mentioning peanut butter because it's so delicious and keeps well unrefrigerated. Other nut butters can be used instead.

Vegan jerky: A few different companies make vegan jerky—processed, yes, but good when you're in a pinch. Turtle Island (makers of Tofurky) makes Tofurky Jurky; Primal Spirit makes a variety of Primal Strips, including Teriyaki, Texas Barbeque, Smoked, and—my favorite—Hot and Spicy Mushroom; Stonewall's makes Jerquee; and Tasty Eats makes Soy Jerky.

Energy bars: Great for a quick refuel, many—if not most—energy bars are vegan. Clif, Luna, Lara, Organic Food, ProBar, Kind Bar, Raw Revolution, 18 Rabbits, and Vega bars are some of the brands to look for.

Olives: A healthful, surprisingly low-cal snack, olives make great road food.

Cereal/granola: Throw your favorite cereal or granola in a bag to enjoy as a hand-to-mouth snack, or even bring along some nondairy milk for the whole shebang. Many nondairy milks now come in small aseptic boxes for travel.

Snack-size applesauce: Individually packaged healthful snacks such as applesauce are available in many stores.

Bagged crisps: Not as healthful as fruit and veggies, but not as greasy as potato chips. Pretzels, tortilla chips, crackers, Veggie Booty (aka Pirate Booty: Veggie) and Tings by Robert's American Gourmet are great treats for the lunch box.

Dark chocolate bars: Good pick-me-ups for a midday snack, there are many healthful vegan bars to choose from. Good brands that carry vegan chocolate bars include Choco-love, Endangered Species, Dagoba, Equal Exchange, Tropical Source, Green & Black, and many more. Choose chocolate labeled "fair trade" as much as possible.

Smoothies and fruit drinks: Certainly you can make your own and transport them in a thermos or portable cup, but many companies make good, healthful bottled smoothies to pack for lunch, including Odwalla, Naked Juice, Bolthouse Farms, and Sambazon.

Better-Than-Egg Salad

YIELD: 4 SERVINGS OR SANDWICHES

Serve as a salad or sandwich—perfect any time of the year.

1½ pounds extra-firm tofu
½ cup eggless mayonnaise
2 red bell peppers, finely chopped
4–5 scallions (white and green parts), finely chopped
2 carrots, finely chopped
3 stalks celery, finely chopped

2 tablespoons fresh parsley, finely chopped
4 teaspoons pickle relish
1½ tablespoons prepared mustard
¾ teaspoon turmeric
½ teaspoon salt, or to taste
Black pepper, to taste

In a large bowl, mash tofu with a fork, potato masher, or your hands.

Add the mayonnaise, bell peppers, scallions, carrots, celery, parsley, relish, mustard, turmeric, salt, and pepper, and combine well.

Serving Suggestions
- Serve on crackers as an appetizer or party dish.
- Serve as a side salad—great for picnics and BBQs.

Wheat-free

Better-Than-Chicken Salad

YIELD: 4 TO 6 SERVINGS

A variation of my Better-Than-Egg Salad uses tempeh instead of tofu. Cube up one or two packages of tempeh, steam the cubes for 10 minutes in a steamer basket, let cool, then add all the dressing ingredients from the Better-Than-Egg salad, except the relish and mustard. Or make a curried version, which combines the eggless mayonnaise with chopped celery, a chopped apple, a handful of raisins, ¼ cup finely chopped walnuts, 2 teaspoons of curry powder, plus salt and pepper to taste.

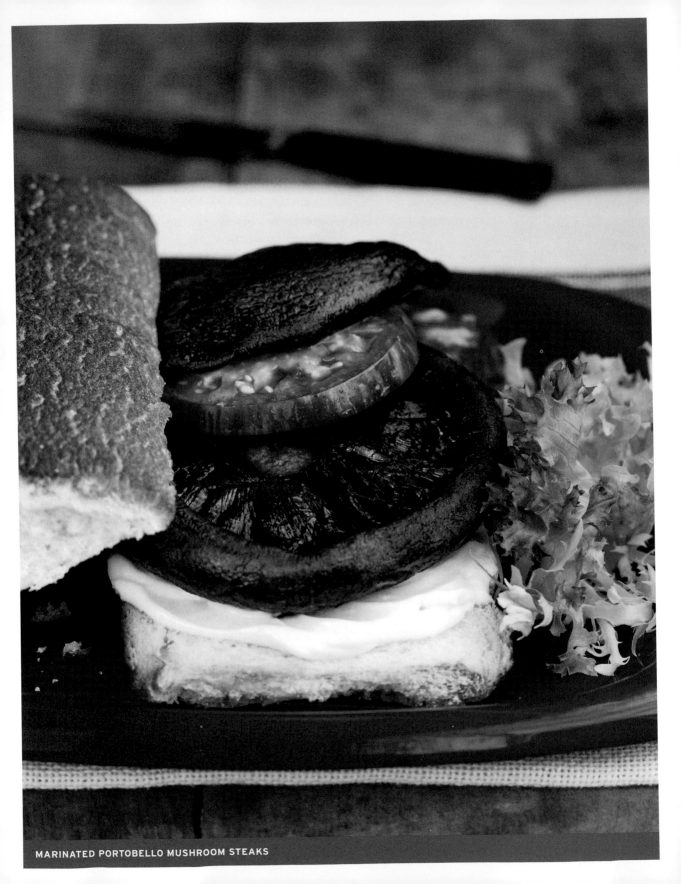

MARINATED PORTOBELLO MUSHROOM STEAKS

Marinated Portobello Mushroom Steaks

YIELD: 4 TO 6 SERVINGS

These can be served as a main dish along with sautéed greens and creamy mashed potatoes or added to a bun with all the fixings!

8-12 large portobello mushrooms
½ cup balsamic vinegar
½ cup tamari soy sauce
½ cup water
2-3 sprigs fresh rosemary (or
   1 teaspoon dried)

2-3 sprigs fresh thyme (or 1 teaspoon
   dried)
2-3 sprigs fresh marjoram or oregano
   (or 1 teaspoon dried)
Freshly ground black pepper
Small amount of olive oil for sautéing

Remove the stems from the underside of the mushrooms and lightly wipe the tops with a damp paper towel.

In a large bowl, combine the vinegar, tamari, water, rosemary, thyme, marjoram, and black pepper. Stir to combine. Add the mushrooms to the marinade, and make sure each one is covered by the marinade. You may need to move them around to give all the mushrooms a chance to be coated by the marinade. Marinate the mushrooms for as little as 30 minutes or as long as overnight.

When ready to cook, add some oil to a large sauté pan, and turn the heat to medium.

Remove the mushrooms from the marinade, but do not discard the marinade. Add as many mushrooms as can fit in the pan, tops down. They will shrink as they cook. Cook for about 3-5 minutes, until lightly browned. Turn and cook for another 3-5 minutes.

Remove the fresh herb sprigs from the marinade and pour the marinade into the pan (reserving some for the next batch of mushrooms, assuming you don't fit all of them into the pan). Cover and cook for 5-7 minutes. Flip the mushrooms, cover, and cook for another 5-7 minutes.

When the mushrooms are fork-tender, remove from the pan, and repeat above steps with remaining mushrooms. To serve the mushrooms hot, simply cook the mushrooms in two different sauté pans on the stove all at once. Serve two mushrooms per person.

Wheat-free

Sloppy Joes

YIELD: 4 SERVINGS

Here's another way to use tempeh instead of tofu, although the latter would work for this recipe, as well. This is a hearty dish that can be served as a main dish or as a sandwich.

One 8-ounce package tempeh
1 tablespoon olive oil
1 yellow onion, finely chopped
1 bell pepper (red, yellow, or orange), finely chopped
One 15-ounce can tomato sauce
1 tablespoon chili powder (more or less to your liking)

½ teaspoon salt
¼ teaspoon pepper
2 tablespoons vegan Worcestershire sauce
1 teaspoon hot sauce (optional)

Steam the tempeh for 10 minutes in a steamer basket placed in a pot filled with a small amount of water. Transfer it to a bowl, let cool, and crumble it with your hands or mash it with a fork or potato masher.

In a large saucepan on medium heat, heat the oil and sauté the onion and pepper until the onion is translucent. Add the tempeh, and sauté for a few minutes, stirring constantly to prevent sticking.

Add the tomato sauce, chili powder, salt, pepper, Worcestershire sauce, and hot sauce. Cover, reduce heat, and simmer for 10 minutes or longer. Serve on toasted buns.

Wheat-free

DID YOU KNOW?
Many versions of Worcestershire sauce contain anchovies. Look for one without.

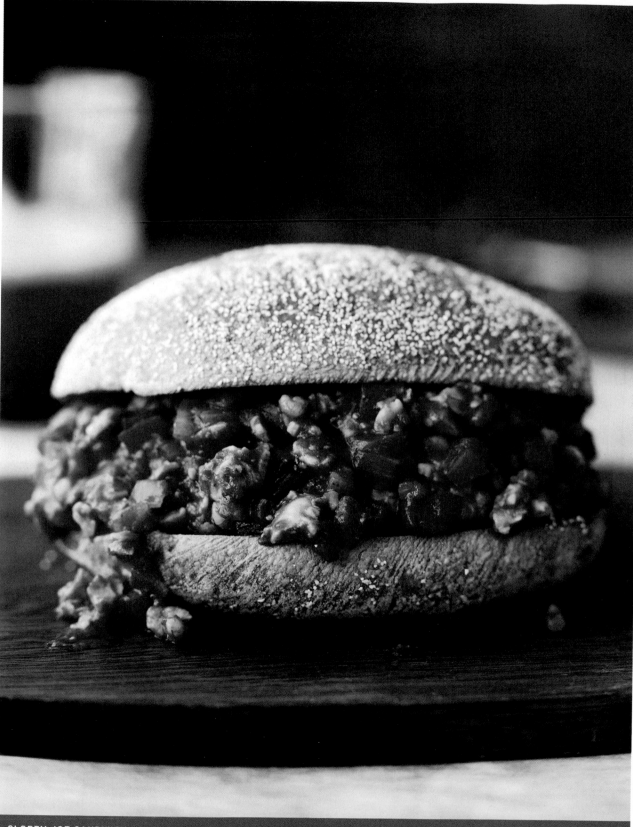

SLOPPY JOE SANDWICH

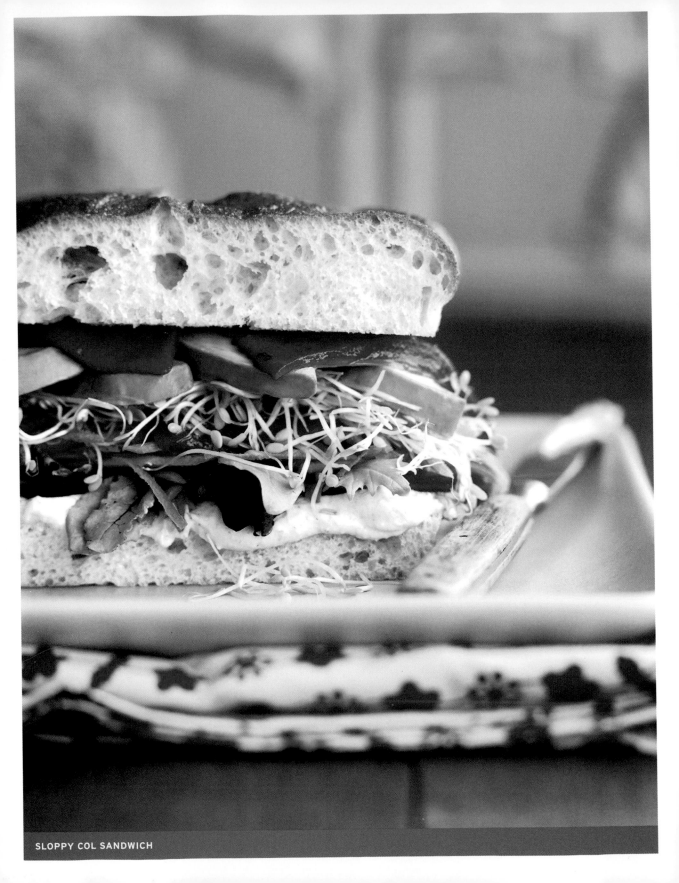

SLOPPY COL SANDWICH

Sloppy Col Sandwich

YIELD: 4 SERVINGS

As versatile as the veggies, bread, and spread you use, this sandwich is so easy to make and absolutely delicious.

Hummus, store-bought or homemade
   (see page 159)
1 loaf focaccia or 4 fresh whole-wheat
   rolls
1 ripe avocado
2 roasted red peppers, sliced

1 bunch alfalfa sprouts
2 or 3 carrots, shredded
2 tomatoes, sliced
1 cup mixed salad greens
Salt and pepper, to taste

Spread the hummus on the bread—or if you prefer, use the avocado as your spread, or both! If you use the hummus as the spread, you can still add the avocado as one of the sandwich fillers.

Create your sandwich. Add the red peppers, sprouts, carrots, tomatoes, salad greens, and any other ingredients you wish. No need to measure anything—just pile on the veggies! It's that easy.

Sprinkle on some salt and grind some pepper on top of the ingredients, and repeat to make another sandwich.

Variations
- Add pesto instead of hummus, and drizzle a little balsamic vinegar over the veggies.
- Use eggless mayonnaise as a spread.

Soy-free

Sesame Soba Noodles with Shredded Vegetables

SERVES 6 TO 8 AS A SIDE DISH

A delicious cold salad with an Asian flair, the brownish soba noodles contrast beautifully with the green onions, orange carrots, and red peppers. Don't skip the toasted sesame seeds; they add wonderful flavor and crunch.

16 ounces dried soba noodles
¼ cup tamari soy sauce
3 tablespoons sesame oil
2 tablespoons seasoned rice vinegar
1-2 tablespoons chili oil

1 red bell pepper, thinly sliced
1 cup chopped green onions
2 carrots, cut into matchsticks
2 tablespoons toasted sesame seeds

In a large stockpot, cook the noodles in boiling salted water until al dente, about 5-7 minutes. Rinse with cool water, drain well, and transfer to a large bowl.

In a small bowl, mix together the tamari, sesame oil, rice vinegar, and chili oil. Pour over the noodles and, using tongs, toss the noodles with the sauce to coat well. Marinate in a covered bowl in the refrigerator for at least 1 hour or up to 24 hours, tossing occasionally.

Before serving, stir in the red peppers, green onions, and carrots, and sprinkle with toasted sesame seeds. Taste, and add more tamari, sesame oil, vinegar, or chili oil, as needed. This salad is best when served cold, not room temperature or warm.

SHOPPING TIP:

Some commercial soba noodles contain eggs, but plenty of brands are egg-free. Just look at the ingredients.

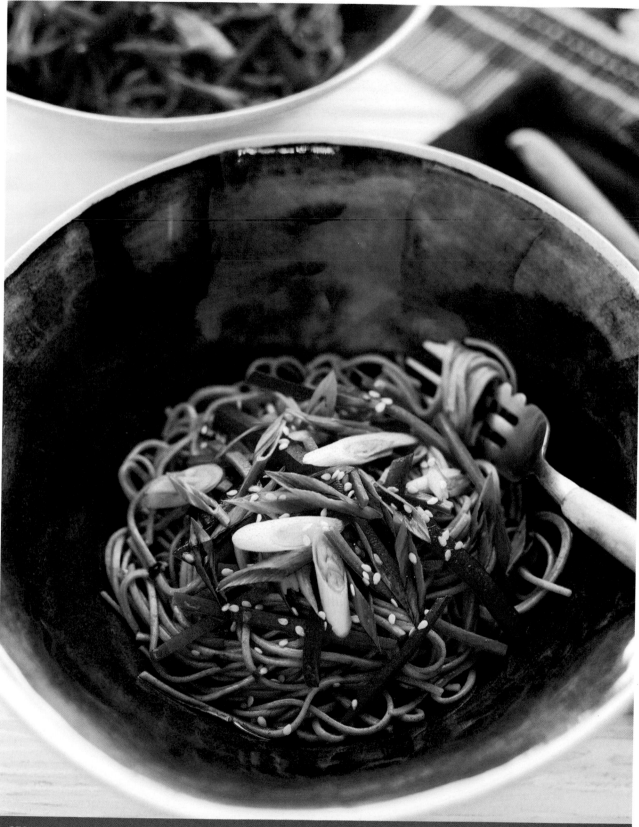

SESAME SOBA NOODLES WITH SHREDDED VEGETABLES

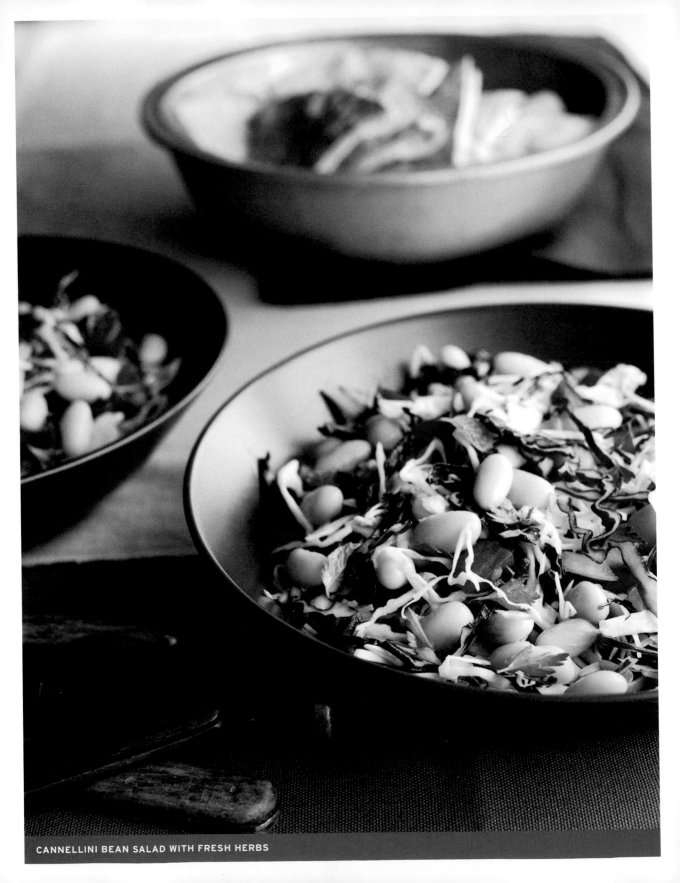

CANNELLINI BEAN SALAD WITH FRESH HERBS

Cannellini Bean Salad with Fresh Herbs

YIELD: 4 TO 6 SERVINGS

Finely chopped parsley and sage also pair well with these beautiful white legumes, which are essentially white kidney beans.

Two 15-ounce cans (3 cups cooked) cannellini beans, rinsed and drained

4 medium tomatoes, coarsely chopped, or ¾ cup cherry tomatoes, halved

1 small red onion, finely chopped

2-3 medium cloves garlic, pressed or minced

Juice from 1 lemon

3-4 tablespoons minced fresh mint

2 tablespoons minced fresh parsley

1-2 tablespoons olive oil

1 cup finely shredded green cabbage

1 cup finely shredded red cabbage

Salt and freshly ground black pepper, to taste

Combine all the ingredients, season as necessary, and let sit for 15 minutes before serving.

Wheat-free

Finding Abundant Food Options While Traveling

Whether you travel frequently for work or periodically for pleasure, you've no doubt observed how easy it is to find junk food everywhere you look. To find good *healthful* food on the road, however, requires a little more effort. Healthful options are available in more places than ever before, but I think it's important to keep in mind that fast-food joints, tourist destinations, airports, and even restaurants—by their very nature—cater to people who are either indulging themselves or are (for whatever reason) choosing convenience over health. The point is, it's not being vegan that makes it challenging to find nutrient-dense food on the road. The problem is that as individuals and as a society, we have not made eating well a priority—whether we're at home or traveling.

CHALLENGE YOUR THINKING:
It's not being vegan that makes it challenging to find nutrient-dense food on the road. The problem is that we have not made eating well a priority—whether we're at home or traveling.

CHANGE YOUR BEHAVIOR:
Take some time to prepare for your trip by bringing food with you and knowing where to go once you arrive at your destination.

The truth is that eating vegan on the road is easy in most places and a little challenging in others. It's just a matter of knowing what to look for and taking the time to prepare, which everyone should do, vegan or not, traveling or not.

We know how important food schedules are for infants and children, but at some point as adults, we stop making this a priority for ourselves. Parents never leave the house without having snacks for their kids, and we need to honor this need in ourselves, too. Instead, we create helter-skelter lives without routine or order, which is exacerbated when we travel. Personally, I eat my meals at the same times every day, which means that I know exactly what's wrong with me if my mood or energy level drops. One of the most stressful components of travel is straying from my eating schedule, so I do everything I can to keep some kind of regular routine when I'm on the road.

No matter how hard I try, when I travel, I accept that I'll be eating less optimally than when I'm in my California home, but I do try to follow some guidelines to make traveling as pleasant as possible.

- I try to keep as close to an eating schedule as possible, and I factor this in when traveling between time zones.

- I try to avoid getting hungry so that my energy level stays consistent and strong.

- I try to eat as healthfully as possible, but I accept that I might have to choose calorie density over nutrient density. In other words, eating a meal of french fries, salted peanuts, an apple, and crackers is better than nothing—if those are my only options. But the truth is there never is a risk of going hungry. There's always *something* to eat somewhere.

CHALLENGE YOUR THINKING: We know how important food schedules are for infants and children, but at some point as adults, we stop making this a priority for ourselves. Parents never leave the house without having snacks for their kids, and we need to honor this need in ourselves, too.

These goals can be reached no matter where you're traveling to or what your mode of transportation is.

AIRPORTS

Depending on the time of my flight, I try to eat before I leave for the airport, even if I know it's a vegan-friendly airport. With food out of the way, I can focus on just getting through security and onto the plane.

However, at some point you will probably need to eat at an airport. When it comes to vegan food, some airports are most definitely better than others, but you'll always be able to find *something*. It might be a bean burrito at Taco Bell (their refried beans are made with vegetable oil, not lard; just ask for no cheese or sour cream) or a vegetable sandwich at Subway (pile on the veggies and ask for oil and vinegar and mustard instead of mayonnaise). Most airport restaurants have pre-made food, but there are often vegan options, some more healthful than others.

Each year, the Physicians Committee for Responsible Medicine puts out a list of the airports with the best vegan options. They evaluated fifteen of the busiest U.S. airports, and you might be surprised to know which airports ranked the highest in terms of offering the most healthful plant-based options. One year it was Orlando International Airport, and another year Detroit Metropolitan Wayne County Airport tied with San Francisco International Airport; a consistent top ranker is Dallas/Fort Worth International Airport. Many vegan options can be found in Denver, Chicago, Newark, Los Angeles, Phoenix, and Minneapolis/St. Paul, among others.

Follow the guidelines in "Day 8: Eating Out and Speaking Up" in terms of finding vegan food in various types of restaurants, but in addition:

- Many cafes sell bagels they will toast for you. Ask if they have peanut butter instead of dairy-based butter, and if not, just spread on some jelly.

- Many kiosks sell bagged nuts, seeds, energy bars, trail mix, fruit leather, baked chips, pretzels, bananas, and apples.

- Many airports have fruit smoothie or fresh fruit juice stands, such as Jamba Juice, whose default milk for most of their smoothies is soy. Just ask them to replace the frozen yogurt or sherbet with sorbet or—better yet—a banana.

AIRPLANES

Free meals on airplanes are virtually obsolete on most airlines, unless you're traveling first-class or on an international flight. If you are, be sure to contact the airline at least twenty-four hours in advance to confirm that your special meal request is in the system. The airlines vary in terms of offerings and quality, but I've had the pleasure of enjoying Amy's burritos and fajitas, decent green salads, and vegan cookies. I've also enjoyed some really good Indian meals, which are often called "nondairy strict vegetarian" or even "Hindu nondairy," depending on the airline.

In the coach/economy cabin, sandwiches and snack boxes are often available for purchase, though most of these are filled with chicken sandwiches and crackers and cheese.

Instead of relying on the airline, I plan ahead and always bring food on the plane with me, much to the envy of the people in my row. Some things travel better than others, as I have learned the hard way. In my travel bag, there are always variations of:

- Peanut butter and jam sandwiches
- Hummus and roasted red pepper wrap
- Baggies of cut-up carrots, celery, and cauliflower (snow peas are also great; bell peppers get too funky)
- A bag of nuts, particularly walnuts, almonds, and pistachios
- A bag of trail mix or granola
- Dates, apples, and bananas
- Energy bars

Other convenient travel foods include dried fruit, fruit leather, whole-grain crackers, homemade popped popcorn, and vegan beef jerky. It's easy to stock up on these things before leaving my home to go somewhere else; the key is making sure to have enough when I'm coming back.

The other two things you will never find me without are my stainless-steel water bottle for cold water and my tea thermos for hot water. Although you cannot bring filled water bottles through the security gate, you can bring empty ones, so I just fill them up with water from fountains once I'm at my gate. As for my tea, I always travel with my favorite white, green, and oolong teas. My tea thermos has a built-in strainer, enabling me to just add tea leaves to the thermos and then fill it with hot water, which the flight attendants are happy to do for me. The other option is to use a spoon strainer that you can get at kitchen supply stores. Fill the strainer with loose tea leaves and steep it in a cup of hot water.

CAR TRAVEL

Day 9 provides a bevy of options for packed lunches and snacks, which can easily be implemented if you're taking a road trip or camping and bringing along a cooler. To have even more options (and if you're not one to build a campfire), consider buying a portable burner that's fueled by butane cartridges. I've used them in my cooking classes for years, and they're incredibly convenient for car trips.

ACCOMMODATIONS

Most chain hotels have something vegan at their breakfast buffet, such as bagels and toast with peanut butter and jam, fresh fruit, and cereal. Unless noted, the pastries, pancakes, and waffles all tend to contain animal products. Some large hotel chains also carry soy milk (just ask), which can be used for the cereals they offer. If the hotel doesn't have nondairy milk for the cereal, order fruit salad with cereal, and stir it all together.

> **CHALLENGE YOUR THINKING:** Never underestimate how postively people will rise to accommodate you, but first you have to ask for what you want—joyfully and with respect.

Bed-and-breakfasts are a different story. Proprietors of bed-and-breakfasts often love to show off their creativity by making delicious vegan breakfasts upon request. Some of the most memorable breakfasts I've ever had were at nonvegan bed-and-breakfasts. Contact them before booking and ask if they can accommodate you. Whenever I contact B&Bs, I always get overwhelmingly positive responses. My favorite experience was when I called a B&B in West Hollywood to ask if they accommodate vegans. The wonderful response on the other end of the line was, "Oh, sweetheart, of course we accommodate you being vegan. So no problem. Now tell me, sweetheart, what is vegan?" How could I not fall in love immediately with someone who says yes first and only then asks what *vegan* means? Now *that's* customer service!

Never underestimate how positively people will accommodate you. But in order to experience this, you have to ask for what you want—and do so with confidence, joy and humility.

Whether you're staying in a chain hotel or a bed-and-breakfast, one thing you always have access to is hot water. Packaged oatmeal, dry soups, packaged dry noodle dishes, quick-cooking oats, or pre-made Indian foods are easy to travel with and great to have on hand. Just add hot water and you have a hot, filling meal for the airport or hotel room.

INTERNATIONAL TRAVEL

The same principles apply whether you're traveling domestically or internationally. It's true that some cultures/countries are more vegan-friendly than others, but you may be surprised by the number of options you will find. Cities will certainly have more vegan-friendly restaurants, but even in rural areas, there are always things to eat. I promise you I've never been at risk for starving while on vacation. Some of the most memorable meals I've ever had have been on the road—and I've also had some that met only one essential need: filling my belly. Sometimes that's good enough.

I think we forget that plant-based foods were once the staples in the diets of people all around the world, so choosing the simple indigenous foods of the countries we're visiting means increasing the chances that they're vegan.

- Tomatoes, corn, and beans in Mexican and Latin American cuisine
- Lentils, root vegetables, and grains in African cuisine
- Tofu, vegetables, and grains in Asian cuisine
- Legumes and rice in Indian and Pakistani cuisine
- Regional vegetables in European cuisine

In the United States, we've come to rely on processed foods—even as vegans—but when you travel abroad, you realize that what would be called "peasant food" (versus the "luxury" animal products) not only is the most healthful, but also tends to be vegan. Natively grown fruits and vegetables abound, depending on where you are, and instead of the fancy, expensive bottled salad dressings we've become accustomed to, we can appreciate lime or lemon juice with a little salt or simply oil and vinegar on salads brimming with vegetables.

In terms of communicating your needs in non-English-speaking countries, I've learned that it's much more helpful to know how to say "without meat, cheese, and eggs" rather than "I'm vegan." Not only do most languages not have a word for *vegan*, some people think chickens and fish are eaten by vegans. It's much more effective to order what looks like a vegan-friendly dish on the menu and then, in the language of the country you're visiting, confirm that it has "no butter" or "no milk" or "no animal fat." So, in addition to learning the words for *fruit, vegetables,* and *beans,* as well as specific types within these categories, I highly recommend learning the words for *meat, fish, cheese, butter, eggs,* and *milk.*

One of the most wonderful things about traveling in Italy, for instance, was that—because Italians value each and every ingredient that goes into making their dishes—restaurant menus would provide a description of exactly what the dish entailed. For example, if the title of the dish was White Beans in Tomato Sauce, underneath it would say "beans, olive oil, tomatoes, garlic, and basil." If it was bruschetta, underneath it would say "tomatoes, olive oil, garlic, and salt" (in Italian, of course). And that was exactly what they gave you, which is so different from in the United States, where cheese is automatically added to everything you order, even if it doesn't say so on the menu. In Italy, I would order something like the White Beans and Tomato Sauce and say, *"No formaggio, vero?"* ("No cheese, right?") And the waiter would look at me like I had three heads, as if to say, *Does it say* formaggio *on the menu? Then why would you think it would be there?* (Yes, living in Italy is on my bucket list.)

Once you get to know the foods native to the region you're in, it's a lot easier. For instance, all over Florence are produce stands as well as street vendors that sell *macedonia di frutta*, which is just fruit salad. In Mexico, street vendors sell corn on the cob with lime juice, and baked plantains. In Spain, horchata (nut milk made with water and sugar) is easy to find all over.

In whatever towns I travel to, one of the first things I do is scope out a health food store, which many large and small cities have. If the hotel doesn't already have nondairy milk, I buy some at the store and ask the hotel to keep it in the fridge. At the health food store, I'd also stock up on nuts, granola, and other healthful snacks. Many towns, large and small, also have farmer's markets and farm stands, from which I've crafted the most delicious meals based on local produce and fresh breads.

Perhaps the only time you would need to work a little harder to make sure you're accommodated is if you're part of some kind of tour package, going on a cruise, or staying at some kind of resort. I do think things are improving all the time, and if you talk to the kitchen/chef/organizers beforehand, you may be pleasantly surprised.

The number of vegetarian- and vegan-only restaurants in cities across the world is rising all the time. These days, you can easily find vegan-friendly restaurants by taking advantage of the many resources available. More than ever, travel books include tips for vegans, but the places to go for the most current information are websites and smart phone apps.

WEBSITES

HAPPYCOW.NET: Search or browse for vegan and vegan-friendly restaurants all around the world. They rely on reviews from users, so help others by adding reviews of vegan-friendly restaurants you've discovered.

VEGGUIDE.ORG: Search or browse by region, country, or city for veg-friendly restaurants. Boasting a simple, clean interface, it also depends on reviews from its users.

VEGDINING.COM: Veg restaurant guide with a focus on international travel.

VEGCOOKING.COM: Click on "Dining Out" in the top menu to access a bevy of helpful information, including Restaurant of the Month, Vegetarian-Friendly Restaurant Guide, and Vegan Eating on the Road (where you'll find a Chain Restaurants Guide so you can see all the vegan options in chain restaurants, from Arby's to Taco Bell).

VEGETARIAN CITY GUIDES: This group of websites, devised and kept updated by local activists, is dedicated to particular cities, with lots of resources about their vegan-friendliness. More are being created every day, but currently, there are:

vegalbany.com
vegaustin.com
vegbaltimore.com
vegchicago.com
vegdc.com
vegdetroit.com
veghawaii.org
vegillinois.com
vegkansascity.com
vegmadison.com

vegohio.com
vegphilly.com
vegportland.com
vegsandiego.com
vegsarasota.com
vegseattle.com
vegsf.com
vegtampabay.com

YELP.COM: This is a comprehensive general website for restaurant reviews.

APPS

These apps are available for different devices, including the iPhone, iPad, iPod Touch, Droid, and Palm Pre.

VEGANXPRESS: This is a brilliant app available for a nominal fee that lists the vegan items on the menus of about a hundred chain restaurants in the country. For instance, if you're in the middle of nowhere and have no options other than the Cheesecake Factory or Olive Garden, you can use this app to discover that you will indeed find food to eat. Fast-food chain restaurants are also included, as is a list of junk food found in movie theaters. This is how I learned that Skittles are now gelatin-free.

VEGOUT: Powered by the folks at happycow.net, this is an app version of their restaurant guide to find veg-friendly restaurants when you're on the road. It carries a nominal fee, and it uses the iPhone's GPS to help you locate a restaurant.

VEGGIE PASSPORT: This is a handy app to have—also at a nominal cost—that communicates your veg needs in thirty-three different languages. You type what you want to say ("I don't eat meat, cheese, or eggs"), and it returns text in the language of your choice. Languages include English, Albanian, Arabic, Bulgarian, Chinese, Chinese (Simplified), Croatian, Czech, Danish, Dutch, Finnish, French, German, Greek, Hebrew, Hindi, Indonesian, Japanese, Korean, Lithuanian, Norwegian, Polish, Portuguese, Romanian, Russian, Slovak, Spanish, Swahili, Swedish, Thai, Turkish, Ukrainian, and Vietnamese.

Rethinking Meat Cravings: Salt and Fat Taste Good

Let's talk about one of the great misunderstandings about humans and meat. I've heard countless well-meaning people say things like "I tried eating vegetarian, but I just craved meat" or "Humans were meant to eat meat—just look at my teeth." And then they point to those dull little eyeteeth that would shame any member of the cat family. Have you ever seen the teeth of a true carnivore? They don't resemble human teeth at all. The teeth of obligate carnivores are meant for piercing flesh; their incisors are meant to strip flesh from bones.

Beyond teeth, when we compare the anatomy of humans with that of herbivorous animals and of carnivorous animals, physiologically we resemble the herbivores substantially more than we do the carnivores. (see sidebar on page 122)

CHALLENGE YOUR THINKING:
When we compare the teeth and anatomy of humans with that of herbivorous and carnivorous animals, we resemble the herbivores substantially more than we do the carnivores.

Not only could we not take down another animal with our jaws and claws and strength (or lack thereof), we don't want to. Most of us are quite disgusted by blood and guts and carcasses and corpses, and I think it's fair to say that no one sees roadkill and starts planning lunch. When we see an animal who has been hit by a car, we tend to feel compassion rather than hunger.

We don't crave the flesh, sinews, tendons, muscles, and blood of animals. Obligate carnivores—including lions and other members of the cat family—do; indeed, they would die without it. They don't grapple with a moral dilemma or find themselves in an ethical quandary when they contemplate their meals. We do.

Humans don't see birds or squirrels or cows and start salivating, but if you've ever watched a domestic cat react when a prey animal is within reach, you'd know what it means to crave animal flesh. They get down on their haunches as their teeth begin chattering; they flit their tails and begin to drool. Is that how you react when you see deer grazing on the side of the road or birds flying overhead? My guess is that you don't. (And if you do, I don't want to know!)

Not only do we humans survive without meat, we thrive without it. We have thousands of plant foods from which to choose, bringing us both pleasure and optimal health. We do not crave the flesh of another animal, but what we do crave is flavor, texture, salt, fat, and familiarity, and all of these are found in plant foods. Unfortunately, we've all been conditioned to think of the *form* of our craving (meat, dairy, and eggs) rather than the *source* of it (salt, fat, flavor, etc.), so when we think we're craving meat, we're most likely craving one or all of these elements.

CHALLENGE YOUR THINKING: We do not crave the flesh of another animal, but what we do crave is flavor, texture, salt, fat, and familiarity, and all of these are found in plant foods.

FLAVOR

We are the only animal who eats other animals who has to cook and flavor meat before eating it. Think of all the things you've used to flavor meat: ketchup, mustard, barbecue sauce, Worcestershire sauce, steak sauce, relish, vinegars, oils, horseradish, hot sauce, chutney, jelly, jam, salsa, soy sauce, wasabi, curry, tahini, pickle, garlic, ginger, onion, lemon, lime, and the endless array of spices and herbs. The flavor is in the plant foods, as evidenced by all the condiments in your kitchen.

TEXTURE

I've heard naysayers of veganism scoff, asserting that because (some) vegans eat "vegetarian meats," it belies a latent desire to eat animal-based meat. I couldn't disagree more. People don't necessarily stop eating animal flesh because they stopped liking the taste; they stop eating animal flesh because they don't want to contribute to violence or because they want to be healthy. There are larger considerations than our own appetites and gustatory pleasures.

Indeed, just because we stop eating animal flesh doesn't mean we don't still desire a hearty, chewy texture. The pleasure of food has as much to do with mouthfeel as it does with flavor. Even the word *meat* doesn't refer only to the flesh of animals. In fact, the original word, *mete,* referred to that which was eaten, in order to distinguish it from that which was drunk. In other words, it simply refers to solid food rather than to beverages. We talk about *nut meat* and *coconut meat,* and I strongly ad-

CHALLENGE YOUR THINKING: People don't necessarily stop eating animal flesh because they stopped liking the taste; they stop eating animal flesh because they don't want to contribute to violence or because they want to be healthy. That doesn't mean they stop wanting a satisfying mouthfeel.

CHANGE YOUR BEHAVIOR: Eat foods that have a hearty, chewy texture, such as thawed tofu, tempeh, seitan, and mushrooms.

vocate the use of the terms *vegetarian meat, grain-based meat,* and *soy-based meat.*

In terms of chewy, texture-rich plant-based foods, there are many options:

- **FROZEN TOFU:** You can read more about tofu in "Day 21: Demystifying Tofu: It's Just a Bean!," but in terms of creating a satisfying mouth-feel with this versatile food, the secret is in *freezing* it.

    Take any tub or vacuum-packed container of any firm tofu (firm, extra-firm, or super-firm—not silken) and throw it intact into the freezer. Here it may remain for as little as twenty-four hours or for as long as six months.

    When you're ready to eat it, remove it from the freezer and thaw it out on the counter for a few hours. Once it's completely thawed, open the package, dump out the water, hold the tofu over the sink, and squeeze out all the water like you would with a sponge. By doing this, you make the tofu very porous, which means it now has room to soak up another liquid, such as a flavorful marinade. Additionally, you change the texture of the tofu completely, making it deliciously *chewy.*

    Now you're ready to prepare it any way you like:

    - Cube it or crumble it and toss it into green salads.
    - Crumble it and add it to bean chili or marinara sauce.
    - Crumble it, add it to a sauté pan, and add taco seasonings. Cook, and fill soft or hard taco shells.
    - Cube it, and add it to a stir-fry.
    - Slice it, and grill, broil, or bake it.

- **TEMPEH:** Whereas tofu is made from boiled and strained soybeans, tempeh (*TEM*-pay) is made by fermenting whole soybeans with a grain, usually rice. Sold as square or rectangular patties/cakes, tempeh is different in flavor and texture from tofu. Its nutty earthiness contrasts with tofu's neutral flavor, and whereas tempeh is firm and chewy, tofu boasts a spongy, fluffier texture. The fermentation process causes

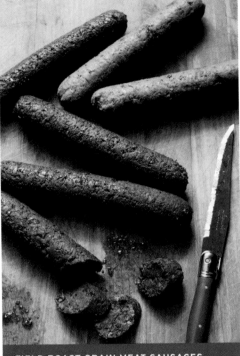

FIELD ROAST GRAIN MEAT SAUSAGES (FROM TOP TO BOTTOM): SMOKED APPLE SAGE AND MEXICAN CHIPOTLE tempeh to be only slightly bitter, but steaming it for 10 minutes before you do anything else to it is the secret to dulling its bitter edge and tenderizing this Indonesian staple.

Once steamed, you can sauté it, grill it, stir-fry it, deep-fry it, marinate it, and bake it, as well as:

- Cube it and fry it up in a little oil. Add to a stir-fry.
- Crumble it into pasta sauce or chili.
- Grate it and cook it with taco or fajita seasonings.
- Cut it into strips and marinate in BBQ sauce; bake for 30 minutes at 350 degrees.
- Make Tempeh Bacon (page 77), Better-Than-Chicken Salad (page 97), or Sloppy Joes (page 100).

Although its texture doesn't change like tofu's does, tempeh can definitely be frozen. Just thaw it completely before using in a recipe. Also, keep in mind that any black specks you see on the tempeh are just a natural part of the fermentation process.

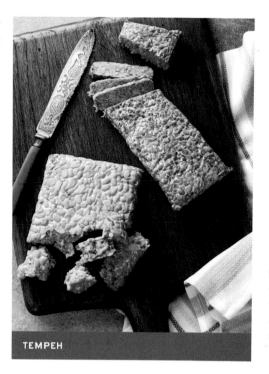

TEMPEH

- SEITAN: Pronounced *SAY*-tan, this wheat-based food goes by many names: wheat gluten, grain meat, wheat meat, and—my least favorite—mock meat. Believed to have originated in China, where seventh-century Buddhists eschewed the consumption of animal flesh, seitan was developed as an alternative to duck meat. The more they kneaded wheat flour and water, the more the starch came out, ultimately resulting in a chewy, protein-rich substance they called *mien chien* or "wheat meat." It's also known as "Buddha's food."

Sauté seitan as part of a stir-fry, grill it, bake it, barbecue it, or fry it. Flavor it however you like, and serve it up.

- MUSHROOMS: Ironically, the very thing that draws some people to mushrooms—their meaty, chewy texture—is what repels others. There are many mushrooms to choose from, and each provides a satisfying mouthfeel, though the ones often compared to animal-based meat

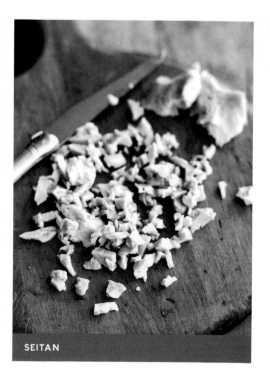

SEITAN

are portobellos. (See Marinated Portobello Mushroom Steaks on page 99.) Whole, marinated, and properly cooked (grilling is my favorite method), they are fantastic placed on a bun with all the fixings.

Focusing on the most common and readily available mushrooms, here are some ideas for incorporating them into your repertoire:

- Baby portobellos—also called brown mushrooms or creminis—can be minced or pureed and, combined with some binding ingredients and delicious flavorings, made into burgers.
- Brown mushrooms are ideal for gravies (see recipe on page 252), left either chunky or made smooth and creamy.
- Brown and shiitake mushrooms pair beautifully with pasta. Stem and slice them, and sauté with a chopped onion, minced garlic cloves, and olive oil. Cook until the mushrooms are just tender, about 10 to 15 minutes. Toss with cooked pasta and season with salt.
- Add mushrooms to your favorite vegetable, miso, or lentil soups.
- Brush with olive oil, roast or grill them, and add them to a veggie burger with caramelized onions.
- Add them to Tofu Scramble. (See page 86.)
- Sauté mushrooms and use them as a topping for pizza or bruschetta.

SALT

Aside from flavor and texture, we probably crave salt more than anything else, especially when we eliminate meat and dairy from our diet. Most of the sodium in people's diets comes from these animal products, so you're doing yourself a huge favor in terms of reducing sodium and blood pressure by getting these things as far away from your mouth as possible.

If you're craving salt:

- Add some table salt to your dish. With meat and dairy out of your diet, you can afford to have some salt on your food; it does bring out the flavor of food.

- Use tamari soy sauce as a flavoring.

- Make Tempeh Bacon (recipe on page 77), and create a tempeh BLT. Many people talk about how much they love bacon, but rest assured, it is not the backside or belly of a pig that makes people go ga-ga for this greasy meat. It tastes good because of fat and salt—and because it is smoked. Liquid smoke or smoked peppers (chipotles) provide the same flavor without harming anyone—you or the pigs—in the process.

FAT

Let's face it: fat tastes good. By now, everyone knows that the fat in plant foods is healthful, whereas the fat in animal products is harmful. So often when people think they're craving "meat," they're really just craving something with fat. The remedy? Eat fat—*whole* plant-based fat.

- Toast pine nuts or walnuts with some salt, pulse in the food processor (or leave whole), and sprinkle over your pasta.

- Add nuts to your oatmeal and sunflower seeds to your salad.

- Blend peanut or almond butter into your fruit smoothie. (See recipe on page 83).

- Top chili with nondairy sour cream or avocado.

- Cook with a little coconut oil, coconut butter, or coconut milk. Though it's true that the fat in coconuts is saturated, it's molecularly different from animal-based saturated fat and doesn't have the same negative effects on the body.

- Add guacamole to your burrito or fajita.

- Add eggless mayonnaise or avocado to your favorite sandwich.

- Lightly brush your favorite veggies with oil, then grill or roast them.

- Snack on some olives, or add them to a green salad.

- Heck, make a peanut butter and jelly sandwich!

HUNGER

Consider that sometimes when we think we're craving something in particular, we might just be hungry. A woman wrote to me once to say that she was vegetarian for seven years and was hungry all the time. I replied, "You were vegetarian for seven years and you were hungry all the time? Why didn't you just *eat*?" Sometimes it's just as simple as satisfying our need to feel full.

If you identify the actual craving rather than jumping right to the familiar food that satisfies your craving, you can better find the thing that will fulfill that need.

Whether you're vegan for 30 days or beyond, sooner or later every vegan runs across the argument that humans are *made* to eat meat. I would never claim that humans are *unable* to eat meat; of course we're *capable* of it, though we're not doing a very good job. (Lions don't get heart disease; we do.) But just because we *can* do something doesn't mean we should. And it is a mistake to conclude that humans are "carnivores" and "supposed to eat meat," simply because we have what we call "canine" teeth. Let's examine this by comparing the physiology of the herbivorous and carnivorous animals of the world and see where humans fit in.

Since the best place to start is the means by which animals come by their food, let's look at the teeth and nails. Herbivores have much shorter and softer fingernails than flesh-eating animals and pathetically small and dull "canine" teeth. In contrast, carnivores have incredibly sharp claws and large incisors called carnassial teeth capable of tearing and slicing flesh. In fact, the word *carnassial* comes from the Latin word *carn*, which means "meat." Herbivores (and humans) have flat molars that enable them to grind fibrous plants; carnivores lack these.

How about the jaw structure? The jaws of carnivores move only up and down, enabling them to slice and tear chunks of flesh; the jaws of herbivores (and humans) move from side to side, enabling them to push food back and forth into the grinding teeth with the tongue and cheek muscles.

What about saliva? Because carnivores do not chew their food, they don't need to mix it with saliva to help the digestion process. Thus, unlike that of herbivorous animals, the saliva of carnivorous animals does not contain digestive enzymes. The saliva of herbivores—and humans—contains carbohydrate-digesting enzymes.

The intestines? In carnivores, the small intestine is only three to six times the body length, and the large intestine or colon is very short and doesn't have pouches. The small intestine of plant-eating animals—and humans—tends to be very long (greater than ten to twelve times body length) to allow adequate time and space for absorption of the nutrients.

In all ways (including even our facial muscles, jaw muscles, mouth size, stomach acidity, and stomach volume), humans resemble herbivores rather than carnivores.

DAY 12 Discovering That There *Is* Life After Cheese

I've guided thousands of people through the "challenge" of becoming vegan and if you're like the vast majority of them, you probably thought that dairy—and specifically cheese—would be the thing you'd miss most. Given the tenacious hold cheese has on people, I'm certain that everyone has muttered a variation of "I could never live without cheese" at some point in their lives. I'm sure *I* did before I went vegan. My short response is "Of course you can live without cheese"—and a healthier, more satisfying life it will be. But I think my longer response gets to the heart of why we give so much power to this thing called cheese and provides the key to finally letting go of it.

No doubt you'll agree that food triggers high emotions in people, and many of us have some serious attachments to certain products that—quite literally—act as a security blanket. With that in mind, it's no wonder that we react so strongly at the thought that these things will be taken away. What I suggest is that it's the *feeling* we get when we eat something like cheese, and not the cheese itself, that keeps us going back for more. Because it triggers an emotional reaction or a pleasant memory, it's that *emotion* we crave—not the cheese itself. Let me explain.

We tend to get attached to the form of something and forget that the form is often just a conduit for the thing we're really seeking. The risk we take in becoming attached to the form is that we overlook what we really want. We may be seeking comfort—and we happen to find it in cheese. Some may find this comfort in chocolate, some in coffee, some in a good book. There's nothing wrong with seeking comfort; it doesn't always have to belie some deep, hidden pathology. But with this perspective, we can see that it's the *comfort* we're seeking, not the *form* of that comfort. Not the cheese. The comfort can be found in so many ways that don't involve cheese. So let's stop giving cheese so much credit. It's just one form we find comfort in. Comfort is the desire; cheese is the form that desire takes.

> **CHALLENGE YOUR THINKING:**
> It's the *feeling* we get when we eat cheese, and not the cheese itself, that keeps us going back for more. Because it triggers an emotional reaction, a pleasant memory, it's that *emotion* we crave—not the cheese itself.

Maybe eating cheese triggers a nostalgic memory for you. Maybe it reminds you of a trip you took, or of your grandmother, who served you her famous mac and cheese when you visited her, or of your family's cheese-centered dinners when you were growing up. I would argue that it is the experiences, the people, and the emotions that are meaningful for you, not the cheese ingredient. It's just acting as a trigger. And because cheese plays such a huge role in our culture, it's no surprise that it plays a role in many of our memories. If you grew up in a culture without cheese or if you grew up vegan, entirely different foods would be the triggers for you. So it's wonderful to embrace the memories, while recognizing that the food we're so attached to is just a memory trigger.

FAMILIARITY

Another thing many of us seek out is the feeling of familiarity. We're fierce creatures of habit, and we crave that feeling of the familiar. Let's face it—not many of us openly embrace change. How many of us go to the same restaurants over and over and order the same thing off the menu? How many of us have rituals when we return home or before we eat dinner or before we go to bed? When I say rituals, I mean those patterns of behavior regularly performed in a set manner, like the order in which we get ready for bed: wash our face, brush our teeth, brush our hair—whatever. We love that feeling of familiarity; it grounds us. It makes us feel like we belong. It gives significance to or increases our anticipation of whatever it is we're about to engage in.

It also adds order to our lives. Have you ever walked out of the house without your keys because on that morning a wrench was thrown into your regular routine? You walked out a different door, or you got a phone call on the way out—something threw off or upset the order of your normal routine.

The need for order and familiarity is very real, but when our habits or rituals become devoid of meaning—or, worse yet, when they contribute harm to ourselves or someone else—it's then I would suggest we need to reexamine these habits.

Food and eating are two components of our lives where we experience ritual and familiarity on a daily basis. We're used to sitting in the same chair at the dinner table. We have a certain glass we like to drink out of. Some of us like our sandwiches cut a certain way. Some of us get used to having a certain dish on Friday night or to eating in front of the TV. Some of us pray before we eat. Some eat food from our plates in a certain order. At the risk of implying that we all have elements of what is now termed obsessive-compulsive disorder, we can't deny that eating is not just a mere act of taking in nourishment for survival. Would that it were that simple!

"But wait," you say. "That all sounds really nice, but *cheese tastes good*! It's not just a matter of seeking comfort or creating rituals or finding the familiar. Cheese tastes good!" So, you think it tastes good, and from *that* standpoint, you think you could never give it up? To that I would say the following: Let's choose awareness over appetite.

AWARENESS OVER APPETITE

I, like many people, stopped eating animals and their secretions not because I stopped liking the taste but because I didn't want to contribute to exploitation of and violence toward animals. Once I learned the truth about dairy cows (and goats and sheep), there was no way I could keep eating any product that was made from the milk of those animals. It was that simple for me. Their suffering took precedence over any desire I may have had for the stuff—even my childhood English muffin pizzas, the ice cream I had on a regular basis, the croissants I loved with my tea, or the Gouda that I practically lived on when I was in Holland. None of it mattered in the face of suffering. Of course, for others the health benefits of cutting out dairy are the motivating factor—and a powerful one at that.

So if you're attached to cheese but are willing to become *unattached,* it may be that simple for you, too. Read, learn, watch videos about what the cows endure. Educate yourself about the artery-clogging and cancer-causing properties of cheese. The least we can do is learn the truth. The bottom line is that if we think we "can't give up cheese," it may be because we're unwilling to. I promise there will come a time when you will not obsess over cheese, but first you have to give your body and your palate time to adjust without it. You have to give yourself a chance *not* to eat it.

> **CHALLENGE YOUR THINKING:** If we think we "can't give up cheese," it may be because we're unwilling to.

FINDING SATISFACTION WITHOUT CHEESE

In terms of the gustatory pleasure we derive from this substance, when we deconstruct it, it comes down to fat, salt, and mouthfeel, just as with meat. Think about it:

- Consider the common habit of sprinkling Parmesan cheese onto pasta. What we really get out of that—besides the fact that it plays into our need for the familiar—is the satisfaction of salt and fat. With that in mind, try toasting some pine nuts or walnuts along with some salt, pulse them in a food processor, and sprinkle them on your pasta instead.

- Think about the habit of adding sour cream to our favorite Mexican dishes and the role it plays: it has a satisfying creamy texture, it provides some fat, but mostly it's used to cool down a spicy dish. With that understanding, we can accomplish the same things with guacamole, mashed avocado, commercial nondairy sour cream, fresh tomatoes, or shredded lettuce. (A quick homemade sour cream can be made by pureeing silken tofu with lemon juice and some salt.)

- Pesto is a great example of something that has been so laden with cheese as to mask the fresh flavors of the garlic, basil, pine nuts, and olive oil. The latter two ingredients give us the satisfaction of fat, and the oil also creates the creaminess. Try my delicious pesto recipe on page 131.

- When ordering pizza in a restaurant, ask for a pie with just sauce and a variety of vegetables and herbs. In fact, the oldest and most authentic pizza you can have is *marinara,* which is simply tomato sauce spread on thin crust, topped with a little basil. If you have a regular pizza place you use, you can always bring nondairy cheese to them and ask them to make a pie for you with your cheese.

COMMERCIAL NONDAIRY CHEESES

Now that I've said all that, commercial nondairy cheeses, which also provide fat, salt, and a satisfying mouthfeel, can certainly play a role in our repertoires, especially when we're first transitioning away from dairy-based cheeses. But the more you build your diet on whole foods, the less you crave concentrated fat, salt, and processed foods. You will even become accustomed to familiar dishes without nondairy cheese, reserving even this cheese for a special occasion.

When you *are* trying nondairy cheeses for the first time, let me make a few suggestions:

- Judge them on their own merit. Do not taste dairy and nondairy sour cream side by side to compare them. They're going to be different, because they're made from different ingredients. More significantly, you'll be biased toward the old standby, not because it's superior but because that's what you're used to. If you were raised on nondairy milk and cheeses, they would be your preference.

- Try nondairy cheese in the context in which it was meant to be eaten. You wouldn't eat dairy-based sour cream from a spoon, so don't do that with nondairy sour cream, either. Add it to a burrito, fajita, or chili, and try it that way.

New cheeses are being introduced all the time; however, here is a list of my current favorites. You should be able to find many of them in large natural food stores and also in vegan stores online.

Grated Cheeses

Parma, by Eat in the Raw: Made from organic walnuts, nutritional yeast, and sea salt, it's essentially a commercial version of what you can easily make at home.

Soymage Vegan Parmesan, by Galaxy Nutritional Foods: A soy-based powdery cheese used for sprinkling on pasta or pizza. Good for people transitioning, though it may not satisfy people looking for an exact replica of dairy-based Parmesan cheese.

For a homemade option, pulse toasted pine nuts or walnuts with salt in a food processor, along with some nutritional yeast (optional).

> **GOOD TO KNOW:**
>
> Nutritional yeast is a non-active yeast that is yellow in appearance. It comes in flakes and powder, though the former is what I recommend. It has a cheesy flavor that's great for sprinkling on popcorn or pasta. See "Creamy Cheeses" (page 129) for more uses.

Slicing and Spreading Cheeses

Dr. Cow's Tree Nut Cheese: Dr. Cow's gourmet nut-based cheeses are outstanding and organic, though not inexpensive. All of the cheeses have been aged for three months and come in various flavors: Aged Cashew, Aged Macadamia (rolled in mixed herbs), Aged Cashew and Brazil Nut, Aged Cashew and Hemp Seed, and more. They provide that fantastic sour flavor many people look for in certain cheeses.

Sheese, by Bute Island Foods: Several creamy, spreadable flavors are available, including Cheddar, Original, Chives, Garlic & Herb, and Mexican. Standard sliceable variations are also available.

Organic Soy Feta, by Sunergia Soyfoods: Their delicious tofu-based cheeses have the perfect crumbly feta texture and come in many flavors, such as Lemon Oregano, Mediterranean Herb, Tomato Garlic, and Soy Bleu.

Cheese Singles: There are a number of companies that make rice- and soy-based American-style cheese slices. Just make sure they are casein-free.

For a homemade option, try Cashew Cheese made from cashews, nutritional yeast, and oil. This is my favorite. It can be kept creamy or made sliceable using agar to act like gelatin to set the cheese. See page 134 for the recipe.

Melting Cheeses

Daiya Cheese: Daiya melts just like dairy-based cheese and contains no common allergens such as casein, gluten, nuts, or soy. Made from tapioca starch, it's available in Mozzarella, Cheddar, and Pepperjack. Prepare for the best grilled cheese sandwiches with this delicious cheese, and if you buy Tofurky's frozen pizza or Amy's nondairy macaroni and cheese, you'll find its made with Daiya.

Teese, by Chicago Soydairy: Teese boasts Mozzarella and Cheddar flavors. Melts well. (Chicago Soydairy also makes Temptation Ice Cream and Dandies marshmallows.)

Cheezly, by Redwood Foods: Available in Cheddar and Mozzarella, Cheezly melts well and can be used for pizza, pasta, and sandwiches. Because it comes in cube form, it can also be sliced and served with crackers.

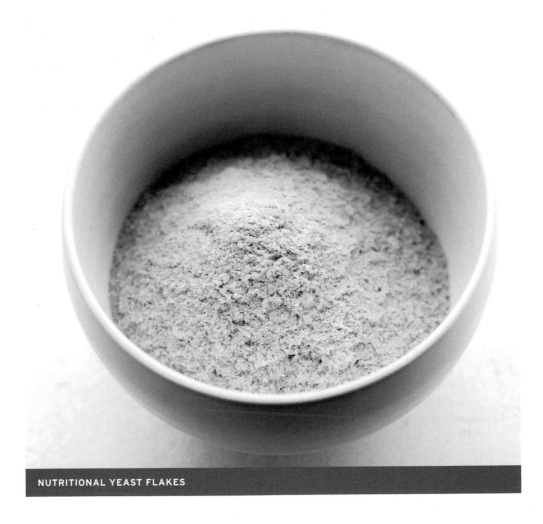

NUTRITIONAL YEAST FLAKES

Vegan Gourmet, by Follow Your Heart: Best when grated first, this soy-based cheese works well for something like burritos or tacos, whether you're using the Cheddar, Mozzarella, Monterey Jack, or Nacho flavor.

Creamy Cheeses

Commercial mac and cheese: A few different brands make boxed and frozen vegan macaroni and cheese, so look for them in vegan stores or natural foods stores.

Homemade mac and cheese: Though you can add agar to the cashew cheese recipe (page 134) to make a block of cheese that you can slice, leaving the agar out yields a delicious creamy cheese that is perfect for macaroni and cheese.

Sour cream: Make your own sour cream by pureeing silken tofu or cashews with lemon juice and salt, or check out the many commercial varieties, such as those made by Tofutti, Wayfare, and Galaxy Foods.

Cream cheese: The commercial versions are very good for spreading on bagels or for making cheesecake! Brands include Tofutti and Galaxy Foods.

Ricotta: Follow the directions in the recipe for Hearty Lasagna on page 137 to make a delicious tofu-based ricotta to use in stuffed shells, manicotti, and lasagna.

Quick (No-Queso) Quesadillas

YIELD: 4 TO 8 SERVINGS

If the combination of Middle Eastern hummus and Mexican tortillas seems strange, just trust me. The result is absolutely delightful and serves as an incredibly fast meal, snack, or appetizer. Kids of all ages love it!

Eight 10-inch flour tortillas (corn is fine, too, but they're usually smaller)
Hummus (store-bought or homemade—see page 159)

½ cup chopped green onions
½-1 cup salsa

Spread a tortilla with 3 heaping tablespoons of hummus and place hummus side up in a large nonstick skillet over medium heat.

Sprinkle with chopped green onions and spread on a thin layer of salsa.

Top with a second tortilla, and cook until the bottom tortilla is warm and turning golden brown, about 3-5 minutes, depending on how high you have the heat. Turn and cook the second side for another few minutes, until it, too, is golden brown. The first one always takes the longest since the pan isn't totally hot yet; this process becomes a lot quicker once the pan is hot, so stay close.

Alternatively, you can spread your hummus on just one half of the tortilla, place the tortilla in the pan, add the other toppings in a thin layer over the hummus, and fold the empty half of the tortilla on top of the filled side. (Just be careful not to overload it, which will make it too difficult to flip it over.) Let it get golden brown on the bottom side, then carefully turn the folded quesadilla over to get golden brown on the other side.

Remove from pan, and serve hot. If using the two tortillas, cut it in half or into pizza-shape triangles to serve as finger food. Repeat with remaining tortillas.

Variations
- Hearty Mexican-style: add some pinto or black beans when you add the salsa.
- Greek-style: instead of salsa and green onions, add spinach, thinly sliced red onions, kalamata olives, and nondairy yogurt.
- Italian-style: instead of salsa and green onions, add roasted red peppers, parsley, and oregano.

Soy-free, wheat-free if using corn tortillas

Basil Pesto

YIELD: ¼ TO ½ CUP

The name *pesto* derives from the tradition of making this sauce in a mortar with a pestle. The following recipe, which I encourage you to use a food processor for, unless you have a few spare hours, proves that you absolutely don't need cheese to make a fantastic pesto. Purchase fresh basil (or grow it yourself) and find a nice fruity olive oil.

3 cups loosely packed fresh basil leaves
¼ cup raw pine nuts
2 or 3 whole garlic cloves, peeled

3 tablespoons extra-virgin olive oil
¼ teaspoon salt, or to taste

Combine the basil, pine nuts, and garlic in a food processor, and blend until the ingredients begin forming a paste, scraping down the sides of the bowl as necessary.

Drizzle in a tablespoon or two of the oil, along with the salt, and process until smooth and creamy. Add more oil and salt as necessary, a little at a time.

Wheat-free, soy-free

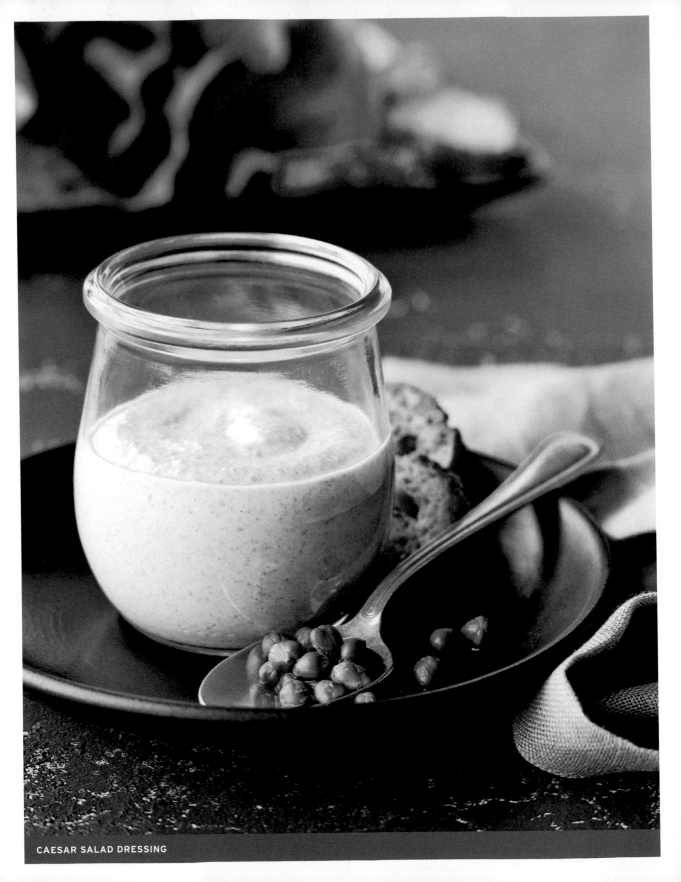

CAESAR SALAD DRESSING

Caesar Salad

YIELD: 4 TO 6 SERVINGS; MAKES 1 CUP OF DRESSING

This healthful version honors Cesar Cardini's original recipe, which did not call for anchovies. This salad delivers all the tangy flavor and creamy texture of the original, with the capers providing the saltiness and a beautiful green hue.

½ cup firm tofu (*not* silken)
4 tablespoons fresh lemon juice
3 whole garlic cloves, peeled
2–3 tablespoons capers, drained
2 tablespoons nutritional yeast
1 tablespoon Dijon mustard

½ teaspoon ground pepper
¼ teaspoon salt
Water or olive oil, as needed, to thin it out
4 heads romaine lettuce
Croutons, homemade or store-bought

In a blender or food processor, blend the tofu, lemon juice, garlic, capers, nutritional yeast, mustard, pepper, and salt. Add water or olive oil, as needed, to thin it out. The consistency should be nice and creamy but not so thick that you can't pour it. Tweak the flavor with the various ingredients to your liking. (You may like it tangier and want to add more mustard, you may like it saltier and want to add more capers, etc.)

Tear the romaine lettuce into bite-size pieces and add to a large bowl. Add the dressing and croutons and toss to combine.

Variations
- Add bits of Tempeh Bacon (page 77) to the salad.
- Reserve some capers to sprinkle on top of each individual serving of salad.

Creamy Macaroni and Cheese

YIELD: 4 CUPS

A delicious recipe based on one in Ann Gentry's *The Real Food Daily Cookbook,* this is quintessential comfort food. The cashew cheese can be kept creamy or formed into a block.

1¼ cups raw cashews
½ cup nutritional yeast
2 teaspoons onion powder
1-2 teaspoons salt, to taste
1 teaspoon garlic powder
⅛ teaspoon ground white pepper
3½ cups nondairy milk (soy, rice, almond, hazelnut, hemp, oat)

3 tablespoons of a thickener such as cornstarch or kudzu root (see variation below)
½ cup canola oil
¼ cup light (yellow or white) miso paste
2 tablespoons freshly squeezed lemon juice (about 1 lemon)
12-16 ounces elbow macaroni, cooked

Add the cashews to the large bowl of the food processor, and using the pulse button, finely grind the cashews. Don't allow the cashews to turn into a paste. Add the nutritional yeast, onion powder, salt, garlic powder, and white pepper. Pulse three more times to blend in the spices.

Combine the milk, thickener, and oil in a heavy saucepan. Bring to a simmer over high heat. Decrease the heat to low-medium, cover, and simmer, stirring occasionally for 10 minutes or until the thickener is dissolved.

With the food processor running, gradually add the milk-oil mixture to the cashew/nutritional yeast mixture. Blend for 2 minutes or until very smooth and creamy. Next, blend in the miso and lemon juice.

Combine the cheese with macaroni and serve. You may also bake it (see p. 135). If you have sauce left over, make more noodles, pour it over broccoli, or serve it as a fondue dip.

The cheese will keep for 4 days, covered and refrigerated.

Variation

The cheese you prepare using this recipe will be creamy, but if you would like to make a hard block of cheese, replace the recipe thickener with 1 cup (about 2 ounces) of agar, which is a vegetarian gelatin sold in natural food stores as flakes. Transfer the creamy mixture to the type of container you'll be using as a mold (rectangular, square, round). Once it sets up (after a few hours in the refrigerator), unmold it, and slice or grate it. Serve with crackers.

Baked Macaroni and Cheese

Preheat the oven to 325 degrees. Transfer the macaroni-cheese mixture to an 8- or 9-inch square baking dish. Cover and bake for 20 minutes, or until heated through. Uncover the dish, and sprinkle ½ cup herbed bread crumbs on top. Continue baking, uncovered, for 15-25 minutes, or until the topping is golden brown and crisp. Serve hot.

Wheat-free, soy-free

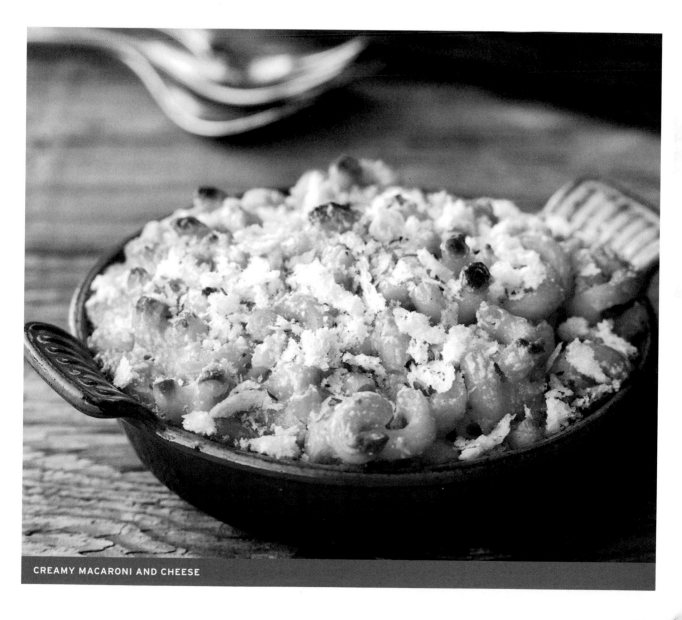

CREAMY MACARONI AND CHEESE

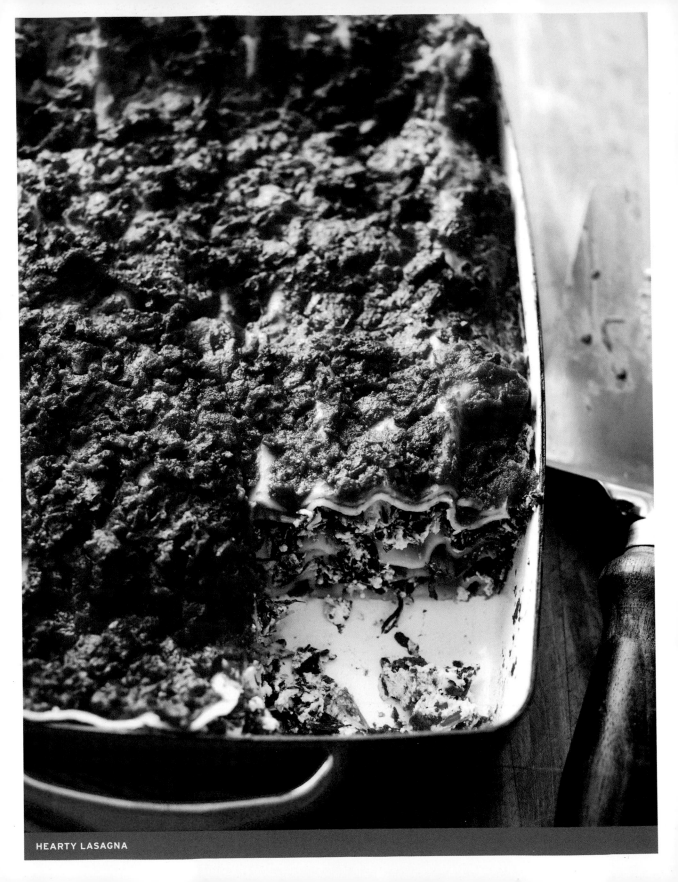

HEARTY LASAGNA

Hearty Lasagna

YIELD: 8 TO 10 SERVINGS

Firm tofu is used to create a beautifully textured "ricotta" cheese for a dish that simply means "layered."

½-1 pound lasagna noodles
Two 10-ounce packages frozen chopped spinach, thawed and drained
16 ounces firm tofu (*not* silken)
1 tablespoon sugar (optional)
¼ cup nondairy milk, more or less as needed
½ teaspoon garlic powder or 2 peeled cloves garlic

Juice from half a lemon (about 2 tablespoons)
2 tablespoons minced fresh basil (about 20 leaves)
1 teaspoon salt, or to taste
4-6 cups tomato or pasta sauce of your choosing

Preheat the oven to 350 degrees.

Cook the lasagna noodles according to the package directions, and drain and set aside. Or use the "no-need-to-boil" lasagna noodles.

Squeeze as much water from the spinach as possible and set aside. (If using fresh spinach, blanch it first, then squeeze out the water. Blanching just means to cook something very briefly in boiling water, then plunge it into cold water to stop the cooking process.)

Place the tofu, sugar, milk, garlic powder or garlic cloves, lemon juice, basil, and salt in a food processor or blender and pulse or blend until smooth. The tofu "ricotta" should be creamy but still have body.

Transfer to a large bowl and stir in the spinach. Continue tasting until you get the amount of salt just right.

Cover the bottom of a 9-by-13-inch baking dish with a thin layer of tomato sauce, then a layer of noodles (use about one-third of the noodles). Follow with half of the tofu filling. Continue in the same order, using half of the remaining tomato sauce and noodles and all of the remaining tofu filling. End with the remaining noodles, covered by the remaining tomato sauce. Bake for 40-45 minutes.

Variations
- Add meatless meat crumbles to your tomato sauce for more texture and flavor.
- Add shredded nondairy mozzarella cheese, such as Daiya Cheese, to each layer.

Herbed Scalloped Potatoes

YIELD: 4 TO 6 SERVINGS

Comfort food galore, this dish is filling, familiar, and fantastically delish.

Olive oil for coating the baking dish
2 pounds yellow potatoes, peeled and
    thinly sliced
2 cups vegetable stock
4 cloves garlic, pressed or minced
2 fresh sage leaves
2 bay leaves

1 teaspoon dried tarragon
½ teaspoon dried thyme
¼ teaspoon dried rosemary
¼ teaspoon freshly ground pepper
Salt to taste
2 tablespoons olive oil, divided

Preheat the oven to 425 degrees. Lightly oil a 2½-quart baking dish.

Layer the potatoes in the dish, and set aside.

In a saucepan, combine the stock, garlic, sage, bay leaves, tarragon, thyme, rosemary, and pepper. Add salt to taste. Bring to a boil over high heat, then immediately remove the pan from the stove. Cover and let stand for at least 30 minutes.

Discard the sage and bay leaves and pour the herbed broth over the potatoes. The potatoes will not be completely covered by the liquid. Drizzle the tops of the exposed potatoes with 1 tablespoon of the oil.

Bake uncovered for 20 minutes. Remove the dish from the oven and turn the potatoes over, pressing down gently to immerse them as much as possible in the liquid. Drizzle the tops of the exposed potatoes with the remaining oil.

Return to the oven and bake for 20 more minutes, or until the potatoes are tender, the liquids are reduced, and the top is nicely browned. Serve at once.

Wheat-free, soy-free

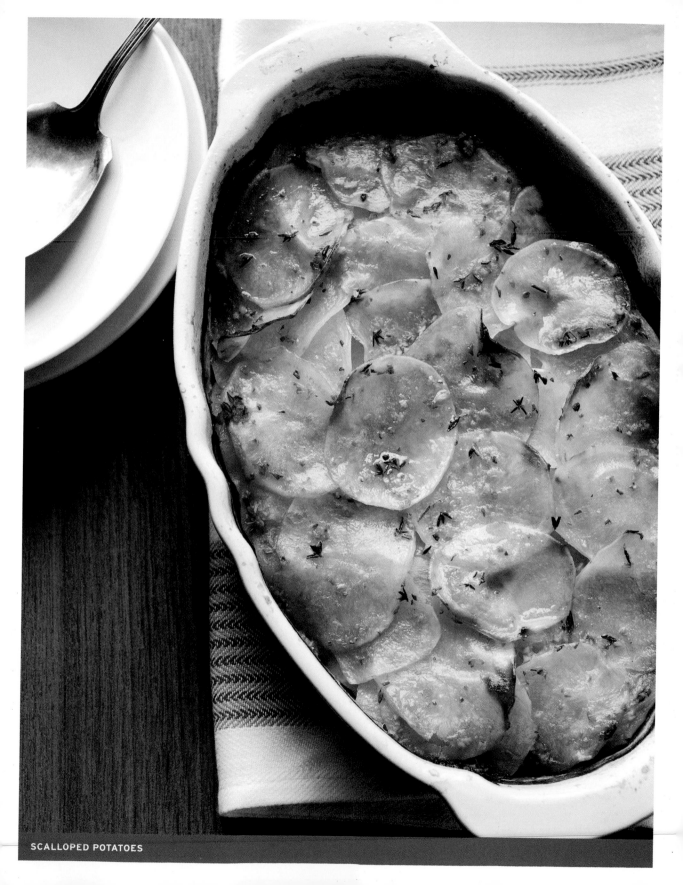

SCALLOPED POTATOES

Cutting Out the Middle Cow and Getting Calcium Directly from the Source

If I were to ask you to tell me the best source of calcium, you would most likely say cow's milk. You wouldn't say horse's milk, or dog's milk, or even human's milk. You wouldn't say kale, collards, or bok choy. From a very young age, we have been sold the idea that cow's milk is an essential and healthful food for humans to consume, lauded for all the calcium it contains.

And it's true. Cow's milk does contain calcium, but why does cow's milk contain calcium? In order to answer that question, we have to ask a few more:

What is calcium? It's a mineral.
Where are minerals found? In the ground.
Why do cows have calcium in their milk? Because they eat grass—or, rather, they're *supposed* to eat grass.

Actually, today, three out of four cows do not eat grass. They're kept on dry lots, which are essentially dirt lots devoid of pasture. In order to ensure that the cows' milk is rich in calcium to live up to the marketing claims, the producers supplement the cows' feed with calcium.

You could supplement *your* feed with calcium. If we look at this entire process simply from a resource perspective alone, we would see how very little sense it all makes.

If you ever pass by cattle grazing in a pasture, you're most likely seeing beef cattle, not dairy cows. In most operations large and small, cows are hooked up to milking machines three times a day. If producers allowed the cows to freely graze, it would be too labor- and cost-intensive to round them up each time they had to be brought to the milking machines. So without grass and foliage, the natural diet of this ruminant whose wild ancestors hark back thousands of years, cows do not consume enough calcium to justify the claims made by the dairy industry.

By now you may be asking another question: if cows get calcium from the grass, wouldn't it make more sense for us to do the same?

Though I'm not suggesting we all start grazing on our front lawns, I am suggesting that we stop going through an animal to get a nutrient we can and should obtain directly from the source: greens!

CALCIUM INTAKE, STRAIGHT FROM THE SOURCE

Part of the reason we are so willing to buy the myth—and the milk—is because we want to be healthy and do the right thing for ourselves and our loved ones. We're told that we need calcium (and we do) and vitamin D (and we do) and that the best source of these nutrients is cow's milk (and it isn't).

It's accurate to say we need calcium; it's inaccurate to say we need cow's milk. For the animals' sake and our own health, the best thing we can do is go straight to the ground where the calcium resides—straight to the green leafy vegetables, where we also benefit from the presence of vitamins, minerals, fiber, folate, and phytonutrients.

Calcium-Rich Greens

> 1 cup cooked collard greens contains 266 mg of calcium; 1 cup raw contains 52 mg.
> 1 cup cooked turnip greens contains 197 mg of calcium; 1 cup raw contains 104 mg.
> 1 cup cooked bok choy contains 158 mg of calcium; 1 cup raw contains 74 mg.
> 1 cup cooked mustard greens contains 104 mg of calcium; 1 cup raw contains 58 mg.
> 1 cup cooked kale contains 179 mg of calcium; 1 cup raw contains 90 mg.
> 1 cup cooked broccoli contains 62 mg of calcium; 1 cup raw contains 43 mg.

CHALLENGE YOUR THINKING: Because cows aren't getting calcium from grass—the source of this mineral—producers supplement their feed with calcium.

CHANGE YOUR BEHAVIOR: Skip the middle cow, and get calcium straight from the source: green leafy vegetables.

Note: The high amount of oxalates present in spinach, Swiss chard, and beet greens substantially decreases our body's ability to absorb their calcium. There are plenty of other reasons to eat these green leafies, but calcium just isn't their star quality.

High-Calcium Foods Outside of the Greens

> 1 tablespoon blackstrap molasses contains 137 mg of calcium.
> 1 cup cooked soybeans contains 175 mg of calcium.
> 1 cup cooked navy beans contains 126 mg of calcium.
> ¼ cup almonds contains 92 mg of calcium.

5 figs contain 90 mg of calcium.
½ cup tempeh contains 92 mg of calcium.

Calcium-Fortified Foods

1 cup calcium-fortified Total cereal contains 1,000 mg of calcium.

1 cup calcium-fortified Special K Plus cereal contains 600 mg of calcium.

1 cup fortified plant-based milk (soy, almond, rice, hemp) contains about 300 mg of calcium.

1 cup calcium-fortified orange juice contains about 250 mg of calcium, the same as 1 cup of cow's milk.

½ cup firm calcium-set tofu contains 861 mg of calcium.*

1 tablet of a typical calcium supplement contains 300 to 500 mg of calcium.

> **CHALLENGE YOUR THINKING:**
> It is quite accurate to say we need calcium. It's quite inaccurate to say we need cow's milk (or any other milk that comes out of an animal).

It's clear that calcium is abundant in plant foods, but intake is just one aspect of calcium status.

CALCIUM ABSORPTION IS AS IMPORTANT AS CALCIUM INTAKE

As with all nutrients that are required from our diet, it is not simply a matter of *taking in* the nutrient. It's also a matter of *absorbing* it and *utilizing* it. *Bioavailability* is the degree to which a particular nutrient can be absorbed and used by the body.

In other words, though it's helpful to know how much calcium is in certain foods, it's also helpful to know how much of that calcium we actually absorb.

Kale: About 50 percent of the calcium in kale is absorbed by our bodies, so it's a very good source.

Broccoli: Over 60 percent of the calcium in broccoli is absorbed by our bodies—very high.

Bok choy: A good amount, 53 percent, is absorbed by our bodies.

Calcium-set tofu: Over 30 percent of the calcium in tofu is absorbed by our bodies. This is about the same bioavailability as the calcium in cow's milk.

Fortified beverages: The calcium used to fortify most juices and plant-based milks has a high bioavailability, ranging from 40 to 60 percent.

* Calcium content in tofu varies according to the brand and type of agent used to set the tofu. When calcium sulfate is used, the calcium content is very high. Calcium sulfate is the most common coagulant used to make firm tofu.

INCREASING CALCIUM ABSORPTION AND DECREASING CALCIUM LOSS

Overall, it's estimated that North Americans absorb about 30 percent of the calcium present in food (even cow's milk), so we want to increase absorption in as many ways as possible.

The best way to increase absorption of calcium is to increase exposure to or intake of vitamin D. Vitamin D supplements are recommended for those who are deficient, those in certain age groups, and for people who lack exposure to the sun. This goes for everyone—not just vegans. Just as the feed of cows is supplemented with calcium, so, too, is their milk fortified with vitamin D during processing. Most plant-based milks are fortified as well. People with light skin would do well to expose their face and forearms to ten to fifteen minutes of warm sunlight a day. People with dark skin may require three times as much.

To determine your vitamin D levels, the Vitamin D Council has partnered with ZRT Labs to make a discounted take-home vitamin D test kit available. See "Resources and Recommendations."

In addition to taking in calcium and increasing our bodies' absorption of calcium, we also want to avoid losing the calcium we take in. The latter has much to do with other characteristics of our diet, namely, our intake of protein and sodium, both of which contribute to loss of calcium from our bones. Plant protein has a lower concentration of sulfur-containing amino acids than animal protein does, but consuming high quantities of protein powders—particularly soy protein—could play a role in calcium excretion. To avoid such losses, keep protein intakes closer to recommendations and sodium intake under 2,400 mg a day. Also, be sure to participate in weight-bearing exercise to keep your bones strong.

> **CHALLENGE YOUR THINKING:** Increasing *absorption* of calcium is as important as *consuming* calcium-rich foods.
>
> **CHANGE YOUR BEHAVIOR:** Increase vitamin D intake by exposing your arms and face to warm sunlight each day, by taking a vitamin D supplement, or by eating fortified foods, which are especially recommended for older people and for people who live in regions with long, dark winters.

DAILY RECOMMENDATIONS FOR CALCIUM

How much calcium do we actually need?

In the United States, the daily recommendations are 500 mg for ages 1 to 3, 800 mg for 4-to-8-year-olds, 1,300 mg for adolescents 9 to 18 years, 1,000 mg for adults 19 to 50 years of age, and 1,200 mg for adults 50+ years of age.

There is absolutely no dearth of calcium-rich foods available to us, and skipping the middle cow (or goat or sheep or llama or buffalo) means that we also skip the harmful saturated fat, dietary cholesterol, animal protein (casein), and lactose.

DEFYING NATURE: LACTOSE INTOLERANCE

All female mammals lactate for one purpose: to provide nourishment and sustenance for their offspring. Though rates of breast-feeding in industrialized countries are much lower than in other parts of the world, and breast-feeding was even discouraged when I was a babe, technically humans can nurse for up to five years or more.

Once we're weaned, we don't need to consume even our own species' milk, and in fact, our bodies stop producing an enzyme called lactase by the time we are past the age of weaning—at about 4 years old. Lactase is the enzyme that enables us to digest lactose, which is the sugar in the milk of mammals, including humans. So by the time we should be weaned, our bodies don't make this enzyme anymore. Although some people around the world adapted genetically to continue consuming animal milk without discomfort, a huge percentage of the world's population suffers from what is called "lactose intolerance," experiencing gas, bloating, abdominal cramping, and diarrhea. According to the *Journal of the American Dietetic Association,* approximately 75 percent of the world's population loses the ability to digest lactose after infancy.

> **CHALLENGE YOUR THINKING:**
> Our bodies stop producing lactase, the enzyme that enables us to digest lactose, because we're not supposed to consume this milk sugar once we're weaned. Lactose intolerance is not a disorder. It's normal!

Lactose intolerance is not a disorder. It's normal! We're not *supposed* to be consuming lactose once we're weaned.

Skipping the middle cow is health- and life-enhancing for everyone, including the cows—and the goats. The goat's milk industry targets lactose-intolerant people, claiming that goat's milk has lower amounts of lactose than cow's milk. And it's true: goat's milk has 6 percent less lactose than cow's milk. Six percent. Not a big difference in my book. The bottom line is that adult cows and goats stop drinking their own mother's milk when they become adults. We should do the same. If you want lactose-free milk, drink plant-based milks!

DYING FOR CALCIUM

Before I realized that cows had to be pregnant in order to produce milk, I also believed that consuming animals' milk didn't contribute to suffering because the cow didn't have to be killed in order for us to take her milk.

I believed it because that's the story we're told and because I desperately didn't want to believe that my consumption of cow's milk, cheese, and butter was harming anyone.

But I was wrong.

Because a cow's life is only as valuable as the offspring and amount of milk she is able to produce, when she is no longer profitable (i.e., when the costs to feed, medicate, and shelter her exceed the revenue derived from her milk output), she is sent to slaughter.

Cows are impregnated every year beginning at two years young; by the time she is four or five, after having endured three or four pregnancies (and the loss of the same number of her calves), she is sold to slaughter. Cattle have a natural life expectancy of twenty or twenty-five years.

In the United States, whether she is used on a small farm, organic farm, "humane" farm, "family-owned" farm, artisan farm, whatever-it's-called farm, she is sent to slaughter when her milk production wanes.

Whether the milk is labeled organic, whole, pasteurized, unpasteurized, homogenized, raw, lactose-free, low-fat, 2 percent, 1 percent, skim, fat-free, rBST-free, or "natural," she is sent to slaughter.

Fifteen percent of the hamburger in this country comes from spent dairy cows. In the United States, of the 9 million cows bred and raised for their milk, 2.5 million dairy cows are sent to slaughter each year.

Make no mistake about it. There is no retirement spa for used-up cows. As much as we want to distance ourselves from responsibility and culpability, there is no such thing as a slaughter-free animal agriculture system. It is not economically viable to feed, shelter, treat, and house animals for the rest of their lives and generate no profit in return.

We have no nutritional requirement for cow's milk, but we do have an ethical imperative to make choices that create as little harm as possible.

So let's just go straight to the source and get our calcium from plants—exactly as the cows do!

CHALLENGE YOUR THINKING: Every dairy cow is killed to be sold for her flesh when she is no longer "profitable"—that is, when she no longer produces enough milk to justify her life. A slaughter-free animal agricultural system is simply not viable.

CHANGE YOUR BEHAVIOR: Make calcium-rich plant-based recipes.

DAY 14 Choosing Plant-Based Milks

You're two weeks into this challenge, and surely by now you've seen all the plant-based milks on the market. If you have yet to give them a try, now is the time to do so! Plant-based milks have been around for centuries and are delicious, healthful, and widely available. Understanding their history as well as how we became so dependent on animal milks will help ground you in your new habit.

People tend to refer to plant-based milks as "alternatives to" or "substitutes for" animal-based milks, and the dairy industry rather scathingly calls them "imitation milks." In fact, the National Milk Producers Federation has been trying for years to make it illegal for nondairy milk companies to use the word *milk*, claiming that it has proprietary ownership of that word. Just try telling a lactating mother that she has to call her milk a "breast *beverage*"! The dairy industry doesn't own the word *milk*.

The words *alternative* and *substitute* imply that the thing they are being measured against is superior—that you choose the substitute when you can't get the real thing. By that definition, when you examine our history and physiology, it's clear that over time animal-based milks displaced human's milk, making animal milks the imposters, the substitutes, and the alternatives to what is indisputably the most natural, nutrient-rich substance for humans to consume in our developing years: human's milk.

> **CHALLENGE YOUR THINKING:**
> Animal-based milk became the imposter, the alternative, the substitute for what is indisputably the most natural, nutrient-rich substance for humans to consume in our developing years: human milk.

All female mammals produce milk for the same reason: to feed and nourish their offspring. At a certain age, depending on the mammal, the infant is able to move on to solid food and is weaned off the mother's milk. In the case of humans, however, after we're weaned, we're sold the idea that we should then switch to the milk of another animal—even though the offspring of that other animal stop drinking their mother's milk once they're weaned.

We don't even drink our own species' milk into adulthood. At the very idea, people wrinkle up their noses in disgust. In fact,

I see similar sneers at the suggestion that humans drink rat's milk or cat's milk or dog's milk. Cow's milk, goat's milk, and sheep's milk? No problem. But dog's milk? That's just disgusting.

Perhaps we have to ask ourselves why we reject consuming the lactation fluid of some species but accept consuming that of others. After all, the milks of rats, cats, and dogs are very nutritious. Why haven't we given them a try?

Could it be because we recognize—instinctively and without marketing manipulation—that rat's milk is made for baby rats, cat's milk is made for kittens, and dog's milk is made for puppies? Could it be because we concede that an animal's milk is *indeed* very nutritious—for the offspring of the respective species?

In other words, *why cow's milk?* For that matter, why goat's milk? Why sheep's milk? For those who live in other parts of the world, why buffalo milk? Why yak milk? Why camel milk? Why horse milk? Is there something special in the milk of these animals that makes humans prone to drink it? What do these animals have in common?

The answer is very simple: they are all herd animals.

Because they move and stay together, herd animals are easy to contain and easy to control. It is this very characteristic that makes these animals targets for domestication, breeding, and confining. In other words, *there is no nutritional component of cow's milk that makes it any more necessary for human consumption than, say, hyena's milk.*

In fact, if hyenas were easy to control, we would have done the same to them. (And hyena's milk is very high in calcium.) The problem is, the hyena would kill you—or at least hurt you pretty badly—if you tried to take her milk. Cows—except for when they're trying to keep you from taking away their babies—are pretty docile animals. As vegetarians, their killer instinct is rather subdued. Hyenas, not so much.

> **CHALLENGE YOUR THINKING:** Cow's milk was chosen because of the nature of the animals—not because of the quality of the milk. Humans have no more nutritional requirements for cow's milk than they do for hyena's milk.

The point is that cow's milk is not manna from the heavens. It is a commercial product that was chosen arbitrarily because of the nature of the animals—not because of the quality of their milk.

LACTATION MACHINES

I remember the day I learned that cows don't just naturally "give milk." I was well into my adulthood, and I remember feeling so stupid. I was an intelligent person. I understood the fundamentals of biology. And yet I had completely wiped out of my mind that in order for mammals to lactate, they have to be pregnant.

Prior to this realization, I had believed that cows were somehow biologically designed to bestow what the dairy industry would call their nutritional gift upon humans. Even our language perpetuates this belief: we don't *take* milk, cows *give* milk—a romanticized vision of what is nothing less than an exploitative process.

In order to get cows to lactate (to produce milk), cows have to be impregnated. In order to keep them lactating to keep the milk production high (and the cows worth keeping alive), they have to be impregnated again and again. Like a human, a cow gestates for nine months. At the end of that time, when she gives birth, all she wants is her baby.

Instead of being able to tend to her offspring, however, the dairy cow finds that her baby is taken from her within days (sometimes a day) of birth, a process that every dairy producer—large or small—will admit is incredibly stressful for both mother and baby. Fiercely protective, a mother cow will do anything to keep her young safe and by her side, but it's a fight she never wins. In the end, her calf is taken from her, and she spends days brooding and bellowing—before being impregnated again.

CHALLENGE YOUR THINKING: The offspring of a dairy cow is merely incidental; he or she is simply the consequence of a pregnancy that is required to keep the animal lactating.

The offspring of a dairy cow (or goat or sheep) is merely incidental. He or she exists only because a cow (or doe or ewe) needs to be made pregnant. The dairy industry is all about stimulating and increasing milk production. The offspring is just the consequence of that pregnancy.

And because the dairy industry is just that—a profit-driven business—the decisions made about the fate of the animals are dictated by motivations for profit, not compassion. If the offspring is a female, she becomes part of the same cycle of impregnation, birth, and loss. If the offspring is a male, having no purpose in an industry that exploits the female reproductive system, he is sold for what is called "veal." His life becomes justified by the profit derived from his death.

Every year, more than 700,000 male calves born to dairy cows in the United States are slaughtered and sold as veal—all for a product that is neither healthful nor necessary for humans to consume.

MILK IS GOOD

By forgoing animal milk, we turn to plant-based milks, which have been around for centuries and which vary according to where you are in the world. Though water is really the only beverage we have a physiological need for (beyond mother's milk when we're young), it is certainly convenient and tasty to be able to make creamy, nutrient-rich milk from nuts (almonds, hazelnuts, peanuts, cashews), grains (oats and rice), legumes (soybeans and peanuts), and seeds (coconut, hemp, or sunflower). Many of these milks are now available commercially, and most can be easily made at home.

Plant-based milks have no saturated fat, no cholesterol, no lactose, and no casein, but they do contain protein, fiber, and other healthful properties.

Whether your decision to wean yourself off animal-based milk stems from your compassion, your health, or both, there are a number of things to consider when choosing the plant-based milk that is right for you:

- All of these milks will taste different to you if you compare them to what you've always known. Give your taste buds a chance to adjust, and resist the temptation to judge them as inferior just because they're unfamiliar to you.

- Variety in our diets is ideal for a variety of reasons, not the least of which is allergy avoidance. Too much of one thing can create an allergy, so don't drink just one type of milk—vary them.

- Different types and brands of milk vary in terms of taste and texture, so if you don't like one, don't throw the baby out with the bathwater and reject the whole lot. Try another.

- All of the plant-based milks can be used interchangeably, though some are creamier than others. The thinnest of the bunch is rice milk. See information on page 151 about coconut milk as a beverage.

- As with cow's milk, most plant-based milks are fortified with calcium, vitamin B_{12}, and vitamin D. Check the package to be sure.

- Most come in plain, vanilla, and chocolate. Some are unsweetened.

- Find plant-based milks either in the refrigerated section of your grocery store or on the shelf, packaged in aseptic cardboard boxes that don't have to be refrigerated until they're opened.

Although I list specific brand names in "Resources and Recommendations," let's take a look at the various options available.

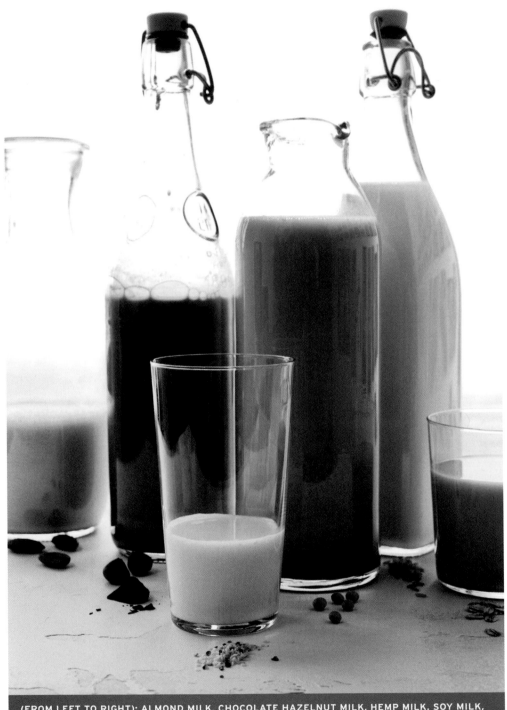

(FROM LEFT TO RIGHT): ALMOND MILK, CHOCOLATE HAZELNUT MILK, HEMP MILK, SOY MILK, RICE MILK, OAT MILK

SOY MILK

Soy milk originated in China, a region where the soybean was native and used as food long before the existence of written records. Soybean or "vegetable milk" is reputed to have been discovered and developed during the Han Dynasty in China, about 164 B.C., and later the soybean was transplanted to Japan. In the East, cow's milk is most definitely the alternative to soy milk; sad to say, however, thanks to the marketing muscle of the North American dairy industry, the consumption of cow's milk now exceeds that of soy milk in Japan.

Soy milk makers are available, so you can make your own at home.

ALMOND MILK

Used widely in the Middle Ages in regions stretching from the Iberian Peninsula to East Asia, almond milk was prized for its high protein content and its ability to keep better than milk from animals, which soured if not used right away. Make your own almond milk in a high-speed blender by combining 1½ cups blanched almonds with 4 cups water. Strain out the almond pulp, sweeten if you like, and refrigerate.

RICE MILK

Most commercial brands of rice milk are made from brown rice. Rice milk is thinner than the other milks, so try a creamier milk when baking.

If you've ever been to a traditional Mexican restaurant, you may have had the pleasure of drinking horchata, a delicious sweet beverage made primarily of rice, sugar, and cinnamon— and often almonds. Mexican horchata is based on the Spanish *horchata de chufa,* which was traditionally made from a grassy plant called the *chufa,* or tiger nut, and has its origin in ancient Egypt and Sudan. Some restaurants serve authentic horchata (no animal's milk), but be sure to ask first if they use cow's milk.

HEMP MILK

The newest commercial milk on the block, hemp milk is made from soaked hemp seeds, yielding a creamy, nutty-tasting beverage. Aside from healthful vitamins and minerals, hemp milk also boasts a high amount of essential fatty acids and poses no allergic threat. People tend to digest hemp milk much better than legume-based milks such as soy.

COCONUT MILK

Coconut *milk* is what we typically call the thick, sweet, milky white substance derived from the meat of a mature coconut. With the exception of a new coconut-milk-based beverage made by Turtle Mountain Foods, coconut milk is often used for cooking and not for drinking. Different from either of these, the juice of the young coconut is referred to as coconut *water* and drunk as a beverage. It's naturally fat-free and low in calories with high nutrition content. You'll often see coconut water served right in the coconut itself with a straw in restaurants specializing in Southeast Asian cuisines (Thai, Burmese, Vietnamese).

COFFEE CREAMERS

Many people are satisfied using any of the nondairy milks in their coffee or tea, but if you're looking for a thicker coffee-creamer-type substance, check out soy and hazelnut creamers or a product called MimicCreme, a gluten-free, soy-free nut-based milk. Also keep in mind that those powdered milks called "nondairy creamers" actually do have dairy in them, but vegan versions exist. See "Resources and Recommendations."

THE SKINNY ON MILK FAT

Through market saturation and advertising and through education materials they give to schools and nutrition policy makers, the dairy industry has skewed our thinking about the best sources of calcium and about what's "natural" for animals and ourselves.

It has also done a great job manipulating people into thinking they're drinking low-fat cow's milk when they choose 1 percent and 2 percent versions. Although it's true that only 2 percent of the total volume of 2 percent milk is fat (after all, milk is mostly water), in reality, relative to total calories, the true percentage of fat in 2 percent cow's milk is 35 percent and in 1 percent cow's milk it is 20 percent.

DAY 15   Putting to Rest the Great Protein Myth

If I had a nickel for every time someone asked me, "Where do you get your protein?" I would be a very wealthy vegan—and so would every other vegan, because it's the most commonly asked question.

I certainly applaud people for asking questions about health and nutrition, but we need to get away from this idea that vegans have to eat one way and non-vegans have to eat another way. The fact is that *everybody* needs to make sure they're getting the nutrients they require, not only to be healthy but also to thrive. Despite all the advanced medical training and technology in developed nations, millions of people are suffering and dying from preventable diseases. There is much we can do to improve our health, so certainly everyone should be asking questions about how to do better—not just once you consider going vegan.

When it comes to protein, the idea that we can't get enough on a vegan diet is simply not true, as emphasized by the American Dietetic Association's position paper on vegetarianism, which states: "Plant protein can meet requirements when a variety of plant foods are consumed and energy needs are met."

Breaking this down, what does it mean to consume a variety of plant foods and meet your energy needs? The first one is pretty self-explanatory. The idea is to enjoy a variety of plant foods throughout the day: vegetables, fruits, grains, nuts, seeds, and legumes. Aside from meeting your protein needs, you will also be taking in a number of other essential and healthful vitamins, minerals, and phytochemicals. Variety is key.

As far as meeting energy needs, that is just a different way of saying you need to take in the adequate number of calories for your body type, weight, and lifestyle, something that pertains to both vegans and non-vegans. I think this is vital to understanding the transition that takes place from eating an animal-based diet to eating a plant-based diet. Because of the nutrient profile of animal products versus plant foods, when you become vegan, you very naturally consume fewer calories because plants are much less calorie-dense than animal flesh and secretions. (Read more about this in "Day 28: Achieving and Sustaining Weight Loss.")

This is not necessarily a bad thing. Many, many people are consuming far more calories than they're expending each day, so they would do well to reduce their caloric intake. And since they're consuming so many calories—the majority of which are from animal products—they're also far exceeding their protein needs, which is not necessarily a *good* thing. So when they switch to a plant-based diet and consume fewer calories and thus less (animal-based) protein, they mistakenly perceive that as a negative. After all, we live in a society where more is better.

What I suggest is that we keep things in perspective and understand that everything is relative. Consuming fewer calories and thus less protein (in the form of animal protein) when you become vegan is natural and—if weight loss is something you strive for—even optimal.

Now, in terms of specific ways in which people would *not* actually meet their protein needs, we see it only in a few scenarios; again, this is the case whether you're vegan or not.

1. YOU STOP EATING. People who suffer from anorexia, depression, poverty, or severe illness, or who are on an extreme diet, don't meet their energy needs because they're not eating! If they're not eating, they aren't getting enough protein—or other macronutrients and micronutrients. Fortunately, these are not concerns for the majority of people.

2. YOU'RE AN ENDURANCE ATHLETE. When you increase your calorie expenditure to the degree that endurance athletes do, you absolutely must also increase your calorie intake to be sure you're getting all of your nutrients, including protein.

Assuming you're taking in adequate calories, not eating low-protein/low-nutrient foods such as potato chips all day, and not eating a fruit-only diet, the risk of protein deficiency is a non-issue.

The simple truth is that people in developed countries tend to suffer not from diseases of deficiency but rather from diseases of excess.

In fact, most people have never even met anyone with serious protein deficiency; they may have seen images of what it looks like on television when they watch late-night appeals for hunger organizations and see children with thinning hair and distended bellies. *They* have protein deficiency because they're not getting enough *food*. There is even a scientific term for this; it's called kwashiorkor. It's a disease we see in countries where rampant poverty prevents people from consuming the calories and nutrients they need to survive and thrive.

In developed nations, we do not have kwashiorkor wards in hospitals, we do not know any kwashiorkor specialists, and we probably do not have any friends—vegan or not—with kwashiorkor. But what we do have are diseases linked to our excess intake of animal protein: cancer, gout, and kidney problems such as kidney stones.

The problem isn't that vegans can't get enough protein; the problem is that most people are consuming way more protein than they need, particularly from animal sources.

COMPLEMENTING YOUR PROTEIN

Regarding protein and a plant-based diet, the American Dietetic Association also states: "Research indicates that an assortment of plant foods eaten over the course of a day can provide all essential amino acids; thus complementary proteins do not need to be consumed at the same meal."

One of the biggest myths about protein is that vegans (and vegetarians) have to complement our protein at each meal; that is, we have to combine certain foods in order to get a complete protein. Unfortunately, this myth started with a book whose intention was to inspire a plant-based diet. The premise of Frances Moore Lappé's 1971 book *Diet for a Small Planet* was that we could feed a hungry world by feeding everyone a plant-based diet, eliminating the intensive, wasteful resources of animal-based agriculture. With the intention of making sure people did this healthfully, she popularized the idea of "complementary proteins."

Her recommendations were based on the fact that every type of protein, whether animal- or plant-based, is made up of amino acids. Some amino acids can be made by the body; those that cannot are known as "essential," and we must get them from food. All plant proteins have all of the essential amino acids; some just have higher amounts of certain ones than others. For instance, beans are lower in methionine, and grains are lower in lysine. So the idea was that we would have to consume beans and grains in one meal to get enough of all the amino acids—to get a "complete protein."

We now know this isn't necessary. We've known this for decades, and yet still the myth persists. Lappé even corrected this notion in subsequent editions of her book. Bottom line: as long as we're eating a variety of foods throughout the day, our bodies are smart enough to assimilate and store the amino acids we need.

HOW MUCH PROTEIN DO WE NEED?

Taking into account our various body sizes and activity levels, you can calculate for yourself your optimal intake. *Experts recommend that adults eat 0.4 gram of protein per day for every pound of healthy body weight.* Infants, children, competitive athletes, and pregnant and nursing women require more protein.

- Healthy 1-to-3-year-old children need 0.48 gram of protein per pound of body weight per day.

- Children 4 to 8 years old should have 0.43 gram of protein per pound of body weight per day.

- The recommendation is 0.43 gram per pound of body weight for 9-to-13-year-olds, and 0.39 gram for 14-to-18-year-olds.

- Pregnant women should aim for about 71 grams per day total.

- A competitive athlete might increase intake to between 0.6 and 0.9 gram per pound of body weight.

PROTEIN IN PLANT FOODS

Though we've all been indoctrinated to believe that meat, dairy, and eggs are the only sources of protein, the fact is that protein is abundant in plant foods. Certainly some plants contain more protein than others, but many grains and vegetables contribute a significant amount of protein to our diets. Unfortunately, we're never taught that broccoli, oatmeal, and carrots have protein, but just think for a moment about the largest, strongest animals on the planet: giraffes, elephants, bulls, and bison. They're all vegetarian animals, and they get plenty of protein–from plants.

Just a glance at the chart on page 157 demonstrates how easy it is to consume a healthful amount of protein each day. I've included some recipes at the end of this chapter that are particularly protein-rich, but that doesn't mean the other recipes in this book aren't also good sources of protein. Bodybuilders and endurance athletes also tend to add additional plant protein in the form of shakes, of which there are a number of options whether you're looking for soy, rice, hemp, pea, or nut protein (see "Resources and Recommendations"). The protein powders used in such shakes tend to average about 23 grams of protein per ⅓ cup of dry powder.

So next time someone says to you, "You're as strong as an ox," you can say, "Well, of course I am. I'm vegan–just like the ox!"

PLANT-BASED FOOD	PROTEIN

Protein shakes
   (soy, rice, hemp, pea)
	amount varies; check label;
	   average 23 g per ⅓ cup

1 cup firm tofu	40 g
1 cup cooked tempeh	30 g
1 cup cooked soybeans	29 g
1 cup cooked lentils	18 g
1 cup cooked pinto beans	15 g
1 cup cooked black beans	15 g
1 cup cooked chickpeas	15 g
3 veggie deli slices	14 g
¼ cup sunflower seeds	8 g
¼ cup almonds	7.4 g
8 ounces nondairy milk	5–10 g
6-ounce container soy yogurt	5–7 g
1 cup cooked corn	5.4 g
1 cup quinoa	8 g
2 tablespoons peanut butter	8 g
1 cup cooked broccoli	8 g
1 cup cooked brown rice	8 g
1 cup cooked oatmeal	7 g
1 bagel	7 g
1 medium baked potato	4.5 g
½ ounce walnuts (7 halves)	4.3 g
1 cup chopped cooked kale	2.5 g
1 cup raw spinach	1.6 g
1 medium raw carrot	0.7 g

Bean Chili

YIELD: 4 TO 6 SERVINGS

Delectable and dramatic, this dish with its many vegetables is a mosaic of colors. It also makes a delicious filling for burritos. Make it a one-, two-, or three-bean chili, depending on the types of beans you have on hand.

3 to 4 tablespoons water for sautéing
3 bell peppers (red, orange, yellow), seeded and cut into ½-inch squares
1 medium yellow onion, coarsely chopped
2–3 cloves garlic, minced
2 tablespoons chili powder
1 teaspoon ground coriander
1 teaspoon ground cumin
1 teaspoon dried oregano
¼ teaspoon cayenne pepper
One 16-ounce can diced tomatoes with juice (or 3 fresh tomatoes, diced, plus ¼–½ cup water)
1 can corn, drained (or 1½ cups fresh or frozen corn, thawed)
1 can kidney beans, drained and rinsed
1 can black beans, drained and rinsed
1 can pinto beans, drained and rinsed
Salt and freshly ground pepper, to taste
½ cup chopped fresh cilantro or fresh parsley (optional)
Nondairy sour cream (optional)

Heat up a few tablespoons of water in a soup pot over medium heat. The water replaces the oil that is often used for sautéing, and you won't know the difference. Just use enough water to coat the vegetables so they don't stick to the bottom of the pot.

Add the peppers, onion, garlic, chili powder, coriander, cumin, oregano, and cayenne, and cook, stirring, for 5 minutes, until the onions turn translucent.

Stir in the tomatoes, corn, and all the beans.

Lower the heat and simmer for 30 minutes. Season with salt and black pepper, and turn off heat. Serve in shallow bowls, top with chopped cilantro or parsley and nondairy sour cream.

Wheat-free, soy-free

Homemade Hummus

MAKES 2 CUPS

Hummus is one of the easiest things to make from scratch, and it is a heap cheaper than the store-bought stuff. Though this recipe happens to be oil-free, it leaves out only the extra calories—not the great flavor.

Two 15-ounce cans chickpeas (garbanzo beans), drained and rinsed

Juice from ½–1 lemon (depends on the size—start with a little, then add more if needed)

2 tablespoons tahini

2 or 3 whole garlic cloves, peeled

1 teaspoon cumin

Water for thinning it out

Salt, to taste

Paprika, as a garnish (optional)

Place the chickpeas in a food processor or blender with the lemon juice, tahini, garlic, and cumin. Process until very smooth, 1-2 minutes, stopping the machine and scraping down the sides as necessary. Add a little water to thin it out. Salt to taste, and sprinkle with paprika.

Variations
- Add roasted garlic instead of raw.
- Add ¼ roasted red pepper.
- For some extra spice, add minced jalapeño peppers to the hummus. Or add a pinch of cayenne.

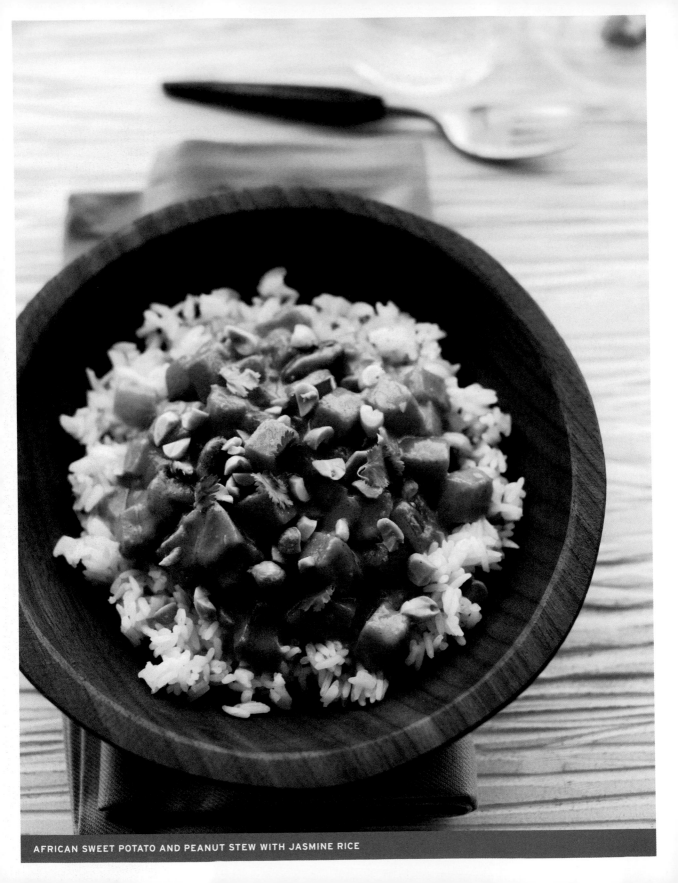

AFRICAN SWEET POTATO AND PEANUT STEW WITH JASMINE RICE

African Sweet Potato and Peanut Stew

YIELD: 6 TO 10 SERVINGS

Light the fire, invite over your closest friends, and cozy up with this hearty, flavorful stew. Serve it over rice, quinoa (which is incredibly nutritious), or couscous (which is a traditional North African accompaniment).

3 tablespoons water for sautéing

2 medium yellow onions, chopped

3 garlic cloves, pressed or minced

2 red bell peppers, seeded and cut into ½-inch squares

3 teaspoons light brown sugar

1 teaspoon grated fresh ginger

1 teaspoon ground cumin

1 teaspoon ground cinnamon

½ teaspoon cayenne pepper

½–¾ cup smooth natural peanut butter (crunchy works great, too)

3 sweet potatoes, peeled and cut into ½-inch cubes (see below)

One 15-ounce can red kidney beans, drained and rinsed

One 15-ounce can diced tomatoes or 2 fresh tomatoes, diced

4 cups vegetable stock

½ teaspoon salt, or to taste

½–1 cup chopped unsalted dry-roasted peanuts (optional)

Chopped fresh cilantro, for garnish (optional)

Heat the water in a soup pot over medium heat. Add the onions and garlic and cook until softened, about 5 minutes. Add the bell peppers, cover, and cook until softened, about 5 minutes. Stir in the brown sugar, ginger, cumin, cinnamon, and cayenne pepper, and cook, stirring, for 30 seconds.

Stir in the peanut butter, and distribute it evenly throughout. You may want to thin out the peanut butter first by mixing it with some water in a small bowl before adding it to the pot. It will make it easier to incorporate it into the stew.

Add the sweet potatoes, kidney beans, and tomatoes, and stir to coat. Add the vegetable stock, bring to a boil, then reduce the heat to low and simmer until the sweet potatoes are soft, about 30 minutes.

Taste and add salt, if necessary. Serve in individual bowls, and top with chopped nuts and cilantro, if desired.

Wheat-free, soy-free

WHAT'S THE DIFFERENCE?

Sweet potatoes and what much of North America calls yams are the same orange-fleshed vegetable (and are different from true yams). You may see varieties of sweet potatoes called garnet yams or jewel yams, which is what I recommend for this stew, though any other variety of sweet potato would also work well.

Better-Than-Tuna Salad

YIELD: 4 TO 6 SERVINGS

Pulsing chickpeas in a food processor (or mashing by hand) yields a wonderful flaky texture reminiscent of the lunchtime staple many of us grew up with.

Two 15-ounce cans chickpeas (garbanzo beans), drained and rinsed (or 3 cups cooked beans)

½ cup eggless mayonnaise (see "Resources and Recommendations")

1 medium red bell pepper, finely chopped

2 carrots, finely chopped

2 stalks celery, finely chopped

2 tablespoons finely chopped fresh parsley

1 cup walnut halves, chopped

1 tablespoon Dijon mustard

Salt and freshly ground pepper to taste

Add the chickpeas to a food processor or blender and grind them down into small flaky pieces. You can certainly make this salad with whole chickpeas, but I find that it makes for a filling that's a little hard to handle in a sandwich. Plus, the flakiness of the ground chickpeas really does resemble the texture of tuna.

In a large bowl, combine all the ingredients except the salt and pepper and mix well. Season with salt and pepper to taste. Serve as a salad on a bed of lettuce or as a sandwich.

Wheat-free

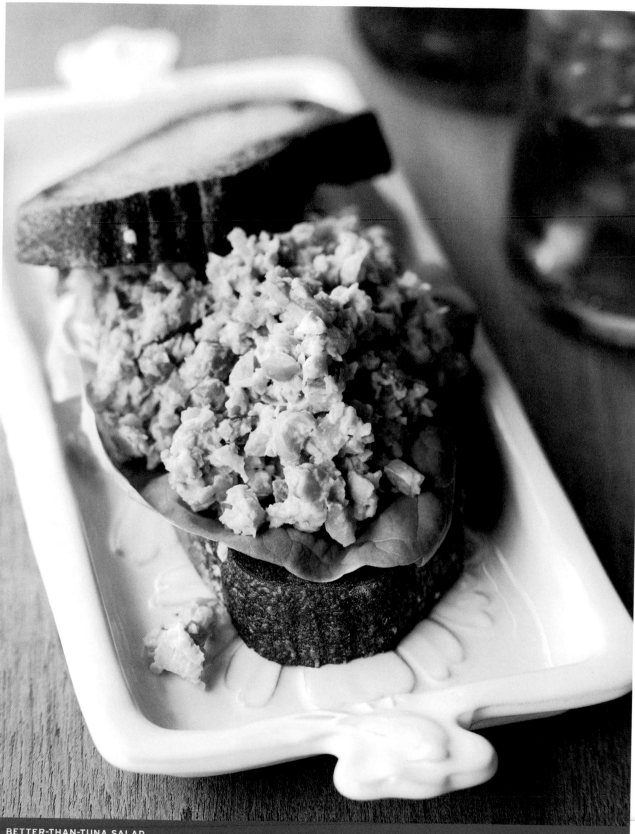

BETTER-THAN-TUNA SALAD

Chickpea Burgers with Tahini Sauce

YIELD: 8 TO 10 PATTIES

Inspired by falafel, my version is much healthier since it forgoes the deep-frying typical of this Middle Eastern staple.

Burgers

One 15-ounce can (or 1½ cups cooked) chickpeas (garbanzo beans), drained and rinsed
1 yellow onion, finely chopped
3 cloves garlic, minced
¼ cup chopped fresh parsley
2 tablespoons tahini
1½–2 teaspoons ground cumin
1 teaspoon ground coriander
½ teaspoon salt
⅛ teaspoon freshly ground black pepper
¼ teaspoon cayenne pepper
1 teaspoon lemon juice
1 teaspoon baking powder
1 cup plain bread crumbs
4 buns or pita pockets

Sauce

One 6-ounce container plain nondairy yogurt
1–2 tablespoons tahini
½ cucumber, peeled, seeded, and finely chopped
1–2 teaspoons lemon juice
1 teaspoon finely minced fresh parsley
Salt and pepper to taste

Preheat the oven to 400 degrees.

Pulse the chickpeas in a food processor until thick and pasty. (You may mash them by hand, but it is a little more labor-intensive and time-consuming.) Transfer to a medium-size bowl.

To the bowl, add the onion, garlic, parsley, tahini, cumin, coriander, salt, black pepper, cayenne pepper, lemon juice, and baking powder. Slowly add the bread crumbs until the mixture holds together. Add more bread crumbs, as needed. Shape into patties.

Place on a nonstick cookie sheet and bake for 10–12 minutes, or until golden brown on the bottom. Using a spatula, flip each patty over, and cook for 10–12 minutes more until the other side is golden brown. Remove from the oven. Alternatively, you may fry the patties with a little oil in a pan on the stovetop.

Meanwhile, in a small bowl combine the yogurt, tahini, cucumber, lemon juice, parsley, salt, and pepper to taste. Chill for at least 30 minutes, and serve with the chickpea burgers, along with lettuce, tomato, and onion on a bun or in a pita pocket.

Soy-free

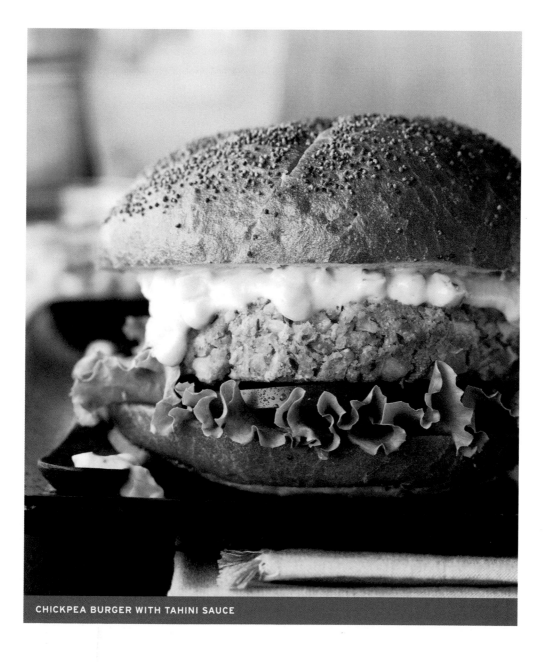

CHICKPEA BURGER WITH TAHINI SAUCE

Simple Bean Burritos

YIELD: 6 SERVINGS

These burritos are perfect to serve at a gathering where you create a build-your-own-burrito bar. Set out all the ingredients, and let people choose their favorite fillings.

Two 15-ounce cans black or pinto beans, drained and rinsed
Water for heating the beans
1 tablespoon chili powder, or to taste
1 teaspoon ground cumin
1 jalapeño pepper, finely chopped
6 large flour or corn tortillas (corn tortillas are smaller, so you may need more)

2 cups cooked brown rice
1 small head lettuce, shredded
1½ cups salsa (use your favorite)
2 avocados or 1 cup guacamole
2 fresh tomatoes, chopped
Nondairy sour cream

In a saucepan, add the rinsed beans and enough water to cover the beans. Add the chili powder, cumin, and jalapeño pepper. Heat over a low flame.

When the beans are heated through, begin filling the tortillas. Spoon a few tablespoons of rice onto a tortilla about 1 inch from the bottom, and spread it out in a horizontal line. Using a slotted spoon, scoop out the beans and add a few tablespoons on top of the rice.

Add the remaining toppings, such as the lettuce, salsa, avocados or guacamole, tomatoes, and sour cream. Do not overfill, or it will be difficult to roll. Begin rolling from the bottom up, tucking the sides in as you go along.

Wheat-free, soy-free

Whole books are written on proper nutrition for athletes—including vegan athletes. If you are doing this Challenge as a high-performance athlete, you're on your way to improving your performance. Many medal-winning, world-class athletes are vegan—and were vegan at their peak, including ultramarathoner Scott Jurek, tennis champions Billie Jean King and Martina Navratilova, Olympian Carl Lewis, NBA champion John Salley, and NFL star Tony Gonzalez.

Because energy output (calorie expenditure) is so much greater for athletes, energy intake (calorie consumption) needs also increase, depending on the performance goals and on the body size and composition of the athlete. Nutrient needs will be met because of the increased calories; if you're lacking energy, the first solution would be to eat more (increase energy intake).

In terms of macronutrients, every sound expert agrees that complex carbohydrates are the preferred fuel for athletes. The American Dietetic Association's position paper on nutrition for physical fitness and athletic performance states: "In general [i.e., for most athletes], it is recommended that 60 to 65% of total energy should come from carbohydrates. Athletes who train exhaustively on successive days or who compete in prolonged endurance events should consume a diet that provides 65 to 70% of energy from carbohydrate."

Complex carbohydrates are abundant in whole grains, vegetables, fruits, legumes, nuts, and seeds. The recommendation for protein for competitive athletes is higher—between 0.6 and 0.9 gram per pound of body weight—than for noncompetitive athletes, for whom the recommendation is 0.4 to 0.5 gram.

Although protein bars and shakes are unnecessary for your average Joe to get sufficient protein, they may be useful for those endurance athletes and bodybuilders who need additional protein. They're also just convenient when you're on the road or in a rush. These are made from soy, rice, hemp, or pea protein. (See "Recommendations and Resources.")

Although individual athletes will hone their diet in different ways, in terms of vitamin and mineral requirements, all the same recommendations throughout this book apply to athletes.

DAY 16   Better Baking Without Eggs

Having enthusiastically noticed the many commercial baked goods on the supermarket shelves, perhaps by now you're anxious to bake some goodies yourself. So grab the flour, sugar, baking soda, and baking powder, and leave the eggs behind. That's right—you do not need eggs to bake.

Even nonbakers suffer from the misconception that baked goods require chicken's eggs, cow's milk, and dairy-based butter. The fact is, to create delicious, decadent, successful baked goods, you do not need animal products at all. What you need is:

- Binding
- Moisture
- Richness/Fat
- Leavening

And all of these things can be better accomplished with healthful, plant-based ingredients. In fact, it's not as if you have to use a replacement for every egg you eliminate. Often, the eggs are totally superfluous and can be left out altogether, with no need for substitutions.

One of the things that led to eggs being used with such abandon was the end of World War II. Prior to and during the war, animal products were considered luxury items, so they were used only sparingly, even in baked goods. Baking without eggs was common and left us with many wartime recipes such as Victory Cake and other eggless desserts. When the war ended, however, Americans had more money than they knew what to do with, and animal products became more available than ever before. To demonstrate their affluence, people purchased meat, dairy, and eggs without thought, and food manufacturers included cow's milk and chicken's eggs in their products, even when they weren't necessary. Animal products equaled wealth—and still do.

Because strongly ingrained habits are hard to change, when you contemplate baking without eggs, you might feel like you'll have to learn to bake all over again. But that's okay. As with any cuisine or technique you're trying for the first time, there's a learning curve, but once you begin practicing these new techniques, new habits will replace the old ones, and you'll never look back.

There are many ways to create binding, fat, moisture, richness, and leavening in recipes; it really depends on the type of baked good. See pages 173–182 for some of my favorite recipes. Once you become familiar with the effect of the different ingredients, you will be able to confidently and successfully veganize any baking recipe.

VINEGAR AND BAKING SODA

When combined with an acidic ingredient, such as vinegar, cocoa, or citrus, baking soda releases carbon dioxide that forms into bubbles in the food. When heated, these bubbles expand and help to rise or lighten the final product.

> RATIO: 1 teaspoon of baking soda with 1 tablespoon of vinegar.
> TYPE: Apple cider vinegar and white distilled vinegar are the two I use most frequently.
> BEST IN: I find this combination works best in cakes, cupcakes, and quick breads.

GROUND FLAXSEEDS

Ground flaxseeds (brown or golden) combined with water result in a thick, gelatinous mixture that provides a perfect medium for adding moisture, fat, and binding. (Read "Day 18: Skipping the Middle Fish: Getting Omega-3s from the Source" for more on flaxseeds.)

> RATIO: For each egg you want to replace, whisk 1 tablespoon of ground flaxseeds with 3 tablespoons of water in a blender or food processor until the mixture is thick and gooey.
> BEST IN: Because flaxseeds have a nutty flavor, they work best in baked goods that are grainier and nuttier, such as waffles, pancakes, bran muffins, breads, and oatmeal cookies.
> TIP: Though you may find ground flaxseeds or flax meal in your grocery store, I recommend buying the whole seeds and grinding them yourself using a coffee grinder. I realize this adds an extra step, but it's better in terms of freshness and flavor.

RIPE BANANA

Mashed bananas are great binding ingredients in baked goods.

> RATIO: Bananas aren't necessarily a measure-for-measure replacement. As a general rule, consider half a mashed or pureed banana as a replacement for one or two eggs.

BEST IN: Bananas are fantastic egg replacers in baking, particularly in breads, muffins, cakes, and pancakes. I don't use bananas, however, when I don't want the banana flavor to dominate.

APPLESAUCE

Applesauce not only acts as a binding agent in baked goods but also is a good substitute for oil when you want to reduce fat and calories.

RATIO: One-fourth of a cup of unsweetened applesauce equals one egg.
BEST IN: Unsweetened applesauce provides the binding and moisture you need in baked goods. It works best when you want the results to be moist, such as in cakes, quick breads, and brownies.
TIP: Buy an organic brand that has no added sugars.

SILKEN TOFU

Silken tofu, often used to make puddings, mousses, and pie fillings, is the softest and creamiest type and is often sold in aseptic boxes, which means you'll find them on the shelves instead of in the refrigerated section of the grocery store. The most popular brand is Mori-Nu. You may store it unrefrigerated for many months until you open it. Silken tofu comes in various textures, soft, firm, and extra-firm, and although recipes tend to specify which to use, a good bet is to go with firm silken tofu.

RATIO: For one egg, whip ¼ cup silken tofu in a blender or food processor until smooth and creamy.
BEST IN: I find the silken tofu "egg" works best when you want rich, dense, moist cakes and brownies, but you can use a little less to create lighter cakes.
TIP: Many general grocery stores carry silken tofu, but you'll definitely find it in a natural foods store. If your local grocery doesn't carry it, request it. Look for vacuum-packed silken tofu on the shelves; it's often in the Asian section of the store.

COMMERCIAL EGG REPLACER POWDER

There are at least two commercial egg replacers, essentially made from potato starch, that provide binding in baked goods. One is called Ener-G Egg Replacer and the other is Bob's Red Mill Egg Replacer. Both last forever in your pantry, providing a convenient and economical alternative to perishable eggs. For instance, one box of Ener-G Egg Replacer makes the equivalent of 112 eggs.

RATIO: Follow the instructions on the box, but in the case of Ener-G Egg Replacer, mix 1½ teaspoons of the egg replacer powder with 2 tablespoons water to produce the equivalent of one egg. The ratio for Bob's Red Mill is like that of flaxseeds: 1 tablespoon of powder mixed with 3 tablespoons of water. I find the results are best for both when you whip it in a food processor or blender to make it thick and creamy.

BEST IN: I find this egg replacer works best in cookies. Because there's no nutritional value, however, opt for ground flaxseeds when you can.

OTHER WAYS TO REPLACE EGGS

Chicken's eggs are often used as a thickener in sauces, gravies, custards, desserts, and beverages. Pastries and breads sometimes use an egg wash to glaze their tops. Here are ways to get the same results without chicken's eggs.

For Thickening

Kudzu: A starch made from the root of the kudzu plant; when added to water and heated, kudzu powder thickens whatever you've added it to. Though it is more expensive than other thickeners, I prefer it for its efficacy and lack of flavor. To prepare kudzu, dissolve 1 tablespoon of kudzu powder in 2 tablespoons of cool liquid, mix well, then stir slowly into whatever sauce you are cooking. Once it begins to heat up, you will notice the liquid starting to thicken. Continue stirring and let it cook for at least 5 minutes.

Agar: Derived from the Malay word *agar-agar*, which means "jelly," agar comes from a type of seaweed that is odorless and tasteless and becomes gelatinous when dissolved in hot water and then cooled. It's ideal when you want a vegetarian gelatin to make terrines, cheese, and Japanese desserts.

Arrowroot: A starch made from the rhizomes of the West Indian arrowroot plant, it's odorless when dry, but it emits a peculiar odor when mixed with boiling water. Because it's so fine, it dissolves well and is a great thickener.

Cornstarch: Cornstarch is ground from the endosperm of the corn kernel and works well as a thickener in puddings or sauces.

Flour: Flour works well as a thickener, though it should always be whisked with water first before adding it to your sauce to avoid clumping.

For Glazing

Onto breads, homemade soft pretzels, or pastries, simply brush on oil, nondairy milk, or nondairy butter.

For Leavening

There are only a few instances where eggs actually act as leaveners in baked goods. (Leavening agents make them rise.) Your main leaveners in baked goods are baking soda and baking powder.

The average American consumes about 250 eggs a year, making the total U.S. egg production about 76 billion eggs. That translates to more than 290 million hens being used for the production of their eggs. Every time we replace chicken's eggs with a plant-based food, we're making a compassionate, healthful choice for ourselves—and the chickens. And as the following recipes attest, we're also making the most delicious choice!

Pecan Balls

YIELD: 3 DOZEN COOKIES, DEPENDING ON SIZE

These melt-in-your-mouth cookies have many names: Mexican Wedding Cookies, Mexican Wedding Cakes, Russian Tea Cakes, Pecan Balls, Snowdrops, and Snowballs. They're often baked during the winter holidays, but they're also popular at weddings and other festive occasions.

2 sticks (1 cup) nonhydrogenated, nondairy butter (such as Earth Balance)

¼ cup granulated sugar

2 teaspoons vanilla extract

2 cups unbleached all-purpose flour, sifted

2 cups raw pecans, finely chopped

2 cups powdered (confectioners') sugar, sifted

Preheat the oven to 300 degrees. Line two cookie sheets with parchment paper or use a nonstick cookie/baking sheet.

With an electric hand mixer or by hand, cream the butter, granulated sugar, and vanilla until light and fluffy, about 1-2 minutes. Add the flour and mix until thoroughly combined. Add the chopped nuts and mix until well blended, about 30 seconds.

Measure out generously rounded teaspoonfuls of dough and roll them into balls. Place the balls about 1 inch apart on the cookie sheet. Bake until they just begin to turn golden, about 30 minutes. To test for doneness, remove one cookie from the sheet and cut it in half. There should be no doughy strip in the center.

Roll cookies in the powdered sugar while they are still hot, then cool on the cookie sheets. Serve when cool.

Variation

Replace the pecans with hazelnuts, almonds, or walnuts.

TIP:

The easiest way to add the powdered sugar to the warm cookies is to put the sugar in a large bowl and gently toss the cookies around in the sugar. You can also use a plastic bag and give them a shake. Just be careful not to knock them around too much.

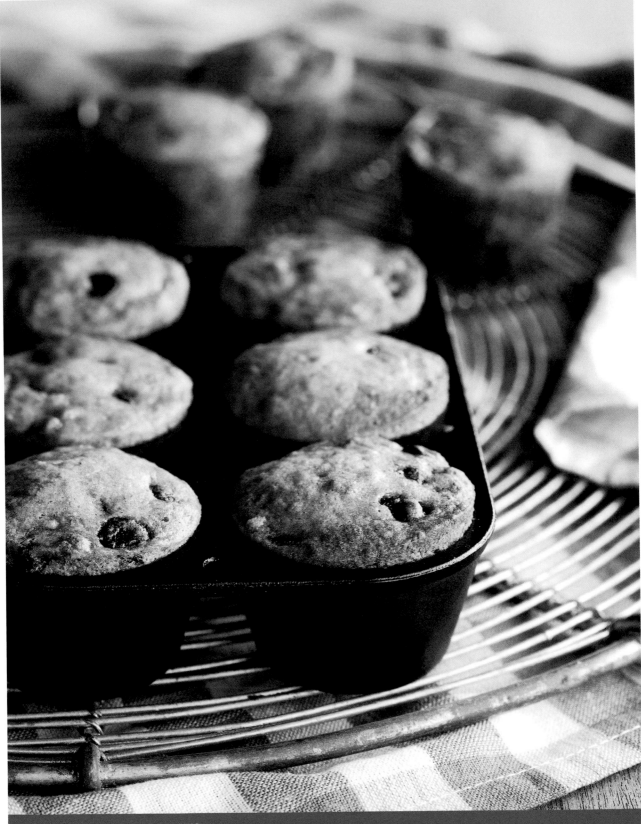

BANANA CHOCOLATE CHIP MUFFINS

Banana Chocolate Chip Muffins

YIELD: 9 OR 10 MUFFINS

Whether you're making them for breakfast (reduce the sugar a little and add walnuts instead of chocolate chips) or as a sweet treat, these muffins will knock your socks off. Bake in a loaf pan to make Banana Chocolate Chip Bread.

2 cups whole-wheat pastry flour or
    unbleached all-purpose flour
1½ teaspoons baking soda
½ teaspoon salt
1 cup granulated sugar
⅓ cup canola or grapeseed oil

4 ripe bananas, mashed
¼ cup water
1 teaspoon vanilla extract
1 cup semisweet chocolate chips (and/or
    1 cup walnuts)

Preheat the oven to 350 degrees. Lightly grease your muffin tins.

Mix together the flour, baking soda, and salt.

In a large bowl, beat the sugar and oil together, then add the mashed bananas. Stir in the water and vanilla and mix thoroughly. Add the flour mixture, along with the chocolate chips, and stir to mix. (Alternatively, you may just peel the bananas, break them into a food processor, and puree them along with the sugar and oil. Add the water and vanilla, then transfer to a bowl. Stir in the flour combo, and add the chocolate chips.)

Fill each muffin tin halfway with the batter. Bake for 20–30 minutes, until they are golden brown and a toothpick inserted into the center comes out clean.

Soy-free

Cinnamon Coffee Cake

YIELD: 12 SERVINGS

Though what I ate growing up was store-bought coffee cake, I feel nostalgic every time I eat this homemade version. It takes no time at all to prepare and will conjure lovely memories for you and your family.

Cake

1 cup nondairy milk (soy, rice, almond, oat, hemp, or hazelnut)

⅓ cup canola oil

1 tablespoon white vinegar

1 cup whole-wheat pastry flour or unbleached all-purpose flour

½ cup granulated sugar

1 teaspoon baking powder

1 teaspoon baking soda

2 teaspoons ground cinnamon

1 teaspoon ground ginger

¼ teaspoon salt

Crumble

¾ cup whole-wheat pastry flour or unbleached all-purpose flour

¼ cup granulated or brown sugar

1-2 teaspoons ground cinnamon

½ teaspoon ground ginger

¼ teaspoon salt

¾ cup chopped walnuts

⅓ cup canola oil or softened nondairy butter (such as Earth Balance)

Preheat the oven to 350 degrees and lightly oil a 9-by-9-inch square baking dish or cake pan.

Combine the milk, oil, and vinegar in a bowl and set aside. In a large bowl, mix together the dry ingredients for the cake: flour, sugar, baking powder, baking soda, cinnamon, ginger, and salt. Add the milk mixture, and stir until just combined. Pour into the prepared baking dish.

For the crumble, in a small bowl combine the flour, sugar, cinnamon, ginger, salt, and walnuts. Add the oil or softened nondairy butter, and use your hands to thoroughly work it into the dry ingredients. If it's too wet, add a little more flour; if it's too dry, add a little more oil or butter. Sprinkle the crumble mixture on top of the batter, covering the entire area.

Bake 40 minutes, or until a toothpick inserted in the middle comes out clean. Let it cool slightly, and serve warm or at room temperature.

Soy-free, if using soy-free milk and butter

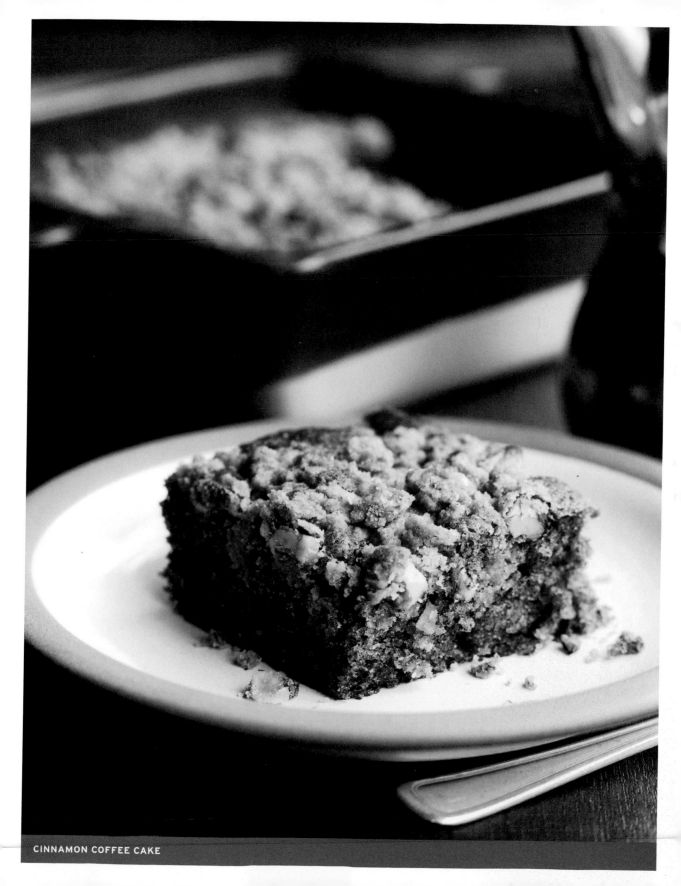

CINNAMON COFFEE CAKE

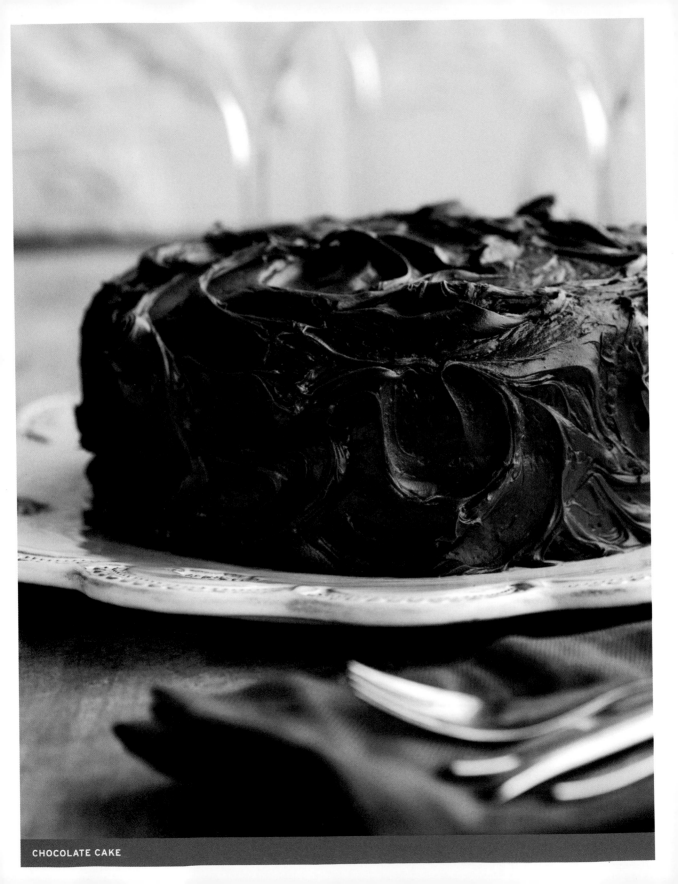

CHOCOLATE CAKE

Chocolate Cake

YIELD: ONE 9-INCH CAKE OR 8 CUPCAKES

A traditional recipe that may look familiar to those of you who recall wartime cakes (those made without eggs), this chocolate cake might be the easiest thing in the world to prepare. It's also incredibly versatile, lending itself to a layer cake, bundt cake, or cupcakes.

1½ cups unbleached all-purpose flour
¾ cup granulated sugar
½ teaspoon salt
1 teaspoon baking soda
¼ cup unsweetened cocoa powder

1½ teaspoons vanilla extract
⅓ cup canola oil
1 tablespoon distilled white vinegar
1 cup cold water

Preheat the oven to 350 degrees. Lightly grease a bundt pan, 9-inch springform pan, or muffin tins.

Combine the flour, sugar, salt, baking soda, and cocoa powder in a bowl until thoroughly combined. Create a well in the center of the dry ingredients, and add the vanilla, oil, vinegar, and water. Mix until just combined. Pour into the prepared pan and bake in the preheated oven for 30 minutes, until a toothpick inserted in the center comes out clean. If making cupcakes, check for doneness after 15 minutes.

Cool on a wire rack. To remove the cake from the pan, run a sharp knife around the inside of the pan to loosen the cake. Cool completely before frosting. (See Chocolate Frosting, on page 182.)

Soy-free

TIP:
If you'd like to make a layer cake or a fuller Bundt cake, this recipe doubles really well.

Oatmeal Raisin Cookies

YIELD: 3½ DOZEN 3-INCH COOKIES

I think the nutmeg makes these cookies extra-special. Moist and crispy at the same time, they will fill your kitchen with a homey aroma.

2 tablespoons ground flaxseeds
   (equivalent of 2 eggs)
6 tablespoons water
½ pound (2 sticks) nonhydrogenated,
   nondairy butter, softened (Earth
   Balance also comes in sticks)
1½ cups packed light or dark brown sugar
¼ cup granulated sugar
2 teaspoons vanilla extract

1¾ cups unbleached all-purpose flour
½ cup oat bran
¾ teaspoon baking soda
¾ teaspoon baking powder
½ teaspoon salt
½ teaspoon ground cinnamon
½ teaspoon ground nutmeg
3 cups rolled oats (not quick-cooking)
1 cup raisins

Preheat the oven to 350 degrees and lightly oil two cookie sheets or line with parchment paper.

In a blender or food processor, whip together the flaxseeds with the water until thick and creamy. The consistency will be somewhat gelatinous. By hand or using an electric mixer, cream together the butter, sugars, vanilla, and flaxseed mixture until well blended.

In a separate bowl, thoroughly combine the flour, oat bran, baking soda, baking powder, salt, cinnamon, and nutmeg. Add to the butter mixture and mix until well blended and smooth. Stir in the rolled oats and raisins until thoroughly combined.

Scoop 2-tablespoon portions of dough onto the prepared cookie sheet and, with lightly greased hands, lightly press to form ½-inch-thick rounds. Bake until the cookies are golden brown, about 12-15 minutes. Remove from the oven and allow the cookies to firm up for a few minutes while still on the cookie sheet. Transfer the cookies to a wire rack to cool.

TIP:

To create uniform-size cookies, spoon the dough for each cookie into a small measuring cup, then pop it out onto the cookie sheet.

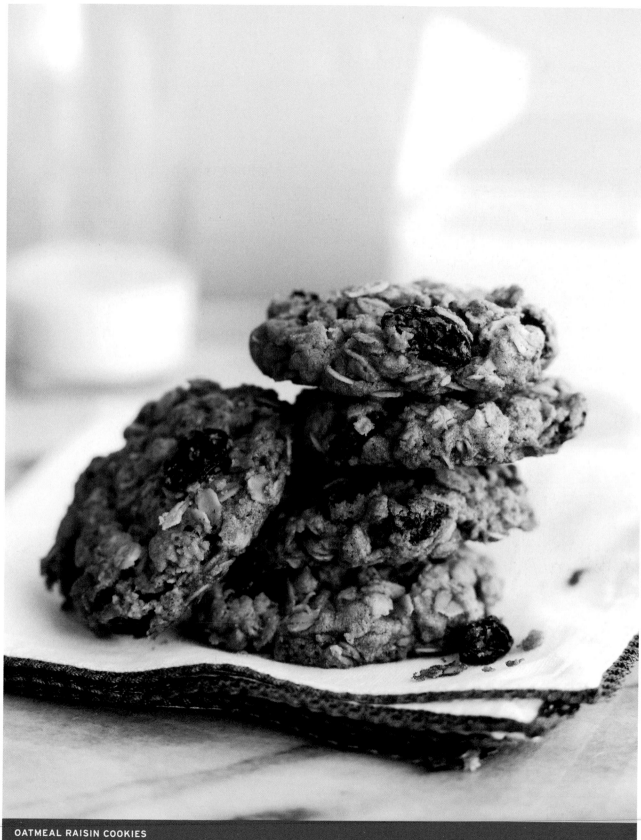

Chocolate Frosting

YIELD: ENOUGH FOR ONE 9-INCH CAKE OR 8 CUPCAKES

This recipe is as easy as it is delicious.

½ cup nonhydrogenated, nondairy butter, softened, such as Earth Balance

3 cups powdered (confectioners') sugar, sifted

⅓ cup cocoa, sifted

1 teaspoon vanilla extract or ½ teaspoon peppermint extract

3-4 tablespoons water or nondairy milk

With an electric mixer, cream the butter until smooth. With the mixer on low speed, add the sugar, and cream for about 2 minutes. Add the rest of the ingredients, and turn the mixer to high speed once all the ingredients are relatively well-combined. Beat on high speed until frosting is light and fluffy, about 3 minutes. Add I or 2 tablespoons more milk if it's too dry. Cover the icing with plastic wrap to prevent drying until ready to use. Store it in a covered container in the refrigerator for up to 2 weeks. Rewhip before using.

Soy-free depending on milk and butter used

Strong Like Popeye: Increasing Your Iron Absorption

Popeye ate spinach. Popeye was strong. Wimpy ate burgers. Wimpy was . . . wimpy. Popeye was on to something. Plant-based iron—not burgers—makes you strong.

Despite the pervasiveness of this muscled pop culture icon, I continue to meet people who claim to have become anemic (i.e., iron-deficient) after becoming vegetarian or vegan. Having diagnosed themselves, most of these folks never actually had their iron levels checked by a doctor; they just assumed they were anemic because they were tired, and friends told them that it was their lack of meat-eating that was making them feel that way.

Having said that, iron deficiency is the most common nutrient deficiency in the United States; the typical North American diet provides only 5 to 6 mg of iron for every 1,000 calories consumed. Worldwide, it's the most prevalent nutritional deficiency, and the groups that are most susceptible are women who menstruate (women of childbearing age), pregnant and lactating women, teenagers, and children 6 months to 4 years. This is true for vegetarians, vegans, and non-vegetarians.

> **CHALLENGE YOUR THINKING:** Popeye ate spinach. Popeye was strong. Wimpy ate burgers. Wimpy was wimpy. Plant-based iron makes you strong—not burgers!

INCREASING ABSORPTION

Studies show little difference in the incidence of iron deficiency between vegans and non-vegetarians in developed countries. In fact, the amount of iron in vegan diets tends to be higher than or at least equal to that in non-vegetarian diets. Why? Because almost everything that crosses a vegan's lips contains iron: beans, nuts, seeds, grains, vegetables, and fruits.

There are two different types of iron in foods: *heme* iron and *nonheme* iron. Heme iron is found in animal products; nonheme iron is found in both plant foods and animal products. After the iron has been absorbed and has reached our cells to be used for building hemo-

CHALLENGE YOUR THINKING:
The body needs to absorb iron, but it doesn't care whether the original source of the iron was heme (animal-based) or nonheme (animal- and plant-based).

CHANGE YOUR BEHAVIOR:
Eat foods rich in iron, eat foods that increase iron absorption, and when eating iron-rich foods, avoid eating them with foods that decrease iron absorption.

globin and other purposes, our body doesn't care whether the iron was originally heme or nonheme. So when people assert that our bodies need heme iron from meat, it's simply not true. The body needs to absorb iron, but it ultimately doesn't care about where it came from in the first place.

Dietary factors most certainly influence our body's ability to absorb iron, and it's these dietary factors we want to increase. Vegans tend to be ahead of the game because of the amount of plant foods they eat—particularly those rich in vitamin C. This is an important vitamin for many reasons, not the least of which is its ability to increase our absorption of iron; in other words, vitamin C increases the iron's *bioavailability* (read more about bioavailability in "Day 14: Choosing Plant-Based Milks"). Furthermore, if you cook vitamin-C-containing foods, such as tomatoes or lemon juice, in cast-iron cookware, some of the iron will make its way into the food.

Eating vitamin-C-rich foods at the same time we eat iron-rich foods is one of the best things we can do. Fruits and vegetables are our main sources of vitamin C, with the richest being tomatoes, citrus fruits (oranges, tangerines, and grapefruit), strawberries, kiwi, papaya, green vegetables (broccoli, kale, collard greens, Swiss chard, Brussels sprouts), bell peppers (yellow, red, orange, and green), and cauliflower.

There is no shortage of iron in plant foods, but some contain higher amounts than others.

HOW MUCH IRON DO WE NEED?

There are some variations for babies, toddlers, and seniors, but the daily recommendation for the United States and Canada is 8 mg for adult men, 18 mg for adult menstruating women, and 27 mg for pregnant women. No one should exceed 45 mg a day, as too much iron can cause an overload.

THINGS THAT DECREASE ABSORPTION

Just as there are things we want to do to increase absorption, there are things we want to do to avoid *decreasing* absorption. When we consume calcium supplements, coffee, or tea at the same time we eat iron-rich foods, we inhibit iron absorption. The bioavailability of iron can be reduced by up to 60 percent by the tannins in black or green teas, for example. So just avoid these things when eating iron-rich foods if you want to increase your iron absorption.

FOOD	IRON CONTENT
Fortified cereals	Varies according to brand; Total, Raisin Bran, and All-Bran are the highest, with up to 18 mg per serving
1½ cups white beans	7.8 mg
1 cup cooked lentils	6.6 mg
1 cup cooked barley	5 mg
1 cup cooked chickpeas	4.8 mg
1 cup cooked pinto beans	4.4 mg
1 tablespoon blackstrap molasses	4 mg
1 medium baked potato	4 mg
¾ cup cooked oatmeal	3.44 mg
½ cup firm tofu	3.35 mg (brands vary; check label)
½ cup cooked quinoa	2.76 mg
1 cup cooked mushrooms	2.7 mg
1 ounce pumpkin seeds	2.5 mg
3½ cups raw broccoli	2.24 mg
12 dried apricot halves	1.08 mg

Also, there are some foods that are high in iron but also high in phytates, which prevent absorption. These iron-rich foods include wheat bran and whole grains. Soaking, sprouting, leavening, or fermentation of whole grains renders the iron more bioavailable by degrading the phytates. While eating whole grains is desirable, we should not be sprinkling wheat bran over all our food.

Finally, the other thing to consider is that vegans have a considerable advantage in the iron department not only because they eat more iron- and vitamin-C-rich plant foods but also because they don't eat dairy. Cow's milk—either the liquid stuff or products made from it—is a poor source of iron. It displaces iron-rich foods from the diet, and the presence of cow's milk or cheese in the diet has been shown to decrease the absorption of iron from a meal by as much as 50 percent.

WHAT TO DO IF YOUR IRON STORES ARE LOW

Many people assume they have anemia just because they're tired, but they might be tired for a number of other reasons, such as not eating enough calories, eating too many high-sugar foods, and possibly not getting enough sleep. This doesn't mean that iron deficiency is not real for some people, but if you're concerned, don't self-diagnose. Check with your doctor and get your iron tested.

Having said that, it's also important to understand a few things about what your iron status means. There are three stages, essentially, of actual iron deficiency:

- The first is just iron depletion—it means your stores are low, but it doesn't affect how you feel.

- The second is iron deficiency, and you may feel tired and have a sensitivity to cold.

- The third is iron deficiency anemia, where your total blood hemoglobin is below the normal range. You are likely to feel exhaustion, irritability, lethargy, and headaches. Your skin may also appear pale.

If you are suffering from the symptoms of iron deficiency, have your doctor measure your iron status. If your doctor thinks your iron stores are too low, he or she may suggest that you eat meat (which is unnecessary) or that you take an iron supplement. You might want to talk to him or her about first increasing your vitamin C intake by taking 100 mg of vitamin C with meals twice a day for 60 days (or increasing intake of vitamin-C-rich foods) and refraining from tea and coffee during meals. If this doesn't work, then—under your doctor's guidance—you may want to take iron supplements.

IS LOW IRON A BAD THING?

Keep in mind that though there is little difference in the incidence of iron deficiency between vegetarians and non-vegetarians, vegans and vegetarians do often have iron stores on the low end of the normal range. However, this doesn't seem to pose a problem. For those in generally good health and with abundant food available, having iron stores at the low end of the normal range is just not a problem. In fact, there are a few potential upsides:

- Low iron stores are associated with higher glucose tolerance and therefore could prevent diabetes.

- High iron stores have been linked to cancer and cardiovascular disease because of increased evidence of free radical damage. Having lower iron stores seems to protect cells from free radical damage.

Consuming too much iron, particularly if you're taking a lot of it in supplement form, can be a problem. Too high an iron level can lead to zinc and copper deficiency and can cause iron overload. (Excess iron is not easily eliminated from the body.) This is one of the reasons many experts recommend taking iron-free multivitamins and getting iron from the diet. (See "Day 20: Are Supplements Necessary?")

WHAT DO VEGANS FEED THEIR DOGS AND CATS?

Once they become vegan, many people begin thinking about the diet of their dogs and cats. With their own diets reflecting compassion and optimal nutrition, they're naturally reluctant to support the slaughter industry by feeding their dogs and cats meat. It's a dilemma for many of us, and I have just one piece of advice: adopt a bunny. They eat lots of produce, and you don't have to worry about this issue at all!

Would that it were that simple.

I want to make it clear that there are many schools of thought about the best diet for our beloved companion animals. Ultimately, you will make the decision that best suits your individual animal. What I want to offer are my thoughts about whether dogs and cats can thrive on a plant-based diet.

In short, dogs are natural omnivores and thrive on a plant-based diet; cats are obligate carnivores and do not. Now, some dogs may have issues with allergens such as corn, soy, wheat, and gluten that are in commercial dog foods, so it's just a matter of finding the right food if that issue arises. But in general, vegan dogs do great, and any vet who tells you otherwise is simply misinformed, especially if your dog is allergy-free and thriving. Whenever you're making food changes in your dog's diet, you'll want to transition him or her slowly, incorporating the new food into his regular food little by little. See "Resources and Recommendations" for recommended brands of vegan dog food.

While there are many anecdotal tales of cats thriving on vegetarian and vegan diets, let's just say I'm not convinced, based on my own research and experience. Cats are physiologically built as carnivores and have very high protein requirements. They do not *require* plant products in their diet, though they do tend to consume some when they eat the stomach contents of their prey, so offering them some veggie food is fine, but the foundation of their diet—at least 75 percent—should be animal-based.

Skipping the Middle Fish: Getting Omega-3s from the Source

Another nutrient that, like protein and calcium, has been touted as strictly animal-based is omega-3 fatty acids. Fish oil supplements are flying off the shelves, and fish is routinely recommended as the best source of omega-3 fatty acids. Apart from the damage this is doing to the oceans and the millions of marine animals killed each year, people are taking in mercury, other heavy metals, and a variety of environmental contaminants (PCBs, DDT, dioxins, etc.). This is especially the case with wild salmon, though you fare no better with farmed salmon.

With East Coast wild salmon all but extinct and West Coast wild salmon endangered, 90 percent of the salmon consumed in the United States is farm-raised in intensive confinement, replete with antibiotics, pesticides, and more than a hundred other pollutants. What's more, their diet of cheap pellets and fish meal consists mostly of wild-caught fish, which contributes to even more animals taken from the ocean. And of course both wild and farmed fish contain unhealthful saturated fat and dietary cholesterol.

CHALLENGE YOUR THINKING:
We absolutely do not need to consume fish to take in the healthful EPA and DHA fats. Even fish don't make these fats; they consume them through the omega-3-rich algae and phytoplankton.

CHANGE YOUR BEHAVIOR:
Do what the fish do and get your omega-3 fatty acids from the plants.

Also added to farmed salmon's feed is something called canthaxanthin (*CAN-tha-zan-thin*), a synthetic petrochemical-based dye manufactured by Hoffman-La Roche, to make salmon flesh pink. Because farmed salmon don't consume their normal diet of crustaceans, they range in color from gray to pale yellow, as opposed to pink. Fish "farmers" and buyers actually choose exactly the shade of pink they prefer the flesh to be using the pharmaceutical company's trademarked SalmoFan, a color swatch similar to those found in paint stores. (This is also done with rainbow trout and even flamingos in zoos to compensate for their unnatural diets.)

Omega-3 fatty acids such as EPA and DHA are absolutely essential for optimal health, but the ultimate question is: do people need to eat fish to ensure sufficient intake of these fats? The answer is *absolutely not.* In fact, fish don't even make EPA and DHA; these special omega-3 fatty acids are made by algae and phytoplankton, not fish. As carnivores, salmon naturally eat other animals, particularly zooplankton, herring, and krill. Krill, a small shrimp-like critter, eats phytoplankton (considered the "grass of the sea") as well as algae. Algae is made up of—among other things—omega-3 fats and carotenoids, the latter of which is responsible for turning krill *and* salmon pink. It is the algae that provides the nutritional benefit, not the fish. In other words, the fish take in these fats from plants, and we can do the same thing.

For the sake of our health, the fishes' lives, and the health of the ocean, we can cut out the middle fish and go straight to the source by

- Consuming plant foods rich in omega-3s
- Increasing our absorption and conversion of these dietary fats into usable DHA (see below)
- Decreasing our consumption of omega-6s.

CONSUMING OMEGA-3-RICH PLANT FOODS

Flaxseeds and hemp seeds are great sources of omega-3 fatty acids; flaxseeds need to be ground first, and I recommend buying them whole in the bulk section of any natural foods store and using a coffee grinder to grind them. Store the ground flaxseeds in an airtight container and place them in the freezer or refrigerator. Whole seeds don't need to be refrigerated until they're ground up. In terms of nutrition, both brown and golden flaxseeds are the same, so choose what is most readily available and most affordable.

Ground flaxseeds are only one option and can be added to your smoothie, oatmeal, cereal, salad, or soup. Hemp seeds and walnuts can also be easily added to your favorite foods. Try to take one of these daily:

- Ground flaxseeds (1 tablespoon per day)
- Shelled hemp seeds (3 tablespoons per day)
- Walnuts (about 14 halves per day)
- Flax oil (1 teaspoon daily)

Note: Although you can bake with flaxseeds (ground or not), you don't want to cook with flax oil. Either take your 1 teaspoon daily directly from a spoon or use it to make a salad dressing. If you like the taste, you can also add it to a fruit smoothie.

INCREASING ABSORPTION OF OMEGA-3S AND DECREASING CONSUMPTION OF OMEGA-6S

Ensuring that we take in a daily dose of omega-3 fatty acids is important, but so is increasing the absorption of these fats. One omega-3 fatty acid is alpha-linolenic acid (ALA), and

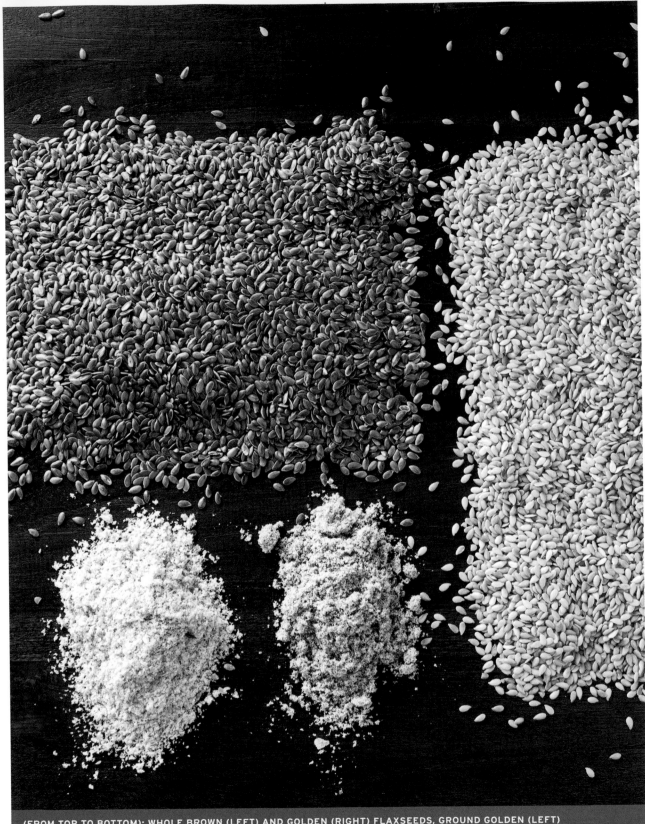

(FROM TOP TO BOTTOM): WHOLE BROWN (LEFT) AND GOLDEN (RIGHT) FLAXSEEDS, GROUND GOLDEN (LEFT) AND BROWN (RIGHT) FLAXSEEDS it's one of the two primary essential fatty acids. The other is an omega-6 fatty acid known as linoleic acid (LA). The word *essential* means our body cannot manufacture it, so it's required in our diet.

Both omega-6s and omega-3s are polyunsaturated fats, and optimal health depends on getting enough of these fats and ensuring a reasonable balance between the two. The problem is that many people do not get sufficient omega-3s but are getting too many omega-6s. They're cooking with omega-6-rich oils—such as corn, sunflower, safflower, and "vegetable oil," which is often just a combination of these other oils—and they're eating a lot of processed, packaged foods, which contain high amounts of shelf-stable omega-6 fats. They're also consuming omega-6 fats in the form of arachidonic acid, found in meat, dairy, and eggs. So one solution to finding balance is eating fewer omega-6-rich oils.

The other is increasing our conversion of omega-3s into a usable form. Two other omega-3 fatty acids are EPA and DHA, which are found mostly in sea vegetables, such as the algae the fish eat. Ultimately, what we want to do is increase our conversion of what are called short-chain omega-3s, such as ALA, into these longer-chain fatty acids, EPA and DHA. We can do this by increasing our consumption of omega-3s through such foods as flax-seeds, flax oil, hemp seeds, and walnuts and by not overeating foods rich in omega-6 fatty acids.

TAKING A DHA SUPPLEMENT

The only problem is that some people don't convert omega-3 fatty acids into DHA sufficiently. These people may be more prone to depression, allergies, and inflammatory skin disease, such as eczema. Also, people with diabetes don't efficiently convert ALA into EPA and DHA. Other factors that inhibit the conversion are excessive saturated fat, cholesterol, and trans fat in the diet. Plus the rate of conversion is limited in infants and declines as we get older.

So, the question we need to ask is: should people in these categories supplement with a direct source of EPA and/or DHA? Should everyone?

As far as the research indicates:

- If you're consuming a high amount of omega-6 fatty acids and thus impeding the conversion to DHA, then you might want to first try lowering the omega-6s and increasing the omega-3s (through flaxseeds, walnuts, etc.).

- If you have diabetes or are over 65, you might want to consider taking DHA directly.

- If you're pregnant or lactating, you might consider going directly to DHA to help pass it on to your infant as well.

If you don't fall into any of these categories—and that's most people—the conversion appears to be adequate when the diet provides a healthy balance of omega-3 and omega-6 fatty acids. Even so, for added insurance, I tend to take a direct DHA supplement for a month once a year. See "Resources and Recommendations" for my recommended brands.

B$_{12}$: A Bacteria-Based (Not Meat-Based) Vitamin

Before you started the 30-Day Vegan Challenge, you might have been concerned about vitamin B$_{12}$ intake, assuming that B$_{12}$ is an animal-based vitamin that you can get only from meat and animal products. Like all other nutrients, B$_{12}$ is not animal-based, but it's not plant-based, either—it's bacteria-based. B$_{12}$ grows on bacteria and fungi, microscopic organisms that reside in the soil and the air.

We used to consume B$_{12}$ from the ground when we ate some soil along with our vegetables, but now that our modern practices dictate that we scrub our veggies because we're (justifiably) concerned about pesticides and toxins, we eat less soil and thus get less B$_{12}$ from that source.

An important water-soluble vitamin, B$_{12}$, also called cobalamin, protects the nervous system and keeps the digestive system healthy; without it, permanent damage can manifest itself in blindness, deafness, or dementia. Symptoms of overt B$_{12}$ deficiency include unusual fatigue, tingling or numbness in the hands or feet, no appetite, nausea, and tongue soreness. Symptoms in the neurological system are one of the biggest concerns, and nerve damage can be irreversible if not caught early enough.

> **CHALLENGE YOUR THINKING:**
> Vitamin B$_{12}$ is not animal-based; it's bacteria-based.

Mild B$_{12}$ deficiency is less easily detectable, though no less significant. Because B$_{12}$ lowers homocysteine levels, it reduces the risk of heart disease and stroke. Vegans and near-vegans who don't supplement with vitamin B$_{12}$ have consistently shown elevated homocysteine levels, so even though you don't have any measurable side effects, it doesn't mean your body isn't affected in ways you can't see or feel.

HOW MUCH IS NEEDED?

One of the things that's so remarkable about this vitamin is how little of it our bodies require; it's such a small amount that it's counted in micrograms. Some new vegans erroneously conclude that because our B_{12} intake requirement is so small and because our body stores it for years, we don't need to worry about B_{12}. Although it *is* true that at the time they become vegan some people have enough B_{12} stored in their livers to prevent overt B_{12} deficiency for a number of years, it is also true that these stores cannot prevent mild B_{12} deficiency, which can produce elevated homocysteine levels.

One of the benefits of our modern era is that we can prevent the nutrient deficiencies of yore by taking advantage of supplements and fortified foods. By consciously ensuring adequate intake of B_{12} and striving for optimal nutrition via the other suggestions outlined in this book, vegans can be shining models of health that everyone will be inspired to emulate.

So how much B_{12} do we need? The U.S. Daily Recommended Intake is 2.6 micrograms (mcg) per day, though research has shown that an optimal range is more like 5 to 10 mcg per day. This is easy to do, since supplements and multivitamins tend to provide large amounts of vitamin B_{12}, over and above the recommendations. This extra amount is nontoxic (as a water-soluble vitamin, unused B_{12} is excreted from the body) but is necessary to make sure everyone is getting the upper amounts and ensures a steady supply to the tissues. It also allows for taking the supplement less frequently.

CHALLENGE YOUR THINKING: Research indicates that B_{12} function cannot be restored to optimal levels by adding small amounts of animal products into the diet, despite professionals and laypeople making these recommendations. Increasing B_{12} through regular supplementation will be the most effective step for maximizing your B_{12} status.

CHANGE YOUR BEHAVIOR: To ensure optimal intake and absorption, take a daily multivitamin that contains B_{12}, along with 1,000 mcg of a separate B_{12} supplement once or twice a week.

There are some concerns about relying on multivitamins for B_{12}, because some of the other vitamins may diminish the efficacy of B_{12}. That said, if a multivitamin is chewable and has 10 mcg or more of B_{12} (as cyanocobalamin) and is taken daily, it is probably sufficient. (Chewables tend to be better absorbed.) To be sure you're getting optimal amounts of vitamin B_{12}, you can take 1,000 mcg twice a week along with your daily multivitamin.

The only time you may need additional supplementation is if you're truly deficient or if you haven't had a regular, reliable source for a while, in which case experts recommend increasing the amount of B_{12} to 2,000 mcg once a day for two weeks, then proceeding with regular recommendations. Individual B_{12} supplements come in tablets, sublinguals (which dissolve under your tongue), lozenges (which dissolve in your mouth), and drops. According to research, sublingual tablets and drops may provide the most rapid response, especially if you're looking to bump stores up right away.

It's worth saying that research indicates that B_{12} function cannot be restored to optimal levels by adding small amounts of animal products into the diet, despite professionals and laypeople making these recommendations. Increasing B_{12} through regular supplementation will be the most effective step for maximizing your B_{12} status.

RECOMMENDED DIETARY ALLOWANCES (RDAS) FOR VITAMIN B_{12}		
AGE	MALE	FEMALE
Birth to 6 months*	0.4 mcg	0.4 mcg
7–12 months*	0.5 mcg	0.5 mcg
1–3 years	0.9 mcg	0.9 mcg
4–8 years	1.2 mcg	1.2 mcg
9–13 years	1.8 mcg	1.8 mcg
14+ years†	2.4 mcg	2.4 mcg

* The Institute of Medicine recommends that infants of vegan mothers be supplemented with B_{12} from birth.
† The RDA for pregnant women is 2.6 mcg and for lactating mothers it is 2.8 mcg.

B_{12} IN FOOD

Some foods such as seaweed, mushrooms, tempeh, miso, tamari, and spirulina have been touted as sources of B_{12}, but this was based largely on faulty testing methods. Though they may contain some amounts of B_{12}, they're not providing reliable or consistent amounts. Although these foods are nutritious for a variety of other reasons, it is not recommended that these foods be relied on as B_{12} sources.

However, many foods are *fortified* with B_{12}, including nondairy milks, vegetarian meats, breakfast cereals, and one type of nutritional yeast, Vegetarian Support Formula (made by Red Star), which grows on B_{12}-fortified molasses. It has a wonderful cheesy flavor (great for popcorn) and can be used to make delicious cheese sauces (see the recipe on page 134). Though it's a delicious addition to any repertoire, it's not recommended that even the fortified version be relied upon as the sole source of B_{12} in your diet, as various factors may diminish its efficacy.

Because I center my diet on whole foods and don't necessarily eat fortified foods every day, I find it easier to simply take a daily supplement.

Before I had stopped eating animals and their secretions, I declared that because I objected to animal cruelty, I would purchase only "free-range" eggs, "organic" milk, and "humane" meat, perceiving myself as an ethical consumer and these products as the final frontier in the fight against animal abuse.

As much as I didn't want to believe that I was the cause of someone else's suffering, my consumption of meat and other animal products was perpetuating the exploitation and violence inherent in the deliberate breeding and killing of animals. Though modern animal factories look nothing like what is idealized in children's books and advertisements, I realized there are also many misconceptions about the practices and principles of a "humane" operation.

As I explored the unpleasant realities of both small and large operations—dairy cows enduring several years of constant pregnancy and loss, "natural turkeys" having to be artificially inseminated because their breasts are so large they're unable to mate in the usual manner, and "free-range" egg farms perpetuating unthinkable cruelty by buying their hens from egg hatcheries that kill millions of day-old male chicks every year en masse—I realized that the fundamental ethical problems we keep running into don't arise merely from *how we raise* animals but *that we eat* animals.

The idea of breeding animals only to kill them is absurd at best, and the unappetizing process of turning live animals into isolated body parts begins at birth and ends in youth since most of the animals sent to slaughter are just babies, whether they are raised conventionally or in operations that are labeled "humane," "sustainable," "natural," "free-range," "cage-free," "heritage-bred," "grass-fed," or "organic." And this end is the same for *all* animals, whether they're used for their flesh, milk, or eggs.

I realized that while I was assuaging my guilt by telling myself that I was eating meat, dairy, and eggs from animals raised "humanely," I was leaving out a huge part of the equation. The slaughtering of an animal is a bloody and violent act, and death does not come easy for those who want to live. Whether done in a chaotic slaughterhouse where desensitized, exploited, stressed-out workers often commit egregious acts of cruelty or on a backyard farm, killing requires a hardening of the heart, and I knew that this is not what I wanted to contribute to.

Once I made this connection, I wanted nothing to do with anyone or anything that hurt animals or that contributed to people being desensitized. If I truly wanted my actions to reflect the compassion for animals I said I had, then the answer was very simple. I could stop eating them.

For me, the bottom line is that as long as we see animals as ours to eat, ours to manipulate, ours to exploit, ours to confine, ours to kill, and their reproductive secretions as ours to take, there's no end to what we can justify doing to them. It's that *mind-set* that simply lends itself to the kind of mechanized system we have today. The answer isn't to change production methods or go backward to the animal farms of the past that we've romanticized and idealized.

The answer is to change our perception of and relationship with nonhuman animals so we can make choices that are truly compassionate, truly healthful, and truly humane.

FORTIFIED FOOD	B_{12} PER SERVING
Product 19 cereal, ¾ cup	6 mcg
Fortified Grape-Nuts Cereal, ¼ cup	1.5 mcg
Nutrigrain Cereal, ⅔ cup	1.5 mcg
Yves Veggie Cuisine Slices, 4 slices	1.2 to 1.5 mcg
Total cereal, 1 cup	6.2 mcg
Yves Veggie Ground Round, ⅓ cup	1.4 mcg
Yves Veggie Wieners or Jumbo Dogs, 1	0.7 to 1.5 mcg
Red Star Nutritional Yeast Flakes, 2 tablespoons	8 mcg
Nondairy milks	~3 mcg
Fortified Raisin Bran or Kellogg's Cornflakes, ¾ cup	1.5 mcg

AVOIDING DEFICIENCY AND INCREASING ABSORPTION

Keep in mind that B_{12} deficiency doesn't occur only in vegans and is typically due to inadequate absorption rather than simply inadequate intake. Because people over 50 tend to lack proper B_{12} absorption, the Food and Nutrition Board recommends that *everyone* (not just vegans) over age 50 should "meet their RDA mainly by consuming foods fortified with B_{12} or a B_{12}-containing supplement."

People with digestive or malabsorption diseases, such as pernicious anemia, even celiac sprue, chronic kidney failure, B_{12} metabolism defects, or cyanide metabolism defects, may also experience inadequate absorption and should consult a health professional to make sure their B_{12} intake and absorption is adequate. In fact, everyone can get their B_{12} levels checked by requesting a test from their doctor. To get the most accurate B_{12} reading possible, a urine MMA test is recommended. You can also get it online through www.b12.com.

Are Supplements Necessary?

By this stage in the Challenge, you should feel empowered enough to understand that a whole-foods, plant-based diet is rich in the nutrients you need to thrive and that B_{12} is really the only vitamin there aren't reliable food sources for. Living as we do in a pill-popping society, however, you may be tempted to ask if there are any other instances when supplements are necessary. You may also be asking if there are ever any risks to taking supplements, if they're just a waste of money, or if it's wise to take a daily multivitamin.

We have been conditioned to believe that all the healthful properties of food can be whittled down into a single magic pill to act as a panacea to counter our poor lifestyle habits, and I'd like to encourage you to think differently. Nature is a complex machine, and the nutrients found in plants come perfectly packaged: the phytochemicals, fiber, vitamins, and minerals all work together to create the benefits we receive.

That said, we live in an industrialized world and eat less nutrient-dense food than ever (before you started this Challenge, of course). But we are fortunate to have at our fingertips everything we need to ensure optimal health, with no nutritional deficiencies.

MULTIVITAMIN

Though the best place to get your vitamins, minerals, and antioxidants is from whole foods, many experts advocate taking a daily multivitamin, if only for insurance. After all, some days you might eat better than others, some days you might be ill and not eat at all, some days you may not absorb certain nutrients as well as others. I encourage you to revisit the chapters on specific nutrients, but let's take a snapshot look at when—if ever—additional supplementation is necessary.

CHALLENGE YOUR THINKING: The healthful properties of food cannot be whittled down into a single magic pill to act as a panacea to counter our poor lifestyle habits. Nature is a complex machine, and all the nutrients found in plants come perfectly packaged to create the benefits we receive.

CHANGE YOUR BEHAVIOR: Take a multivitamin that contains B_{12} as insurance against deficiencies, but rely on whole plant foods—not single supplements—as the source of your nutrients.

Vitamin B$_{12}$

It's likely that getting optimal amounts of B$_{12}$ from a multivitamin is sufficient. However, because other vitamins may inhibit its efficacy when taken at the same time, some experts recommend taking additional single B$_{12}$ supplements of 1,000 mcg once or twice a week. Additional supplementation is also recommended if you haven't had a regular intake of B$_{12}$ for some time. If you have a true deficiency due to lack of absorption, you can determine and treat this with your health professional.

DHA

Many people efficiently convert omega-3 fatty acids into DHA and will get enough DHA by consuming 1 tablespoon of ground flaxseeds a day, 3 tablespoons of shelled hemp seeds, or 1 teaspoon of flax oil. However, the following groups of people may not convert these fats so well and may wish to consider taking a direct DHA supplement:

- People with diabetes
- People over 65
- People who consume a lot of saturated and trans fats
- Pregnant and lactating women
- Premature, non-breast-feeding infants

There is evidence that low levels of DHA are associated with several neurological and behavioral disorders such as depression, attention deficit/hyperactivity disorder (ADHD), schizophrenia, and Alzheimer's disease, so if you suffer from any of these or know someone who does, it may be a good idea to take DHA directly. Taking it for just a few months tends to increase stores.

Calcium and Vitamin D

Although you can find everything you need to know about the best food sources of calcium and how you can increase absorption of calcium through vitamin D in "Day 13: Cutting Out the Middle Cow and Getting Calcium Directly from the Source," there is a little more to say, especially about the latter. Vitamin D deficiency is prevalent in the United States in both vegans and non-vegans. The best source is the sun, but many people spend most of their time indoors or in their cars or—justifiably—wear sunscreen, which blocks the absorption of vitamin D. People living in northern climates or in states with long, cloudy winters miss out on this "sunshine vitamin."

Also, although most light-skinned people can make enough vitamin D by exposing the face and arms each day to five to fifteen minutes of warm sunshine, people with darker skin need at least a half hour.

If you are limiting unprotected sun exposure, a vitamin D$_2$ supplement of 1,000 IU is recommended. (Vitamin D$_3$ is derived from sheep's wool or fish oil; vitamin D$_2$ is obtained from yeast and is vegan.) The Daily Value is:

- 600 IU (15 mcg) per day for children and adults up to 70 years of age
- 800 IU (20 mcg) for people over 70

WHEN *NOT* TO SUPPLEMENT

Other than a multivitamin and the considerations above, there really is no need for additional supplementation unless you're under the care of a doctor. This is especially true when it comes to single antioxidants, which can be ineffective at best and harmful at worst.

According to surveys, 10 to 20 percent of the adult population of North America and Europe (that's 80 to 160 million people) consume single antioxidant supplements.

Recently, a group of researchers thoroughly examined the effect of antioxidant supplements—particularly vitamin A, vitamin E, vitamin C, selenium, and zinc—in terms of mortality and published the results in the *Journal of the American Medical Association*. From their detailed analysis, they concluded that people who take beta-carotene, vitamin A, and vitamin E in single supplements or in combinations don't live any longer than those who don't take them. In fact, those who take the supplements, particularly vitamin A, have an increased risk of death.

The researchers emphasized that their findings should not be translated to potential effects of fruits and vegetables. They're talking about synthetic supplements.

So what is a conscious consumer to do? Most multivitamins contain vitamin E and vitamin A and/or beta-carotene. Before you panic, take a look at the label on your multivitamin bottle. Most likely, the amounts of these antioxidants fall just under or at the recommended Daily Value. You can determine that by looking at the column that reads "% Daily Value." For instance, the Daily Value for vitamin A is 5,000 IU, and your multivitamin probably contains that much, so it will say 100 percent.

Although you're probably fine at those levels, once you're ready to switch to a new multivitamin, look for one that doesn't include vitamin A. See "Resources and Recommendations."

Outside of the amount in your diet, the main concern is taking these single antioxidants over and above what you get in your multivitamin. Unless you're in treatment for a specific deficiency and under the care of your doctor, there is no need to take them as isolated supplements.

Note: *Skipping the supplements doesn't mean you should skip the vitamin A and beta-carotene in your diet!* Beta-carotene is just one of over six hundred carotenoids and is prevalent in sweet potatoes, carrots, kale, mango, spinach, turnip greens, winter squash, collard greens, cilantro, and thyme.

Vitamin E

In terms of vitamin E supplements, there's no evidence they're good, and there is some indication they may be harmful. For a while, professionals were recommending vitamin E supplements because of their supposed efficacy in reducing heart disease and cancer, but whereas vitamin E from foods has been shown to have this positive effect, nearly all the clinical trials on vitamin E from the past few years have yielded negative, inconclusive, or neutral results.

The best food sources of vitamin E are mustard greens, turnip greens, collard greens, kale, chard, spinach, almonds, and sunflower seeds. Also great are olives, avocado, wheat germ, Brussels sprouts, asparagus, and other nuts and seeds.

The daily value for vitamin E is 15 mg (30 IU) for adults, so consider the fact that 1 ounce of raw almonds has almost 7 mg, 1 medium avocado has about 2.5 mg, and 1 medium sweet potato has almost 6 mg. So just from those foods alone, you will not have a problem getting your daily value of vitamin E.

Vitamin C

The researchers found no harm in taking vitamin C supplements, but they also found it wasn't necessarily helpful. If you're taking vitamin C separate from your multivitamin (and if you're not doing it for a specific medical reason), it's your call. There doesn't seem to be anything harmful about taking vitamin C supplements, but experts are also not sure there is really any benefit, either, and you might be able to put your money to better use. The only thing they noticed is that a little extra vitamin C may reduce the duration and severity of the common cold, so if you feel one coming on, you can always bump up vitamin-C-rich foods in your diet.

The Daily Value of vitamin C is a mere 90 mg for adult males and 75 mg for adult women. When you eat a plant-based diet, you take in huge amounts of this water-soluble vitamin—well over the recommended Daily Value, but that's no problem when it comes from food. The best food sources are broccoli, bell peppers, kale, cauliflower, strawberries, lemons, mustard and turnip greens, Brussels sprouts, papaya, chard, cabbage, spinach, kiwi fruit, snow peas, cantaloupe, oranges, grapefruit, limes, tomatoes, zucchini, raspberries, asparagus, celery, pineapples, lettuce, watermelon, fennel, peppermint, and parsley.

Just to give you a little perspective: ½ cup chopped raw bell pepper contains about 140 mg of vitamin C, 1 cup whole strawberries 82 mg, 1 medium orange 70 mg, and ½ cup cooked broccoli 58 mg.

Selenium

The researchers' findings regarding the antioxidant selenium was that there doesn't seem to be a reason to take this antioxidant as a supplement; if it's in your multivitamin, that's plenty. The Adequate Intake ranges from 15 mcg for babies to 70 mcg for adult men and women.

Selenium levels in foods vary according to the soil content, so it's hard to know exactly how much selenium is in a particular food. Nevertheless, the best sources are whole grains (about 19 mcg in 1 cup cooked brown rice), nuts (4 Brazil nuts contain 270 to 360 mcg), and seeds (23 mcg in 1 ounce of sunflower seeds).

As with calcium, which is absorbed better with vitamin D, and iron, which is best absorbed with vitamin C, selenium is better absorbed with vitamin E.

Zinc

As with vitamin C, people tend to take zinc because they've heard it's good for shortening or curing colds, but there is no convincing evidence of this. The amount of zinc in most multivitamins is fine, but there is no need for additional supplementation.

The Daily Value varies:

Children 1 to 3 years 3 mg	Adult men 11 mg
Children 4 to 8 years 5 mg	Adult women 8 mg
Children 9 to 13 years 8 mg	Pregnant women 11 mg
Males 14 to 18 years 11 mg	Lactating women 12 mg
Females 14 to 18 years 9 mg	

As for food sources, 3½ ounces of toasted wheat germ provides 17 mg of zinc; 3½ ounces of cashews yields 6 mg; 3½ ounces of tahini offers 4.6 mg; 1 cup of cooked chickpeas provides 2.8 mg.

Folate/Folic Acid

Folate is a water-soluble B vitamin that occurs naturally in food. The word *folate* comes from the Latin word *folium,* which means "leaf," so it's easy to think of folate-rich foods: they're the green leafy vegetables such as spinach, kale, and collards. *Folic acid,* however, is the synthetic form of folate that is found in supplements and added to fortified foods such as breads, cereals, pastas, and rice. Some experts are concerned that people are getting too much folic acid.

The Daily Value for folate is:

- 150 mcg for children ages 1 to 3
- 200 mcg for children 4 to 8
- 300 mcg for children 9 to 13

Everyone already has a lot to say about how you should do things when you're pregnant, so it's really no different when you're vegan during this process. Everyone will have their opinion on what you need to do and will no doubt express concern about the fact that you're not eating animal flesh and fluids while your baby grows. Having said that, proper nutrition is critical during pregnancy, but that applies to both vegan and non-vegan women.

CALORIE INCREASE

Energy needs increase by about 10 to 15 percent during pregnancy (about 200 to 300 additional calories—the equivalent of a banana with one piece of whole-wheat bread topped with some almond butter), which will result in healthful, necessary weight gain. Depending on your current weight and frame, a weight gain of between 25 and 40 pounds is to be expected. A few ways to gain weight by adding nutrient-dense calories include:

- Making healthful fruit shakes with additional flax oil or ground flaxseeds
- Increasing the consumption of nuts and seeds (and their butters) as well as avocados
- Eating high-fiber, healthful baked goods, such as muffins, fruit crisps, and cookies

PROTEIN

The average-size woman needs 45 to 55 grams of protein per day; average-size pregnant women would do well to take in 65 to 75. Here are a few easy ways to add an extra 20 grams:

- ½ cup firm tofu (may vary according to brand and texture)
- 5 tablespoons peanut butter
- 3 ounces peanuts
- 1½ cups cooked beans (chickpeas, kidney beans, baked beans, pinto beans, refried beans, lentils, black beans)
- Two to three 8-ounce glasses nondairy milk

are doubled to 27 mg/day for pregnant women, which can be met by taking (see "Recommendations and Resources" for my recommended prenatal see "Day 17: Strong Like Popeye."

ZINC

The recommended intake for zinc during pregnancy is 11 mg/day and during lactation it is 12 mg/day. Most prenatal supplements will include this much, and "Day 20: Are Supplements Necessary?" provides ideas for food sources.

CALCIUM AND VITAMIN D

Pregnant women should meet the Daily Value of 1,000 mg for calcium and 15 mcg (600 IU) for vitamin D. (See "Day 13: Cutting Out the Middle Cow and Getting Calcium Directly from the Source.")

VITAMIN B_{12}

The RDA is 2.6 mcg for pregnant women and 2.8 mcg for lactating women, though B_{12} supplements, multivitamins, and prenatal supplements will have substantially more than that.

FOLATE/FOLIC ACID

As explained on "Day 20: Are Supplements Necessary?" folate is the naturally occurring nutrient prevalent in green leafy vegetables; folic acid is the synthetic form of folate. Many experts are concerned that people are getting too much folic acid because it's in multivitamins as well as fortified foods. The RDA is 600 mcg for pregnant women and 500 mcg for lactating women. Nutrient-rich vegan diets provide plenty of folate without relying on folic acid supplements. In addition to the folate-rich foods mentioned on pages 203 and 206, here are a few others:

- 4 spears of 5-inch-long broccoli total 180 mcg
- 2 cups romaine lettuce totals 150 mcg
- 4 spears of cooked asparagus have 85 mcg
- ½ cup cooked green peas equals 50 mcg

ESSENTIAL FATTY ACIDS

Many experts recommend pregnant vegans take a direct source of DHA, aiming for 200 to 300 mg/day. Read "Day 18: Skipping the Middle Fish."

- 400 mcg for anyone over 13 years of age
- 600 mcg for pregnant women and 500 mcg for lactating women

In addition to leafy green vegetables, asparagus, broccoli, and green peas are all fantastic sources of folate. Just ½ cup boiled spinach provides 100 mcg (1 cup of raw spinach is 60 mcg). And ½ cup great northern beans has 90 mcg.

DAY 21 Demystifying Tofu: It's Just a Bean!

I hope that by this time in the 30-Day Vegan Challenge, you're experimenting with new foods and exploring new vegetables, fruits, and grains. You're probably aware that tofu is an option, and maybe you've ordered it in restaurants but are intimidated by the idea of cooking it yourself. Perhaps you've tried tofu but didn't like it. If so, I encourage you to try it again. Many who don't like it are put off by its texture but don't understand that not all tofu is created equal. There are many different brands and many different textures.

Eating tofu is certainly not a prerequisite for being vegan, but if you've been holding off preparing it yourself, I want to try to demystify this wonderful and yet misunderstood food!

DEMYSTIFYING THE BIG WHITE BLOB

Tofu is a food that is made in much the same way as dairy-based cheese. First, you start with milk. In the case of dairy-based cheese, the origin of animal milk is a pregnant female, but the origins of tofu are much more simple, humane, and healthful. You start with a soybean and make soy milk by soaking, grinding, boiling, and straining dried soybeans.

Once you have your soy milk, next you add a coagulant. When you coagulate something, you cause it to curdle. In other words, you transform it from a liquid into a soft semisolid or solid mass. Most of us have seen curdling when cow's milk starts to go bad and you see little white lumps floating around. Those are curds. That particular process of curdling indicates that the milk is spoiling—that it's turning sour.

But there are other ways to sour milk intentionally that don't involve spoiling. You do this by adding an agent that will produce the souring, such as vinegar or lemon juice. In effect you're making buttermilk (which can be useful if you've got a recipe that calls for this—just squeeze some lemon juice into nondairy milk, and voilà!—you've got buttermilk).

The commercial tofu industry, however, uses other coagulants to curdle their milk, and we'll get to those in a moment. First, for the purposes of comparison, let's look at what is used to curdle cow's milk for the making of dairy-based cheese: rennet. Rennet is essentially a bunch of enzymes produced in the stomach of mammals to help the respective offspring digest his or her mother's milk. One of these enzymes causes the milk to coagulate—to curdle or separate into solids (curds) and liquid (whey).

What's actually happening is that the milk proteins, called caseins, are tangling up into solid masses or curds. What remains are whey proteins. In cow's milk, 80 to 87 percent of the proteins are caseins. Considering how much cow's milk and dairy-based cheese people are consuming, these findings should compel us to sit up and take notice.

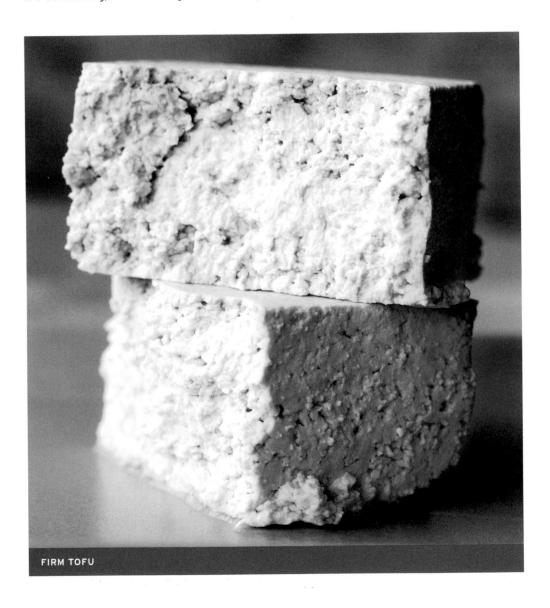

FIRM TOFU

According to T. Colin Campbell, Jacob Gould Schurman Professor Emeritus of Nutritional Biochemistry at Cornell University, casein is the *number one carcinogen* (cancer-causing substance) that people come in contact with on a daily basis.

Though vegetarian rennet is sometimes used in the production of kosher cheeses, nearly all of them are produced with either microbial rennet or genetically modified rennet. Microbial rennet is produced by using certain fermented molds that result in a slightly bitter-tasting cheese, which is unappealing to many. However, with the development of genetic engineering, scientists started using calf genes to modify bacteria, fungi, or yeast to make them produce chymosin, one of the first artificially produced enzymes to be registered and allowed by the FDA in the United States. In 1999, about 60 percent of U.S. hard cheese was made with genetically engineered chymosin.

And people turn their noses up at tofu! If you're eating animal-based cheese, you're either consuming enzymes extracted from dead baby calves or you're consuming genetically engineered enzymes based on calf genes.

If you eat tofu, you're eating neither.

> *Salt coagulants:* Two types of coagulants are used to make tofu: one salt-based, the other acid-based. An example of a salt-based coagulant is calcium sulfate, which is essentially tasteless. Tofu that's made with calcium sulfate is obviously rich in calcium. Other salt coagulants used are nigari salts, such as magnesium chloride and calcium chloride. Calcium chloride is a common coagulant for tofu in North America. You'll recognize this coagulant on the list of ingredients, because it will most likely say *nigari*. And—scary though the name is—glucono delta-lactone (GDL), a naturally occurring organic acid, is used as the coagulant for silken tofu, helping it produce a very fine-textured tofu that is almost jellylike.

Tofu producers may choose to use one or more of these coagulants, as each plays a role in producing a desired texture in the finished tofu. So when you notice a different taste or texture in tofu depending on the brand, a lot of this depends on the coagulant used.

Once you've got your curds, you press them. The curds are processed differently depending on the form of tofu being made. For silken and soft tofu, the soy milk is curdled directly in the tofu's selling package. For standard firm Asian tofu, the soy curd is cut and strained of excess liquid using muslin and then lightly pressed to produce a soft cake. Firmer tofus are further pressed to remove even more liquid.

TEXTURE VARIETIES

People's heads tend to spin as they scan the shelves of silken, soft, medium, firm, extra-firm, and super-firm tofu. What about these varying textures and when do you use which one?

Soft/Silken

The texture of soft and silken tofu is similar to that of very fine custard. You use this type of tofu when you want to make something creamy, such as puddings, mousses, and pie fill-

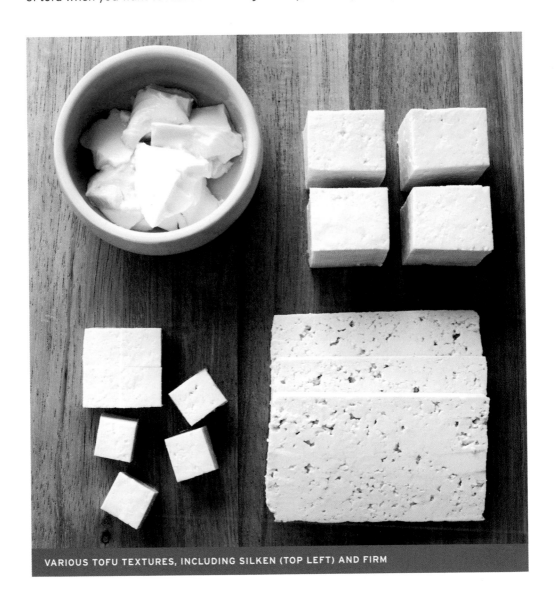

VARIOUS TOFU TEXTURES, INCLUDING SILKEN (TOP LEFT) AND FIRM

ings. (See Chocolate Mousse, page 216.) You can also use it for salad dressings and sauces, and silken tofu also works great in baked goods instead of using chicken's eggs (see "Day 16: Better Baking Without Eggs").

In the grocery store, you'll find silken tofu in an aseptic box, most likely in the Asian foods aisle—*not* in the refrigerated section with the fresh tofu. Mori-nu is the most common brand of this type. It can be stored in your cupboard for up to a year until you open it; then it needs refrigeration.

It can start to get confusing when you look at the little box of silken tofu and notice that even though it says "silken," it will also say "soft," "firm," or "extra-firm." These are just degrees within the texture of silken tofu itself. But heed my warning: even if it says "extra-firm" on the box, this is not the type of tofu you're going to grill or stir-fry; it's much too soft and crumbly for such a purpose.

Soft tofu is similar to silken and is found in water-filled tubs in the refrigerated section of the grocery store.

Firm/Extra-Firm Tofu

Choosing the texture that is appropriate for the dish you're making is the key to enjoying tofu. It needs to satisfy the mouthfeel you're aiming for, whether it's creaminess or chewiness. The more you cook with tofu, the more you understand what textures and brands work best for your purposes. Certainly you can just adhere to what type of tofu recipes call for, but to really learn the nuances between firm tofu and extra-firm tofu, the secret is first thinking about what your ultimate goal is.

- If you want hearty tofu steaks that you marinate with BBQ sauce and throw on the grill, the firmest tofu you can find is best (extra- or super-firm).

- If you're making Tofu Scramble (page 80), you will want to use firm or extra-firm tofu. You don't want it so chewy as to be rubbery; you want it to be soft like the scrambled chicken's eggs you're accustomed to but still have body.

- If you're making Better-Than-Egg Salad (page 97), you want it textured like hard-boiled eggs, such as from extra-firm or super-firm tofu.

- If you are sautéing tofu as part of a stir-fry, you want to use extra-firm or super-firm tofu to hold up to the spatula abuse the tofu will take during the sautéing process.

- Extra- or super-firm tofu is also best for Thai curry.

- For the tofu ricotta (for the Hearty Lasagna on page 137), a firm or extra-firm tofu is ideal.

The tricky part is finding the brand you like, which might require a little trial and error. My favorite local brand is Hodo, and I recommend it if you're ever in the San Francisco area. My favorite national brand of tofu is Wildwood. All of their soybean-based foods—yogurt, milk, aioli (mayonnaise), tempeh, and tofu—are stellar and all are made from organic, non-GMO, U.S.-grown soybeans. Within their firm tofu category, they offer the standard firm, medium-firm, and extra-firm, but one of the things that makes Wildwood unique is their super-firm tofu; it absolutely satisfies the quest for a hearty, dense texture.

When you can't find a super-firm tofu (or even when you can), there is still a way to create a chewy, dense texture with the extra-firm tofu you find in any store: freeze it.

FREEZING TOFU

You can do this with any variation of firm tofu (firm, extra-firm, or super-firm—not silken) that is packed in water. Once you arrive home from the grocery store, instead of putting the tofu in the refrigerator, put it in the freezer unopened. For best results, let it freeze for at least twenty-four hours. (It can last in the freezer for up to six months or longer.)

When you're ready to use it in a recipe, thaw it out on the counter for four to five hours. (It thaws faster on the counter than in the refrigerator). Now the magic begins.

When it's completely thawed, open the package, hold the block of tofu over the sink, and squeeze out all the water. As with a sponge, water will come oozing out of the tofu once you've thawed it. Now it's ready to be eaten and/or cooked.

There are several advantages to freezing and thawing tofu.

1. Because you've squeezed out so much water, you make the tofu very porous. In fact, all the pores will be visible to your naked eye, and all of these pores create room for another liquid—in particular a marinade—to penetrate the tofu and create more flavor.

2. The other thing you've done is change the texture completely. Tofu already has great texture when it's super-firm, but it's even chewier after having been frozen and thawed. Now you can grill it, bake it, sauté it, cut it up and add it to a green salad, or crumble and salt it and use it like feta on a Greek salad.

Although frozen-and-thawed tofu can be used in virtually every way you use tofu that hasn't been frozen, there are some instances in which you wouldn't want this super chewy texture. For instance, you want the Caesar dressing on page 133 to be creamy and thick but not chunky and chewy; and you wouldn't want your Tofu Scramble (page 80) to be so chewy it's rubbery.

As you ask yourself what your end goal is in terms of texture, you'll become more adept at choosing the right tofu for each instance. The following recipes utilize both firm and silken, but many more are found in other chapters, such as Hearty Lasagna (page 137), Tofu Scramble (page 80), and dressing for Caesar Salad (page 133).

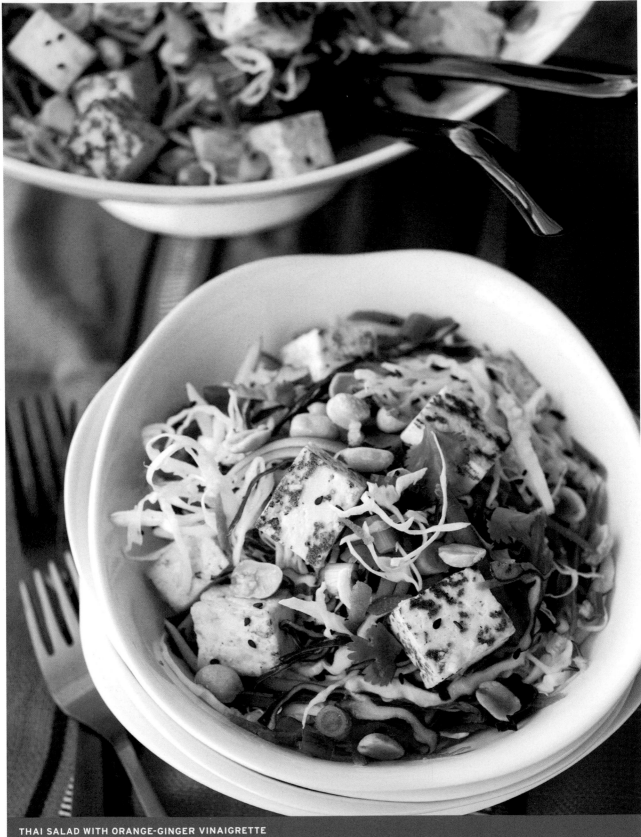

THAI SALAD WITH ORANGE-GINGER VINAIGRETTE

Thai Salad with Orange-Ginger Vinaigrette

YIELD: 8 TO 10 SERVINGS

A beautifully colored dish, this can be served as a side dish or a main.

Salad

1 small head green cabbage, shredded

½ large or 1 small head red cabbage, shredded

1 cup shredded carrot

1 red onion, thinly sliced

½ cup chopped green onion

1 cup roasted, unsalted peanuts

¼ teaspoon red pepper flakes, or more if you like it spicy

1-2 teaspoons black sesame seeds, toasting optional

½ cup chopped parsley or cilantro

16 ounces extra- or super-firm tofu, cubed and sautéed in sesame oil

Orange-Ginger Vinaigrette

¼ cup orange juice

¼-½ cup seasoned rice vinegar

3 tablespoons maple syrup

2 tablespoons minced ginger

2 tablespoons toasted sesame oil (optional)

2 teaspoons garlic, minced

Combine the cabbages, carrot, red onion, green onion, peanuts, red pepper flakes, sesame seeds, parsley or cilantro, and tofu in a large bowl. In a medium-size bowl, thoroughly combine the vinaigrette ingredients, and combine this mixture with the veggies. Stir well and serve. (Because the salad can get soggy if it sits in the dressing overnight, if you plan on preparing it in advance, keep the salad ingredients separate from the dressing until about an hour before ready to serve.)

Variation

You can leave out the tofu if you want, since this delicious salad is perfect on its own, but adding tofu (sautéed in sesame oil) will add additional flavor and texture.

Wheat-free, soy-free without tofu

Chocolate Mousse

YIELD: 6 SERVINGS

This is a quick and delicious dessert. You won't miss the dairy in this rich and creamy mousse that's also perfect as a pie filling.

1 cup semisweet or other nondairy chocolate chips
12 ounces silken tofu (soft or firm)

½ cup nondairy milk
½ teaspoon vanilla extract
Fresh berries for serving (optional)

Place the chocolate chips in a microwave-safe bowl and microwave for 1 minute. Give the chips a stir and heat for another 1 minute. They should be melted at this point; just give it another quick stir. (You can also melt the chips by creating your own double boiler. Place the chips in a small saucepan. Set this pan in a larger pot that is filled with ¼-½ cup water. Heat over a medium flame on the stove and stir the chips in the small pot until they are melted.)

Pour the tofu into a blender or food processor. Add the melted chocolate, nondairy milk, and vanilla. Process until completely smooth, pausing the blender or food processor to scrape down the sides and under the blade, if necessary.

Chill the mixture in serving bowls—or in a low-fat graham cracker or cookie crust—for at least 1 hour before serving.

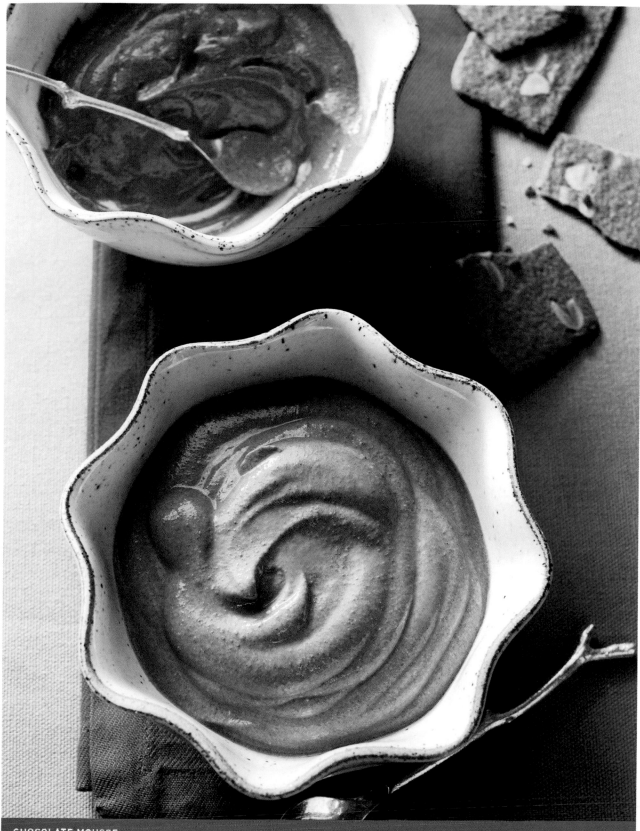

CHOCOLATE MOUSSE

SOY IS NOT EVIL

Soy was once the darling of health food proponents, but lately a few individuals have been evangelizing their anti-soy rhetoric far and wide; the way they talk, you'd think the innocent soybean was threatening the very survival of the human species. Soy naysayers have claimed that soy causes thyroid problems, birth defects, male reproductive problems, nutritional deficiencies, certain cancers, and cognitive dysfunction. In summary, *the negative claims about soy don't hold up in peer-reviewed studies. The overwhelming scientific research on soy is positive and concludes that soy is either neutral or helpful—not harmful.*

From a broader perspective, let's remember this:

1. **SOY IS NEITHER A MIRACLE FOOD NOR A POISON.** We're talking about a bean. It's not a toxin. It's not a chemical. It's not a weapon. It's also not a panacea. It's a bean, a legume, a plant food. It's a bean that, like other plant foods, contains health-promoting nutrients.

2. **YOU DO NOT HAVE TO EAT SOY FOODS TO BE VEGAN.** There are thousands of edible plant species available if you dislike soy or have an allergy or sensitivity to soy.

3. **EAT FOODS—ALL FOODS, INCLUDING SOY—IN THEIR WHOLE STATE.** One of the problems is that concentrated soy protein is being added to a number of processed foods—everything from Clif bars and cookies to ice cream and pudding. Extracting a single beneficial component from a food, sticking it in a product, and calling it healthful is problematic. The complexity in whole plant foods extends far beyond what we can replicate in a lab, and the health benefits of these whole foods stem from the combination of all of their components eaten at once in their *whole* state.

In other words, the problem isn't soy. The problem is processed food. There's a big difference between eating processed foods made with soy isolate protein (that's what it will be called on ingredients labels) and eating whole or minimally processed soy foods, such as soybeans, soybean sprouts, edamame, tempeh, miso, tofu, and soy milk. Yuba, essentially the skin of steamed soy milk, can also be enjoyed in a whole-foods diet, as can tamari soy sauce as a condiment.

Does this mean we should never eat soy cheese on our pizza or Clif bars on a hike? In my opinion, no. However, I do recommend making whole foods the *foundation* of our diet and eating processed foods in smaller amounts.

CREATING THE FEAR

It's important to point out that many of the soy detractors are meat-advocating organizations and individuals. Scaring people about soy, they also create fears about veganism. If you hear something negative about soy, it is likely from the meat- and dairy-promoting Weston A. Price Foundation or Mercola.com.

Finally, an environmental argument against soy is that rain forests are being cut down to grow soybeans. This is true—but only because they're making room for cattle grazing and for growing soy crops for livestock—not human consumption. The companies whose soy foods I recommend grow their soybeans in the United States according to organic standards and for human consumption—not for the meat industry.

Keeping Things Moving with Fiber

At this stage in the Challenge, you're no doubt already experiencing the benefits of a fiber-rich diet, which may mean more skipping to the loo, but rest assured these changes are contributing to a lighter and healthier you.

Although our bodies don't digest fiber, it's essential for optimal health, related to treatment and prevention of diabetes, colorectal cancer, gastrointestinal disorders, high cholesterol, heart disease, and obesity. High-fiber foods help move waste through the digestive tract faster and easier, so possibly harmful substances don't have as much contact with the gastrointestinal tract. Fiber-rich diets are also associated with weight loss, because the fiber helps create a feeling of fullness, helping to shut down appetite and preventing us from overeating.

Everyone knows we need to consume fiber, but not many people could tell you why. And most likely there are more people who could tell you the difference between a Big Mac and a Whopper than can tell you the difference between soluble and insoluble fiber!

The two different types are equally important, and most foods provide a mixture of both.

Soluble fiber dissolves in water and is found in a variety of fruits, vegetables, legumes, and grains. It cuts cholesterol, adds to your feeling of fullness, and slows the release of sugars from food into the blood. These actions reduce your risk for health problems including heart disease, obesity, and diabetes. Think about how oatmeal or ground flaxseeds get gooey in water; in your body, toxins and cholesterol quite literally attach to these sticky substances and get moved out of the body. Good sources of soluble fiber are oats, oat bran, oatmeal, apples, citrus fruits, strawberries, beans, barley, rye flour, potatoes, raw cabbage, and pasta.

As you may have guessed, **insoluble fiber** does not dissolve in water and is found in grain brans, fruit pulp, and vegetable peels and skins. It is the type of fiber most strongly linked to protection against cancer and improved waste removal. Think about the toughness of apple skins or the rigidity of sesame or sunflower seeds. Acting as a natural laxative, they help give stool the bulk it needs to move quickly out of the gastrointestinal tract, speeding the passage of food removal and thus contributing to a reduced risk of colon cancer. Good sources of insoluble fiber are whole grains (including barley and rye berries), whole-wheat products, cereals made from bran or shredded wheat, raw crunchy vegetables, fruits, nuts, and seeds. Wheat bran is the most concentrated source.

You may have noticed there are no animal products listed. That's because there is *no* fiber outside of plants. There is *no* fiber in meat, dairy, or eggs. None. Fiber exists only in plant foods.

> **CHALLENGE YOUR THINKING:**
> Fiber exists only in plants. There is no fiber in meat, dairy, or eggs. Zero. Zilch. Zip.

HOW MUCH DO WE NEED?

Fiber is a good example of a nutrient that non-vegans tend to be deficient in. Most Americans consume *far less* fiber than is recommended.

The World Health Organization recommends an intake of 27 to 40 grams per day for most adults. The USDA recommends 25 grams per day for women and 38 grams per day for men. (The recommended intakes for children range from 12 to 25 grams per day.) However, according to recent USDA surveys, the average intake of dietary fiber by women 19 to 50 years of age is about 12 grams. Intake by men of the same age is about 17 grams.

On the other hand, vegans consume an average of 40 to 50 grams of fiber per day. The rural Chinese, with their high consumption of vegetables and grains, consume as much as 77 grams of fiber per day. These high-fiber diets are believed to be at least partly responsible for the numerous health benefits of plant-based diets.

Here's what the American Dietetic Association says: "Incidence of lung and colorectal cancer is lower in vegetarians than in non-vegetarians. Reduced colorectal cancer risk is associated with increased consumption of fiber, vegetables, and fruit. The environment of the colon differs notably in vegetarians compared with non-vegetarians in ways that could favorably affect colon cancer risk."

COOKED VERSUS RAW

There are a lot of opinions about whether it's better to eat more cooked veggies or more raw veggies, and I think I can settle this once and for all: eat *both*. A combination of raw and cooked fruits and vegetables makes for a healthful, varied diet—full of all the nutrients we need and can best absorb.

How much raw should we eat in proportion to cooked? Because people do tend to eat fewer raw fruits and vegetables, it would behoove them to increase their consumption of green salads, fruits, and raw veggies. Three-quarters raw and one-quarter cooked is a good ratio in the warm months, but it might change to about 50/50 in the wintertime, and that's fine. The main thing is to take in a variety of raw and cooked foods. For a detailed analysis of raw foods, I recommend reading *Becoming Raw* by Brenda Davis and Vesanto Melina.

FIBER FROM FOODS, NOT SUPPLEMENTS

The prevalence of our low-fiber diets can be seen in the popularity of over-the-counter digestive aids, laxatives, fiber supplements, and concentrated bran. Instead of increasing healthful plant foods, people tend to continue consuming their regular diet of fiberless meat, dairy, and eggs and then rely on aids to treat the symptoms. Coping with daily constipation may be uncomfortable, but it may also be a step on the road to a much more serious problem. Prevention—*not* Band-Aids—is what's called for.

And it doesn't take much. A group of researchers recently reviewed a number of studies and concluded that if Americans ate an additional 13 grams of fiber a day *from food sources*, about a third of all colorectal cancer cases in the United States could be avoided. That's a significant risk reduction for a small change, and I hope you're already seeing how easy it is to add 13 grams of fiber to your daily repertoire. You're most likely already doing that just by taking this Challenge.

- That 1 cup of kidney beans you're now eating for lunch gives you 13 grams.

- The 1 tablespoon of ground flaxseeds you're now adding to your morning smoothie or oatmeal yields nearly 7 grams. One cup of oatmeal alone will give you 12 grams!

- A midday snack of raspberries (8 grams in 1 cup) and an apple (5 grams for a medium fruit) will give you that additional 13.

Remember, this additional fiber has to come from *food,* not supplements—and not concentrated bran fiber. As discussed in "Day 20: Are Supplements Necessary?" you cannot extract something beneficial from the whole package and expect it to work the same way the whole package works. The key is consuming the fiber via the whole food. If you're concerned about how to find more comfort digesting this additional fiber, see "Day 27: Dealing with Changes."

Eating by Color

When it comes to living ethically, my message is simple: live according to your own values of kindness and compassion. When it comes to my message of eating healthfully, my message is equally simple: eat by color.

And when I say color, I mean naturally occurring color—not artificial color, not color on a flashy cereal box. I mean the natural color in plants. After all, the greatest number of healthful compounds can be found in the most colorful foods; more than that, though, some of the healing power of plants actually comes from their color.

The pigments that give fruits, vegetables, and flowers their distinctive hues are called phytochemicals. More than nine hundred different phytochemicals have been identified, and experts estimate that hundreds more are still undiscovered. Although phytochemicals are not technically classified as nutrients, which are defined as "life-sustaining substances," they've been identified as containing properties, such as the ability to act as an antioxidant, that appear to play a role in disease prevention and treatment.

Different phytochemicals operate in various ways on a molecular level, including helping to prevent cell damage, preventing cancer cell replication, decreasing cholesterol levels, and causing cancer cells to self-destruct. In the grander scheme, they strengthen the immune system, create healthy blood sugar levels, slow the aging process, keep the brain functioning optimally, and reduce inflammation.

Because these substances perform so many different beneficial functions, experts recommend eating a wide variety of colorful plant foods. The more variety you consume, the more color you consume, and different body parts are affected depending on the color. For instance, lycopene, a phytochemical prevalent in tomatoes, concentrates itself in the prostate gland of men. Lutein and zeaxanthin, found in spinach and corn, concentrate themselves in the retina and lens, contributing to reduced risk of cataracts and macular degeneration.

You don't have to be a scientist, memorize charts, or become obsessed with learning all the complicated phytochemical names. All you have to do is follow nature's helpful map for making the most healthful choices possible. That map is *color.* We can detect the highest concentration of the different phytochemicals just by looking at the color of plants:

- Blueberries made blue by anthocyanins
- Carrots made orange by beta-carotene
- Beets made red by betacyanins
- Corn made yellow by lutein

Now, that doesn't mean that these plant foods don't contain other phytochemicals. Other phytochemicals are intrinsic throughout; you just can *see* these because the most concentrated phytochemicals are the most visible and prominent. Bananas, for instance, though white in appearance, also contain the blue anthocyanin pigments, just at a lower level. Eating an abundance of fruits, vegetables, legumes, grains, nuts, seeds, mushrooms, herbs, and spices means that we accumulate a variety of healthful compounds bit by bit.

Each time we choose an animal product, we are *not* choosing a healthful plant food and thus not benefiting from the nutrients that nourish us and increase our health. Keep in mind that there are no naturally occurring phytochemicals in meat, fish, dairy, or eggs. *Phyto-*, after all, means "plant." Phytochemicals, antioxidants, and fiber—all of the healthful components of plant foods—originate in plants, not animals.

It's only when animals eat plants that they take in these and other nutrients. Cattle consume calcium and protein from the grass and foliage they eat; salmon turn pink from the plant-eating animals they eat; and egg yolks turn yellow from the lutein-rich plants the chickens eat (and from the synthetic lutein added to their feed).

By going directly to the plants, we skip the unnecessary and unhealthful animal-based saturated fat, protein, lactose, and dietary cholesterol, all of which work against the benefits of the fiber, phytochemicals, vitamins, minerals, and antioxidants prevalent and inherent in plants.

Also, when we let color be our guide, we rather effortlessly choose whole rather than processed, packaged foods. The colors of these whole foods span the rainbow, but even those in more muted tones and noncolors (white, tan, brown, black) are packed with nutrition!

So create your shopping list based on color:

Red: tomatoes, beets, raspberries, cherries, cranberries, pomegranates, rhubarb, watermelon, strawberries, guava, red bell peppers, red chili peppers, red plums, red apples, red potatoes, red lentils, red beans, pink grapefruit, red miso.

Blue/purple: blueberries, blackberries, prunes, beets, eggplant, plums, pluots, purple cabbage, purple onions, purple potatoes, mulberries, figs, purple cauliflower, purple carrots, purple pole beans, kohlrabi, raisins, purple grapes, purple kale, radicchio

Orange: butternut or winter squash, oranges, cantaloupe, yams, nectarines, mangos, carrots, pumpkin, persimmons, tangelos, mandarins, kumquats, apricots, peaches, orange bell peppers

Yellow: corn, pineapples, lemons, plantains, yellow potatoes, yellow onions, squash, yellow bell peppers, grapefruit, papaya, quinces, sweet potatoes, ginger, saffron, yellow miso, yellow split peas, yellow watermelon

Green: spinach, broccoli, peas, asparagus, kiwi, green grapes, avocados, green bell peppers, zucchini, cabbage, lettuce, cucumbers, turnip greens, edamame, green tea, kale, collard greens, artichokes, Brussels sprouts, green beans, okra, limes, celery, honeydew melon, pistachios, beet greens, chard, basil, parsley, mint, green olives, fennel, rosemary, green split peas, pumpkin seeds

White/tan: garlic, white onions, coconut, cauliflower, white potatoes, pears, bananas, jicama, turnips, white tea, peanuts, white beans, oats, cashews, quinoa, barley, sesame seeds, bulgur wheat, couscous, farro, parsnips, soy beans, tofu, tempeh

Brown: whole grains, legumes, chocolate/cocoa, flaxseeds, coffee, dates, chestnuts, almonds, walnuts, pecans, brown lentils, pinto beans, brown mushrooms, shiitake mushrooms

Black: black beans, black sesame seeds, black kale, black carrots, black turnip, black tea, forbidden rice, black quinoa, wild rice, black mushrooms, black olives, black currants, black vinegar, nori seaweed, arame seaweed, wakame seaweed, black walnuts

Although all of the recipes included in the 30-Day Vegan Challenge are nutrient-rich and colorful, the following recipes are noted for their concentration of certain pigments:

- Red in the Muhammara and in the Fresh Strawberry Pie with Chocolate Chunks
- Orange in the Carrot-Ginger Soup
- Green in the Kale Chips, Garlic and Greens Soup, Basil Pesto, and Split Pea Soup
- Yellow in the Polenta Squares

CHALLENGE YOUR THINKING: There are no naturally occurring phytochemicals in meat, fish, dairy, or eggs. *Phyto-* means "plant." Only when animals eat plants do they take in phytochemicals, antioxidants, and other nutrients. Cattle consume calcium and protein from the grass and foliage they eat; salmon turn pink from the plant-eating animals they eat; and egg yolks turn yellow from the lutein-rich plants the chickens eat.

CHANGE YOUR BEHAVIOR: Eat a variety of plants using color as your guide.

Carrot-Ginger Soup

YIELD: 2 TO 4 SERVINGS

This silky, creamy soup is a staple in the Patrick-Goudreau household, as it is incredibly easy to make, delicious to eat, and beautiful to behold.

2 tablespoons water for sautéing

1 large or 2 small yellow onions, coarsely chopped

2 teaspoons garlic, finely chopped

6-7 carrots, peeled and sliced into rounds

2 medium yellow potatoes, peeled and quartered (Yukon Gold is my favorite)

2½ teaspoons finely chopped fresh ginger

½ teaspoon white pepper

½ teaspoon salt

4-5 cups vegetable stock or water with vegetable bouillon cube

Heat 2 tablespoons water in a large saucepan over medium-high heat.

Add the onions and garlic and sauté until the onions are translucent, about 5 minutes. Add small amounts of stock or water if the pan gets too dry. Add the carrots, potatoes, ginger, pepper, salt, and enough stock and/or water to cover the vegetables, about 4-5 cups.

Reduce heat to medium and cook until the carrots and potatoes are soft and easily pierced with a fork.

Transfer to a food processor and puree the soup until creamy. Return the pureed soup to a pot to heat up. Add salt as needed.

Wheat-free, soy-free

Muhammara
(Roasted Red Pepper and Walnut Spread)

YIELD: 1 CUP

This is most certainly my favorite spread. Make it the day before serving to allow the flavors to mingle.

2-3 whole roasted red bell peppers
   (fresh or from a jar)
²/₃ cup bread crumbs
1 cup walnuts, raw or toasted
4 large whole garlic cloves, peeled
½ teaspoon salt

1 tablespoon fresh lemon juice
2 teaspoons agave nectar
1 teaspoon ground cumin
¼ teaspoon red pepper flakes (or more
   for added spice)

In a blender or food processor, combine the peppers, bread crumbs, walnuts, garlic cloves, salt, lemon juice, agave nectar, cumin, and red pepper flakes. Puree to a smooth consistency. Scrape down the sides of your blender/food processor, and make sure all of the ingredients are thoroughly combined.

Serve with pita triangles, fresh bread, crackers, chips, carrots, mushrooms, cucumber, or other raw veggies—or use as a spread for your favorite vegetable sandwich.

Soy-free

Polenta Squares

YIELD: 6 SERVINGS

Creamy polenta is fantastic, but once it's allowed to set up, the polenta can be made into any shape you want using a cookie cutter. To create simple squares or polenta fries, just cut them with a sharp knife.

4 cups water

1½ cups coarse cornmeal or polenta

¼ cup nondairy milk (soy, rice, almond, hazelnut, hemp, oat)

1 teaspoon salt (may need more, but add gradually)

2–3 tablespoons nutritional yeast flakes

½ cup sun-dried tomatoes, finely chopped

2 tablespoons fresh basil, minced

2 tablespoons fresh parsley, minced

1 tablespoon olive oil

Add the water to a 4-quart saucepan, and heat to boiling.

When the water has boiled, slowly add the cornmeal, whisking frequently as you pour it in. If you don't whisk, it will clump up. Reduce the heat to medium-low and continue stirring for about 5 minutes to allow the polenta to absorb the water and thicken up. Slowly add the nondairy milk, salt, and nutritional yeast, and stir until the liquid is absorbed and the polenta thickens, about 5–10 minutes.

Add the sun-dried tomatoes, basil, and parsley, stir for 1 more minute, and remove from heat.

Taste, and add additional salt, if necessary.

At this point, the polenta will be thick (and getting thicker). Once you remove it from the heat, you can serve it immediately, or, to form it into shapes, you will want to let it set up.

To let it set, pour it into a 9-by-13-inch glass or nonstick pan, and spread evenly with a rubber spatula. Place in the refrigerator for at least an hour or overnight. When ready to serve, cut into squares or punch out other shapes using a cookie cutter, and set aside.

Heat the olive oil in a skillet on medium heat. Sear the polenta squares until golden on both sides and heated throughout. Serve with hot marinara sauce.

Variation

Instead of pan-frying the polenta, as long as it is nice and firm, it can also be grilled. Brush the squares first with olive oil, and grill until seared on both sides and heated throughout.

Wheat-free, soy-free, depending on milk used

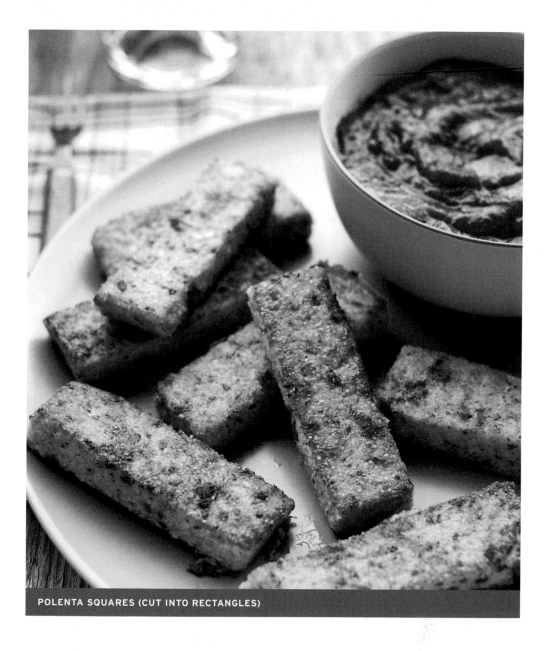

POLENTA SQUARES (CUT INTO RECTANGLES)

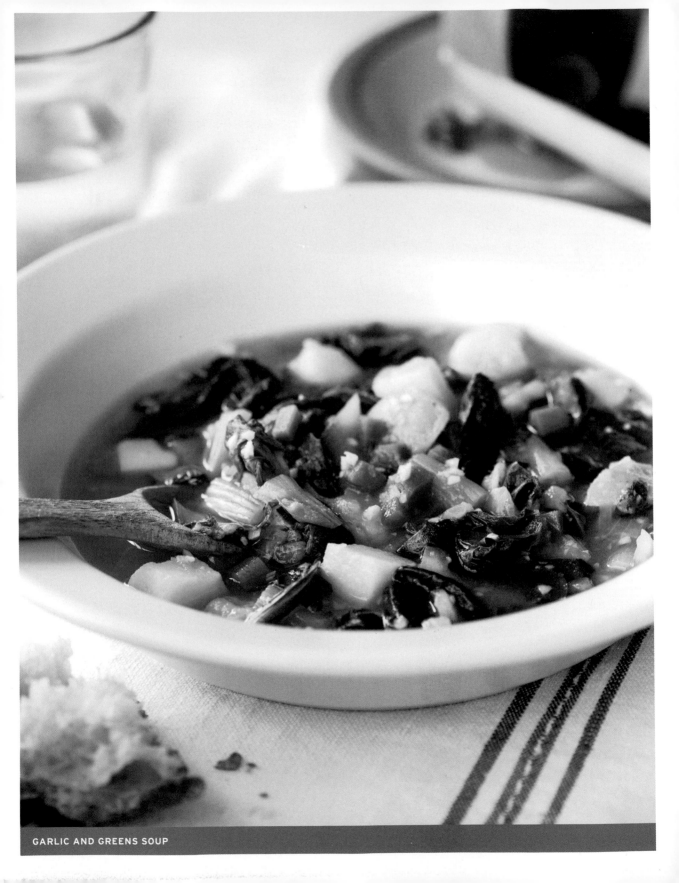

GARLIC AND GREENS SOUP

Garlic and Greens Soup

YIELD: 4 SERVINGS

This soup packs a wallop, starting with a whole head of garlic, making the kind of robust, assertive goodness you want on a cold winter day. At the start of even the slightest cold, rely on this soup to heal what ails.

1 head garlic, separated into cloves, peeled, and minced or pressed

1 large yellow onion, finely chopped

1 tablespoon olive oil or water for sautéing

1 bunch kale, bok choy, or chard, chopped into bite-size pieces

3 yellow potatoes, such as Yukon Gold, diced (not peeled)

8 cups vegetable stock

1 tablespoon seasoned rice vinegar

Salt and pepper to taste

In a large soup pot, sauté the garlic and onion in the oil or water until the onion turns translucent, about 5 minutes.

Add the greens, potatoes, and vegetable stock to the soup pot and bring to a boil. Simmer everything together for about 25 minutes, until the potatoes can be pierced easily with a fork.

Just before turning off the heat, add the rice vinegar, and add salt and pepper to taste.

Variations

- Add 1 cup cooked barley to the soup about 5 minutes before it is finished cooking.
- Add 2 finely chopped carrots to the soup at the same time the potatoes are added.

Soy-free, wheat-free

Kale Chips

I strive to eat kale every day, and here it is in one of my favorite forms.

1 bunch curly kale (green or purple)   **Pinch of salt**
1 teaspoon olive oil   **Pinch of nutritional yeast (optional)**

Preheat a toaster oven or regular oven to 350 degrees.

Tear or cut the leaves away from the thick stems, and tear the leaves into bite-size pieces. Wash and thoroughly dry the leaves.

Transfer the kale to a large bowl, drizzle it with the olive oil, and sprinkle with the salt. With your hands, toss the leaves until they are well coated.

Lay the leaves out on a baking sheet in a single layer, sprinkle them with nutritional yeast (if using), and bake until the leaves are crisp but not burnt, 10-15 minutes, checking every 5 minutes or so. (See note below about removing ones that are already done.)

Variations
- For a bit of a bite, toss with a little chili powder.
- Try it with garlic salt instead of regular salt.

Soy-free, wheat-free

TIP:

I cannot emphasize enough how little salt and oil you need for optimal flavor. When you make these again and again, like I do, you'll find just the right ratio for you. I also cannot emphasize too much how critical the baking time is. If you bake them too little, they are just limp pieces of kale; if you bake them too long, they will burn. You may need to check halfway through the cooking time to remove the pieces that are already crispy. Continue cooking, and keep a close eye on the remaining leaves. The other trick is not piling the kale leaves on top of one another on the baking tray. If you do, the leaves on the top will cook, but those on the bottom will stay moist. Make sure they're all laid out in a single layer, even if you have to cook them in more than one batch. Since the leaves shrink so much when cooking, you may want to double the recipe for a higher yield.

Split Pea Soup

YIELD: 4 TO 6 SERVINGS

This is perfect comfort food, whose cooking time offers a good excuse to relax with loved ones. To boot, it's filling, packed with protein, brimming with fiber, and, despite its creaminess, low-calorie and low-fat. It also freezes well. What more could you ask for?

2 cups green (or yellow) split peas
6-7 cups water or vegetable stock
1 medium yellow onion, diced
2 creamy yellow potatoes (such as
   Yukon Gold or fingerlings), diced
2 or 3 garlic cloves, pressed or
   minced
2 carrots, diced

2 stalks celery, diced
½ teaspoon dried marjoram
½ teaspoon dried basil
½ teaspoon dried parsley
¼ teaspoon ground cumin
¼ teaspoon black pepper
½ teaspoon liquid smoke
Salt and pepper to taste

Rinse the split peas, checking for any impurities, such as stones or residue.

Place all of the ingredients, except the salt and pepper, in a soup pot, and bring to a simmer. Cover loosely and cook until the peas are tender, 1 hour or longer. Check it every so often to make sure the liquid isn't evaporating too quickly. The flame should be low-medium.

The resulting soup should be thick and creamy, with the split peas quite broken down and mushy. Add salt and pepper to taste, and serve hot.

Variation
If you would like creamier soup, you can puree it in a food processor or blender.

Wheat-free, soy-free

Fresh Strawberry Pie with Chocolate Chunks

YIELD: 8 TO 12 SLICES

This delicious, easy-to-prepare seasonal pie requires no baking and calls for the ripest, sweetest strawberries, which you can find at your local farmer's market in the summertime.

4 cups ripe strawberries, sliced
1 cup ripe strawberries, whole
5 pitted dates, soaked 10 minutes in
   warm water and drained
2 teaspoons fresh lemon juice

Dark chocolate chunks, preferably from
   a good, organic, fair-trade bar
   (optional)
No-Bake Pecan Crust (see page 235)

Have your crust ready.

Arrange the sliced strawberries on top of the crust and set aside. In a food processor or blender, combine the remaining 1 cup of strawberries with the 5 soaked dates and lemon juice. Puree until smooth. Pour this mixture over the sliced strawberries. Arrange the chocolate chunks on the top of the sauce (optional), and refrigerate for 1 hour before serving. (You will need to refrigerate even if you don't add the chocolate. This will help the pie set and make it perfect for slicing.)

TIP:

Because of the freshness of the ingredients, this pie is best when served within an hour or two of preparing it.

No-Bake Pecan Crust

YIELD: ONE 8- OR 9-INCH PIE CRUST

This is an incredibly simple crust that requires absolutely no baking and pairs well with a no-bake fresh fruit pie.

2 cups raw pecans or almonds
¾-1 cup pitted dates, preferably Medjool
Canola oil for greasing pan

Place the nuts in a food processor and grind them until they are a coarse meal. Add the dates and process until thoroughly combined. Press the mixture into a nonstick or very lightly oiled 8- or 9-inch tart pan or springform pan.

TIP:

You will create the prettiest outcome by using a pan that has a removable bottom, such as a tart pan or a springform pan. That way, the pie can be admired from the side as well as the top.

DAY 24 Eating Confidently and Joyfully in Social Situations

As you enjoy the last week of the 30-Day Vegan Challenge, no doubt you're learning what every vegan knows: that making your own dietary changes can make other people uncomfortable. I often say that the food is the easy part of this lifestyle change—you learn some new recipes, you restock your kitchen, you read labels as though it were second nature.

But then you're in a social situation and you're asked to defend your new way of eating. You get asked the same questions over and over—about protein, about how to replace cheese, about what the Bible says about eating animals. Next, someone begins pointing out all the areas in your life where you're not perfect, calling you a hypocrite for not solving world hunger. You tell someone you're vegan, and you're expected to have advanced degrees in nutrition, philosophy, anthropology, animal husbandry, ecology, and the culinary arts. You tell someone you're vegan, and that person takes it personally, becoming defensive about his or her own eating habits.

To be honest, I think this pressure takes its toll on new vegans—especially if they are naturally shy or reticent about their opinions—and I believe it's why many people just give up and revert back to eating meat, dairy, and eggs. I think it's why many wind up feeling isolated and shy away from coming out of the "vegan closet," if you will. I think it's why many people resist becoming vegan in the first place. And although we can't change how people are going to react to us, we *can* change how we represent our vegan-ness.

When you state "I am vegan," you aren't simply saying "I eat vegetables." You are a physical representation of someone who is living a conscious life with an awakened mind and heart. You're authentically manifesting what it means to truly eat healthfully and compassionately. And people know this. They feel it, and it rocks their world because *you're* doing what they say they want to do but don't follow through on. For this reason, they would rather you just keep it to yourself and stop "making meat-eaters feel guilty," an accusation leveled at many vegans who often say nothing more than "I'm vegan."

I call this phenomenon "being the vegan in the room," which I think is a powerful and privileged position to be in. It can also be pretty scary for those who don't want to look at their eating habits or consider changing them.

GIVING PEOPLE THE BENEFIT OF THE DOUBT

To avoid discomfort, many vegans figure it's a lot easier not to say anything at all, so they don't stand up for what they believe in, they don't reveal themselves as they truly are, or they compromise and eat an animal product just to make someone else happy. And although I understand that it is indeed easier to blend in and conform, the question we have to ask ourselves is "At what cost?" At the cost of our own health? At the cost of our own values?

We often say we're a culture that values individuality, but I'm not so sure. I think we value conformity a lot more. *Nonconformity* is a dirty word in many people's vocabulary. For fear of "being different," many people continue to eat animals and their secretions because they're afraid they won't look like everyone else.

It reminds me of an old Arabic folktale about a witch who visits a kingdom one night and poisons the central well with seven drops of a potion that drives people mad. The next morning all who drink from that well go mad. The king, however, knew about this in advance and, like all self-respecting kings with their own water source, did not drink from the communal well. The next day, those who had drunk the poisoned water came to the king and accused him of being mad. The king, aware of what had transpired, was faced with a dilemma: drink from the well and lose his sanity like the rest of his subjects, but remain king; or not drink, remain sane, but be swept from power by those who would view his very sanity as madness.

Though the stakes may not seem as high as those in this story, I think they *feel* that way to many people. Though they may not have a kingdom to lose, many people are afraid of losing their social status, their friends, or their comfort level, and all of these things may be valued as highly by an ordinary citizen as a kingdom is by a king.

We all say we want to make a difference. We all say we want to leave our mark on this world, do something meaningful, live a meaningful life, help others, effect change, contribute something important. And I do think people mean it when they say it, but I wonder sometimes if this all means as much to them as *not appearing different*. We all say we want to make a difference, but in order to make a difference, we may have to do something different. It's only people willing to assert their individuality, their personal beliefs, who actually make a difference. It's easy to go along with the status quo, but the question we have to ask ourselves is what it is we really want at the cost of our own values.

But let's be clear. Reflecting your values—whether they are motivated by health or by ethics—in your behavior doesn't mean you have to constantly rock the boat. It's really just as simple as being authentically *you*. For instance, anyone who meets me knows where I stand on certain things, namely, my belief that animals are here for their own sake and not for my pleasure. That's not something I have to apologize for. That's not something that changes according to who invites me to dinner, who can handle it, or whom it might make uncomfortable.

And if you think about it, it would be pretty self-centered of me to try to control other people's reactions—being afraid to tell someone I don't eat animals because it might make that person uncomfortable. Who am I to guess what someone's reaction is going to be? Who am I to protect someone from the very thing that might open up his or her own repressed feelings about animals? Who am I to deny someone the chance to show me he or she cares about me? In truth, I've never seen people at their most beautiful or generous as when they learn I'm vegan and either begin sharing their own stories and feelings about animals, asking me questions about food and nutrition, or offering to make a special dinner just for me. That's their choice, and I always appreciate it.

Frankly, I think we don't give people the benefit of the doubt enough. I think we underestimate our friends and family, and as long as we think we're "protecting them" from any discomfort, we're not only denying our own ethics, harming our own health, and perpetuating the abuse of animals, but we're also potentially denying other people their own transformation, because how else does this occur except through honest interaction and communication with others? By speaking our truth, we give others permission to speak theirs.

ASKING FOR WHAT YOU WANT

I highly recommend revisiting "Day 8: Eating Out and Speaking Up" and taking a close look at the communication strategies I recommend. Being a joyful vegan in a non-vegan world is the art of walking the line between being humble and speaking the truth. The power of example is the most profound gift we can give. If we are confident and joyful in our veganism, others will respond in kind.

For instance, my husband works for a company that provides breakfast for the employees every day. They bring in bagels and cream cheese and sundry other animal products, but for David—and the now handful of vegans in the office—the people in charge of the food prepare a special vegan breakfast—from fruit smoothies to tofu scramble. (They also started bringing in nondairy yogurts, nondairy milks, and nondairy cream cheese for the bagels.) When they found out David was vegan (because he spoke up and told them he was), they simply asked him what he wanted for breakfast, he made some suggestions, and wouldn't you know other people began coveting the vegan breakfasts as well? No problem. No bother. No big deal. He also tells me stories of how they bring in vegan pizza (no cheese, lots of veggies), or vegan sandwiches when they have in-house lunch meetings, and everyone winds up gravitating to the more healthful vegan options.

The same rules apply for any situation you're going to be in: going to a friend's house for dinner, the boss's house for brunch, a wedding, a summer barbecue, an office outing. Simply letting the host know in advance, offering to help with the food, and offering to bring food are all simple ways to make the situation pleasant and comfortable. It's just a matter of speaking up with truth, graciousness, and integrity.

I think it's important in all our relationships to know where we begin and another person ends. What a mess I'd be if my behavior were determined by how it would make other people react. In other words, if my being vegan *does* make someone uncomfortable, that's not mine. Whatever someone does with my values isn't mine to worry about. I'm not saying that we be demanding or rude or ungracious, but what I am saying is that we need to speak our truth without being attached to what that truth will do to other people.

So don't drink from the poisoned well. Stay sane. Stay true. Because if you don't stand up for what you believe in, you might as well not have any opinions at all. What's the point of having values if we don't manifest them in our behavior?

DAY 25 Celebrating the Holidays

Whether you're vegan or not, holidays can be stressful. Self- and family-imposed expectations, unexpected expenses, and cross-country travel can take their toll on even the most balanced individual. Add food to the equation, and it can be a recipe for disaster. Though food exists in our lives for mere utilitarian reasons—to provide the sustenance we need to survive—it plays a complicated and emotional role for many, many people.

Though transitioning from an animal-based diet to a plant-based one seems like it's just about choosing broccoli over beef, it's so much more profound than that. It's about questioning assumptions, reexamining our values, aligning our behavior with our principles, and shifting the paradigms with which we grew up. This can be a little unnerving to those who are closest to us, especially when they feel their own traditions are being threatened— especially during the holidays. Within the familial microcosm, most likely everyone has been cooking the same favorites year after year, making a ritual of carving the holiday bird, and passing down recipes from years past.

For the larger society, by eschewing turkeys on Thanksgiving, lambs on Christmas, eggs during Passover, corned beef on St. Patrick's Day, fried foods during Hanukkah, and ham on Easter, vegans are seen as flying in the face of tradition and essentially upsetting the natural order of things.

The strong response people have to vegans not eating the "standards" on certain days of the year seems to belie the unfortunate fact that we place more value on tradition than on health or compassion. And yet those things need not be mutually exclusive. We can most certainly eat in such a way that it reflects our values and honors tradition at the same time. Holiday meals are an opportunity to demonstrate to our loved ones that we are not rejecting *their* traditions but rather embracing *your* values. Communicating this distinction to them can work wonders in alleviating tension.

It's also important to point out that as much as we romanticize the notion of tradition, our attachment to it is not as tenacious as we think. The truth is we cherry-pick from the lot and decide which traditions and customs we want to uphold and which ones we want to leave behind, for reasons of convenience, modernity, or ethics. This is especially true when it comes to the quintessential American holiday: Thanksgiving.

THANKSGIVING

Much of what informs our consciousness about the first Thanksgiving is myth—based on romanticized notions rather than informed facts, having been contrived and developed over the last few centuries. This is especially true when you look at what we consider the traditional Thanksgiving menu.

The animals killed for that first Thanksgiving in 1621 were most likely ducks, geese, and various kinds of fish. If cranberries were served, they would have been used for their tartness or color—not in the form we eat them today. (It would be fifty more years before berries were boiled with sugar.) Potatoes were not available, and thus mashed potatoes were not enjoyed, and because it's improbable that the colonists had flour for pie crust or an oven in which to bake it, pumpkin pie was most likely absent. And forks were not used.

As Thanksgiving approaches each year, every vegetarian or vegan is accused of "breaking tradition" for not eating turkeys. And yet, if we hold historical accuracy as the standard for being true to tradition, then all of us who eat mashed potatoes, pumpkin pie, sweet cranberry sauce, biscuits, or any of the other things that were not on the table of the first Thanksgiving are breaking tradition. Are we not also breaking tradition by eating with forks?

Our emotional attachment to tradition is very powerful, so we justify our consumption of turkeys at Thanksgiving by attempting to sanctify it in terms of historical accuracy, which is simply absent here. The fact is we eat turkeys because that's what we were taught, that's what we've enjoyed, *and* because of a woman named Sarah Josepha Hale.

Hale, who lived from 1788 to 1879, was the editor of a popular magazine and began a forty-year quest in 1827 to make Thanksgiving a national holiday. She wrote romantic accounts of the first Thanksgiving, taking liberties to appeal to her readership and including recipes for roasted turkeys, stuffing, and pumpkin pies—none of the things that would have been on the table of the first Thanksgiving, but all of the things we eat today.

Though the holiday traditions Hale created share few similarities with the original feast, I think most of us would admit that we are not as interested in creating an exact replica of the first Thanksgiving as we are in having customs and traditions we can point to that help

CHALLENGE YOUR THINKING: We can eat in such a way that it reflects our own values and honors tradition at the same time. They need not be mutually exclusive.

CHANGE YOUR BEHAVIOR: Demonstrate to your loved ones that our food choices aren't about rejecting *their* values but rather about embracing *your* values.

us feel connected to something bigger and older than ourselves. We shape our traditions out of our ideals. This is why it's just as traditional *not* to have turkeys on the table. We pick and choose which traditions we want to celebrate.

Even as the myths started by Hale began to permeate the culture's consciousness, turkeys were still not widely accepted as the quintessential Thanksgiving dish until the mid-twentieth century. Wild turkeys–dark-feathered and thus dark-skinned–became unappetizing to consumers. To make turkey meat more appealing, the Beltsville white was bred in 1947 at the behest of the National Turkey Federation. Turkey consumption increased manifold and has been increasing ever since. In fact, according to the USDA slaughter numbers, an average of 240 million turkeys are killed each year–21 million of which are killed each November.

Though she did a great disservice to turkeys–curious, playful, social birds–Hale did have noble ideas about the significance of this holiday. She envisioned that it would be about charity and generosity, writing: "Let us consecrate the day to benevolence of action, by sending good gifts to the poor and doing those deeds of charity that will, for one day, make every American home the place of plenty and of rejoicing."

For the fifty-two English colonists who gathered for a three-day harvest feast in 1621 along with ninety Wampanoag Indians, it was a celebration of food, feasting, and praising God and the Three Sisters (corn, beans, and squash), respectively. Before Hale's mythologizing of that first Thanksgiving, it was considered to be a simple regional holiday that was celebrated solemnly through fasting and quiet reflection. Quite a bit different from the gluttonous and commercial celebrations of today.

Creating a beautiful Thanksgiving menu that draws from all the riches of the autumn's harvest is easy and not very different from what most of us grew up with. The side dishes remain the same with just a few tweaks (nondairy butter, vegetable stock instead of animal-based, nondairy milk, etc.), but when it comes to the main dish, I believe that what people are attached to is not a lifeless animal but rather a *centerpiece* on the table, a focal point on the plate, and this can be accomplished in so many ways using plant-based foods.

- **STUFF IT:** Stuff eggplants, bell or jalapeño peppers, mushrooms, winter or summer squash, potatoes, olives, peapods, or corn husks. (See Harvest-Stuffed Acorn Squash on page 254.)

- **CONFINED AND REFINED:** Create a main dish using ramekins, custard cups, or individual bowls, or make miniature pot pies for each person.

- **SHAPELY:** Use cookie cutters to press polenta, tortillas, or pancakes into eye-catching shapes.

- **A MEATY MAIN:** Tofu, tempeh, seitan, and portobello mushrooms are all great options to serve as the main dish. They are hearty, meaty, and protein-rich, which is one of the criteria by which people tend to judge main dishes. (See Marinated Portobello Mushroom Steaks on page 99.)

- **LOAF IT:** Anything made as a loaf, patty, timbale, mold, or burger also serves as a great main-dish item.

- **ROLL IT:** Phyllo dough can be prepared with a million different fillings, then layered, folded, or rolled to make the perfect focal point for a plate.

Options for side dishes abound:

- Mashed potatoes and Mushroom Gravy (see page 252)
- Green beans sautéed in garlic and tossed with almond slices
- Traditional bread stuffing using vegetable broth and nondairy butter
- Cranberry relish
- Fresh or frozen corn
- Mashed rutabagas
- Roasted Brussels sprouts or root vegetables
- Cornbread
- Drop Biscuits (see page 259)
- Green salad

And of course dessert options are never lacking, ranging from pies, cakes, and cobblers to crisps, cookies, and breads.

These are some of the dishes my husband and I enjoy at the annual Thanksgiving meal we host in our home. All of our friends pick a different dish to bring, and it's a veritable feast. For those years we've gone back east to celebrate the holidays with our families, we've been so grateful to our parents, who have allowed us to enjoy a vegan holiday with them as well. We cook (with their help), and everyone enjoys delicious, seasonal harvest fare. Don't underestimate how your family will respond. Give them the benefit of the doubt, and don't forget: if you agree to cook, it means they don't have to, so they're usually pretty open to the idea.

HALLOWEEN

Another holiday connected to autumn and the harvest is an ancient Celtic holiday called Samhain (pronounced *SAH-win*). Its descendants can be found in our modern-day Halloween and in the Catholic holiday All Souls' Day. Many European cultural traditions hold that Halloween is one of the times of the year when spirits can make contact with the physical world, and this is also seen in the Mexican holiday Día de los Muertos (Day of the Dead), whose emphasis is on honoring the lives of those who died and celebrating the continuation of life.

Like Thanksgiving, Halloween is a food-centered holiday, though in this case the food is *junk*. Many parents, having transitioned to or contemplated veganism, worry about how their children will participate in the most popular of Halloween rituals: trick-or-treating. Fear not. It turns out that a lot of candy given out during Halloween is vegan. It's junk, but it's vegan junk. So don't worry. Your kid can be a normal kid, just like everyone else, and get to eat junk, including Blow Pops, Cracker Jack, Dots, Skittles, Airheads, Hubba Bubba, Jolly Ranchers, jujubes, Mary Janes, Pez, Now and Later, Sour Patch Kids, Swedish Fish, SweeTarts, and Twizzlers, plus nonsugary treats such as corn chips, potato chips, nuts, pretzels, and crackers.

There are also a few things you can do to make trick-or-treating a little less tricky:

- Make it clear that the rules are to eat no candy until they get home. Though it was for reasons of safety and temperance (and not about being vegan), this was certainly my parents' rule when I was little.

- Find other vegan parents and kids to trick-or-treat with, so that your children have like-minded people they can relate to.

- Make your children part of the process of sorting through the non-vegan candy they receive.

- If they tend to get a lot of non-vegan candy, have alternatives waiting for them at home. They can swap the non-vegan stuff for the vegan candy and pick exactly what they want.

Halloween might seem like it's about the candy, but it's also about the quest—the excitement of going from house to house and collecting the booty! It's about dressing up in exotic or scary costumes, and it's about being with friends and having fun. Try to put an emphasis on these things more than on the candy. Besides, these days Halloween parties seem to have replaced trick-or-treating, anyway, so you can also throw a fabulous costume party and serve up lots of vegan treats.

EASTER

Although Easter is a holy Christian holiday, it falls in the spring, a time of rejuvenation and renewal, with many symbols dominating the celebration, particularly the eggs of birds.

Growing up, I relished our family's annual egg-decorating ritual and the egg hunts that followed, but my fond memories have less to do with the eggs themselves and more to do with the fact that the whole family was together, we children were given license to be creative, and we participated in an exciting quest with all the neighborhood kids.

There are so many ways to celebrate the true meaning of this holiday—birth, renewal, rejuvenation—while creating a familiar, festive ritual without the chicken's eggs, which are themselves just symbols.

- Paint wooden eggs or leaves with a hole in the top to enable you to enjoy the artwork all year round or during the winter holidays, when they can be hung on the tree.

- Host an egg hunt using plastic eggs filled with goodies and wooden eggs your children decorated.

- Create a special Easter basket filled with daffodils, Easter lily bulbs, egg- or bunny-shaped cookies, carrot cake, chocolate bunnies and eggs, books and coloring books, stickers, and a stuffed animal.

- Plant an herb or vegetable garden. What better way to celebrate the cycles of life and rebirth?

PASSOVER

A Jewish holiday observed by most Jews, Passover (Pesach) commemorates their exodus out of Egypt, from slavery to freedom. A vegan Seder is not only traditional in its own right, but it more accurately reflects the principles of freedom and mercy that signify this holiday.

Matzoh

The most significant observance involves the removal of leavened foods and the serving of matzoh commemorating the fact that the Jews leaving Egypt did not have time to let their bread rise. Matzoh, unleavened bread made from flour and water, can be used as flour (for cookies and cakes), meal (for bread crumbs), farfel (a noodle or bread cube substitute), and full-sized matzohs (as bread). Matzoh is eaten three times during the Seder.

Seder Plate

The Seder plate is a special plate containing six symbolic foods used to retell the story of the exodus.

- Charoset, a mixture of fruit and ground nuts soaked in wine, represents the mortar used to cement bricks when the Jews were slaves in Egypt. (See recipe on page 257)

- Parsley, celery, or other green herbs dipped in salt water symbolize spring and new life, as well as the tears of the Jewish slaves.

- Freshly grated horseradish, sometimes mixed with cooked beets and sugar, symbolizes the harshness of slavery.

- Bitter herbs, such as the bitter-tasting roots of romaine lettuce, are also used to signify the bitterness of slavery.

- Jewish vegans replace the egg, a symbol of fertility and new creation, with a flower or roasted nuts. Some even use a miniature white egg-sized eggplant whose stem has been removed.

- Jewish vegans replace the shank bone, meant to symbolize the sacrificial lamb, and point out that even the Talmud explicitly allows for roasted beets to be used in its stead.

VALENTINE'S DAY

Valentine's Day also revolves around food, and for thousands of years many plant foods have been eaten for their aphrodisiac qualities, inspired by their sensory characteristics or even by their internal effects.

Some of the effects are strictly visual and can easily be incorporated into your menu. The color red, for instance, has always been associated with passion and can be found on Valentine's Day menus in the form of beets, cherries, and cranberries. The sensual pomegranate has long symbolized fertility, and the asparagus has been enjoyed as an aphrodisiac because of its (ahem!) shape.

Some aphrodisiacs are considered such because of their texture. Agave nectar, derived from a cactuslike plant, oozes a thick sweet syrup. The romantic effect of champagne has more to do with the bubbles than with the alcohol. And apricots, mangoes, peaches, and tomatoes (the last also known as "love apples") are on the list of sensual foods primarily for their built-in succulence.

Many foods cause real physical changes in the body, both positive and negative, making them either ideal for a romantic meal or destined to douse the fire. Choosing foods that keep the blood flowing to all of our organs is optimal, and plant foods do this in spades—some more than others, such as hot peppers and garlic. Meat and other animal products, on the other hand, constrict the blood vessels, decreasing blood flow and thus potentially decreasing the libido.

Turning up the heat—in terms of both temperature and spiciness—can have a powerful effect. My favorite romantic after-dinner elixir is Mexican hot chocolate, which simply entails adding chili powder to hot cocoa or melting chili-laced chocolate bars in almond milk. If you want to add even more chocolate decadence to your romance, check out the amazing fudge, brownies, cookies, and cocoa from Allison's Gourmet (www.allisonsgourmet.com).

The idea is to excite the senses, not overload or dull them. Overeating and excessive alcohol may leave you lethargic rather than libidinous, and even the most sensuous food or beverage can backfire if consumed in excess. To paraphrase Shakespeare: it may provoke and unprovoke; it may provoke the desire, but take away the performance.

NEW YEAR'S EVE

Depending on your religious and cultural heritage, the New Year is celebrated anytime between January and December and is often tied to the reaping of the harvest and the planting of new crops. Plant-based foods play a significant role in celebrations around the world. Many of the global traditions that ring in the New Year can be done vegan-style.

- In many cultures, it's the custom to conceal a token inside bread or a dessert, ensuring prosperity in the coming year to the one who finds it. Armenians bake a coin into their traditional flatbread, Italians hide a bean in their torta della befana, and Greeks serve vasilopita with a coin tucked inside. Scandinavians stir an almond into their rice pudding, while Mexicans hide a doll inside their king's cake, the recipient of which becomes king for the day.

- The Spanish good-luck ritual of eating twelve grapes at midnight—one each time the clock chimes—is shared by the people of Portugal, Mexico, and the Philippines. In Peru, the same custom is practiced, but a thirteenth grape is eaten for good measure.

- A water festival is a common New Year tradition in Thailand, Burma, Cambodia, and Laos. Symbolizing renewal, the water is often colored pink, red, or yellow to signify the hope for a "colorful future."

- Legumes serve as a symbol of good luck in many countries' festivities. In Italy, it's believed that eating lentils will bring good fortune all year long. Argentineans say that eating beans signifies that you will keep your job or find a better one. In the southern United States, black-eyed peas and turnip greens represent coins and dollars.

- Although the Buddhist custom of releasing captive animals in East and Southeast Asia is rarely practiced in modern times, it's a New Year ritual born out of compassion. In Poland, homemade animal-shaped breads symbolize good fortune and are given away as gifts to friends and family.

Also, many traditional foods served during the New Year celebrations are naturally vegan or can easily be made so. Incorporate them into your menu for an unforgettable way to ring in the New Year.

- Dolmas (stuffed grape leaves) from Armenia
- Marzipan ring cake from Denmark
- Baklava from Iran
- Zouni (vegetable soup), soba noodles, and mochi from Japan
- Bannock (oat cake) and whiskey from Scotland
- Kutya (boiled wheat with raisins and poppy seeds) from Ukraine
- Champagne from around the world

In reexamining our traditions, we will find that we can still celebrate what is important to us while remaining true to our values. We may also find joy in creating new traditions that everyone can take part in.

The recipes on the following pages include an entire menu for harvest holidays, such as Thanksgiving, as well as a traditional Passover dish called charoset. Other recipes featured throughout the various chapters, particularly the many salads, are particularly appropriate for the spring holidays.

Butternut Squash Risotto with Toasted Sage

SERVES 4 TO 6

Nothing says comfort more than a plate of creamy risotto. It requires a little attention on the stovetop, but it's worth every minute. And it's even better the next day!

7 cups vegetable broth
   or half water and half broth
2½–3 cups butternut squash (about
   1 medium), peeled and cut into
   1-inch cubes
2 tablespoons olive oil
2 tablespoons minced garlic
2 tablespoons minced fresh sage

2 cups arborio rice
½ cup white wine (optional)
Salt and freshly ground black pepper
   to taste
Fresh flat-leaf parsley or sage for
   garnish, minced

Add the broth to a large saucepan, adjusting the heat to maintain a gentle simmer. Add the squash and allow it to cook in the simmering broth. The squash is done when easily pierced with a fork; do not overcook or it will be mushy.

(Alternatively, you could just heat the broth up on its own and roast or steam the squash separately. The main idea is to have the squash cooked before adding it to the rice.)

Warm the olive oil in a large sauté pan over medium-low heat. Add the garlic and sage and sauté for a few minutes until the garlic turns golden brown.

Add the rice to the pan (do not rinse the rice first), and stir until the rice is less opaque, about 3 minutes. Add the white wine, if using, and cook until it evaporates, just a few minutes.

Add about 1 cup of the simmering broth to the rice (without adding the squash), and stir until the broth is absorbed. Continue to add broth, one ladleful at a time, until the rice kernels are al dente in the center and creamy on the outside, 20–25 minutes in all.

Finally, when the broth is almost gone from the original saucepan and the rice is the perfect texture, add the cooked squash to the rice along with the last addition of broth.

Add salt and pepper to taste, sprinkle some parsley or sage on top, and serve right away.

Wheat-free

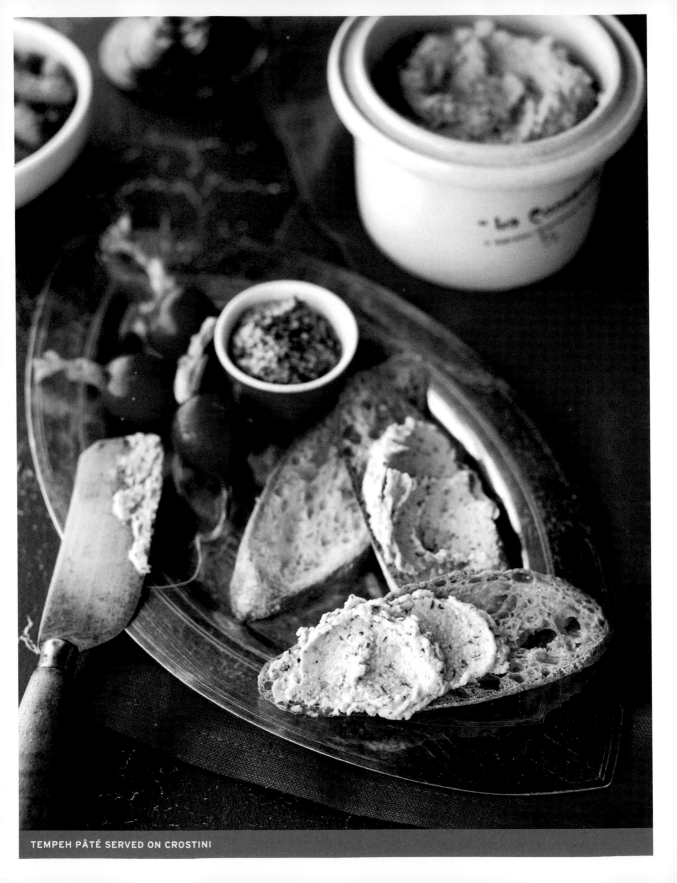

TEMPEH PÂTÉ SERVED ON CROSTINI

Tempeh Pâté

YIELD: 1¾ CUP

Though people often think of duck or goose livers when they think of pâté, the definition is much broader (and kinder) than that: *pâté* simply means "paste" in French. Our use of steamed tempeh provides the perfect texture for a delicious spread—without harming anyone in the meantime.

One 8-ounce package tempeh
½ cup eggless mayonnaise, or more
   to taste
½ cup finely chopped green onions

¼ cup finely chopped fresh dill
½ teaspoon minced fresh ginger
2-4 tablespoons tamari soy sauce

Break the tempeh up and add to steamer basket. Steam for 10 minutes, until its nutty aroma fills the air and it turns a lighter color. Transfer to a bowl and let cool.

Add the steamed tempeh to a food processor and process until it is pastelike. Add the mayonnaise, green onions, dill, ginger, and just 2 tablespoons of the tamari. Mix well. Taste and add additional tamari or mayo, as needed. Serve on crackers or crostini.

Wheat-free

TIP:

The fresh dill is the secret weapon in this recipe. Dried dill will not be an adequate substitute.

Mushroom Gravy

YIELD: 3 CUPS

Perfect for mashed potatoes, stuffed squash, or biscuits and gravy. Puree it to make a smooth, creamy concoction, or leave it chunky. As the latter, this gravy is fantastic as a side dish, served over quinoa, or as a topping for Salisbury tofu or tempeh.

2 teaspoons nonhydrogenated, nondairy butter, such as Earth Balance
1 yellow onion, chopped
1 pound cremini mushrooms (about 20 mushrooms), thinly sliced

2 cups vegetable stock
3 tablespoons flour or other thickener such as cornstarch or arrowroot
2-3 tablespoons tamari soy sauce
1/2 teaspoon dried thyme
Freshly ground black pepper

Heat the butter in a large skillet and sauté the onion over medium-high heat, stirring frequently, until the onions begin to turn translucent, about 5 minutes. Add the mushrooms and cook for about 5 minutes more, until they soften and turn golden brown.

In the meantime, in a separate bowl, whisk the flour into the stock along with the tamari, thyme, and black pepper. When there appear to be no lumps, add it to the onion mixture and cook over medium-low heat, stirring constantly until thickened, 5-10 minutes.

For smooth gravy, puree it in a blender or food processor. You may want to play a little with the flavor and add more tamari or pepper to taste. Reheat the mixture if necessary on low heat in a saucepan.

Wheat-free, if using cornstarch as thickener

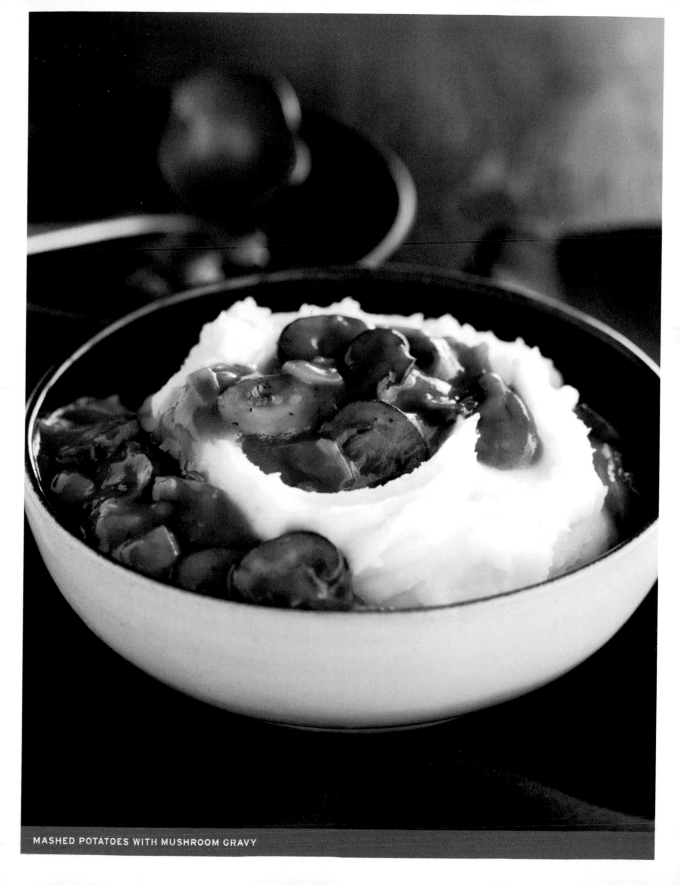

MASHED POTATOES WITH MUSHROOM GRAVY

Harvest-Stuffed Acorn Squash

MAKES 8 SERVINGS

The foundation of this attractive dish is antioxidant-rich fruits and vegetables, whole grains, and nuts. The earthy colors make for a beautiful autumn dinner centerpiece.

4 acorn squash, halved lengthwise,
   seeds and membrane removed
2 medium yellow onions, chopped
1 tablespoon olive oil
4 stalks celery, diced
2 cups cooked brown rice (cooked with
   a veggie bouillon cube for flavor)
1 cup toasted pecans, coarsely chopped
   (or walnuts, almonds, or chestnuts)

½ cup dried diced apricots and/or raisins
1 teaspoon ground ginger
1 teaspoon ground cinnamon
½ teaspoon ground cardamom
½ teaspoon salt or to taste
Freshly ground pepper to taste

Preheat the oven to 375 degrees.

Place the squash halves, cut side down, onto one or two nonstick cookie or baking sheets. There is no need to oil the squash. Bake for 30 minutes. The squash may not be fully fork-tender, but it will eventually be returned to the oven to cook all the way through.

Meanwhile, in a sauté pan, cook the onion in olive oil until it becomes transparent. Add the celery and sauté a couple of minutes. Remove from heat and add to a large mixing bowl, along with the cooked rice, pecans, apricots and/or raisins, ginger, cinnamon, cardamom, salt, and pepper. Adjust seasonings as necessary.

Remove the squash from the oven, spoon out some of the cooked squash, and combine this squash flesh with the rest of the ingredients. Be sure to scrape only a little; you want to leave some squash in the shells, too.

Press the rice mixture into each squash cavity, mounding the rice as much as possible. (Depending on how large the squash are, you may end up with some leftover rice mixture, which makes a great side dish by itself.)

Cover with aluminum foil and bake for 30 minutes or until squash flesh is thoroughly tender. Remove the foil for the last 10 minutes of baking.

Wheat-free, soy-free

Roasted Brussels Sprouts with Caramelized Onions and Toasted Pistachios

SERVES 4 TO 6

The combination of the roasted Brussels sprouts, the sweet onions, and the toasted pistachios puts this dish over the top in terms of flavor. These are a great side dish for a Thanksgiving feast or any fall dinner.

1½ pounds (about 40) Brussels sprouts, ends trimmed and sprouts cut in half if large
3 tablespoons olive oil
½ teaspoon salt
½ teaspoon freshly ground black pepper
2 tablespoons nonhydrogenated, nondairy butter, such as Earth Balance

4 small-medium yellow onions, thinly sliced
1 teaspoon sugar
½ cup pistachios

Preheat the oven to 425 degrees.

Place the Brussels sprouts, olive oil, salt, and pepper in a large bowl. Toss to coat. Pour onto a baking sheet and place on the center oven rack.

Roast in the oven for anywhere from 20 to 40 minutes, shaking the pan every several minutes for even browning. The Brussels sprouts should be dark brown when done.

Meanwhile, in a large skillet or sauté pan, melt the nondairy butter over medium-low heat. Add the onions and sugar; cook, stirring occasionally, until the onions turn dark golden brown and are caramelized, about 30 minutes.

While the onions and Brussels sprouts are cooking, toast the pistachios in a 200 degree toaster oven for 4 minutes. Let cool, and coarsely chop.

When the onions and Brussels sprouts are done cooking, toss them together, along with the toasted pistachios. Serve hot or at room temperature in a pretty serving bowl.

Variation
Use toasted pecans or walnuts instead of pistachios.

Wheat-free, soy-free

Apple Cobbler

YIELD: 6 TO 8 SERVINGS

Cobblers may very well be my favorite type of dessert. They're so easy to make, and so many different options are available, depending on the season and your fruit preference.

Filling

5 cups tart apples, peeled and sliced
¾ cup granulated sugar
2 tablespoons unbleached all-purpose flour

½ teaspoon cinnamon
¼ teaspoon salt
1 teaspoon vanilla extract
¼ cup water

Cobbler Biscuit Dough

1⅓ cups unbleached all-purpose flour
2 tablespoons sugar
1½ teaspoons baking powder
½ teaspoon salt
5 tablespoons nonhydrogenated, nondairy butter, melted

½ cup nondairy milk
1-2 tablespoons nondairy milk or melted nondairy butter
1 tablespoon sugar

Preheat the oven to 375 degrees. Have ready an ungreased 9-inch-square baking pan at least 2 inches deep.

In a large bowl, combine the apples with the sugar, flour, cinnamon, salt, vanilla, and water. Spread evenly in the prepared baking dish and set aside.

Prepare the cobbler dough. Thoroughly combine the flour, sugar, baking powder, and salt. Add 5 tablespoons melted butter and ½ cup milk. Stir just until you form a sticky dough.

Using a tablespoon, scoop the dough over the fruit. Either leave the dough in shapeless blobs on the fruit or spread it out. There will be just enough to cover the fruit. Brush the top of the dough with the remaining 1-2 tablespoons of milk or butter and sprinkle with the 1 tablespoon of sugar. Bake until the top is golden brown and the juices have thickened slightly, about 35-40 minutes. Let cool for 15 minutes before serving.

Charoset

YIELD: 8 CUPS CHUNKY OR 4 CUPS FINE

Also called charoses or haroset, this is an integral part of every Passover Seder. An Eastern European recipe mixing apples, almonds, spices, and red wine, Charoset can also include a variety of other ingredients native to their area, including bananas, apricots, coconut, oranges, dates, exotic nuts, and a wide variety of spices.

6 apples, chopped (unpeeled for optimal nutrition)
1 cup raisins
¾ cup chopped toasted almonds
Freshly grated zest of one large orange
3 tablespoons freshly squeezed orange juice

3 tablespoons sugar or agave nectar
2 tablespoons red wine
1 teaspoon ground cinnamon
Pinch ground ginger

Mix together all of the ingredients. For a coarse, chunky mixture, simply refrigerate until ready to serve. For a smoother, more "mortarlike" mixture, blend very well by hand, or pulse in a food processor or blender. Chill until ready to serve, or serve at room temperature. Don't refrigerate for more than 2 hours before serving, or the charoset will become too wet.

DID YOU KNOW?

The color and texture of charoset are meant to recall the mortar with which the Israelites bonded bricks when they were enslaved in ancient Egypt. The word comes from the Hebrew word *cheres*, which means "clay."

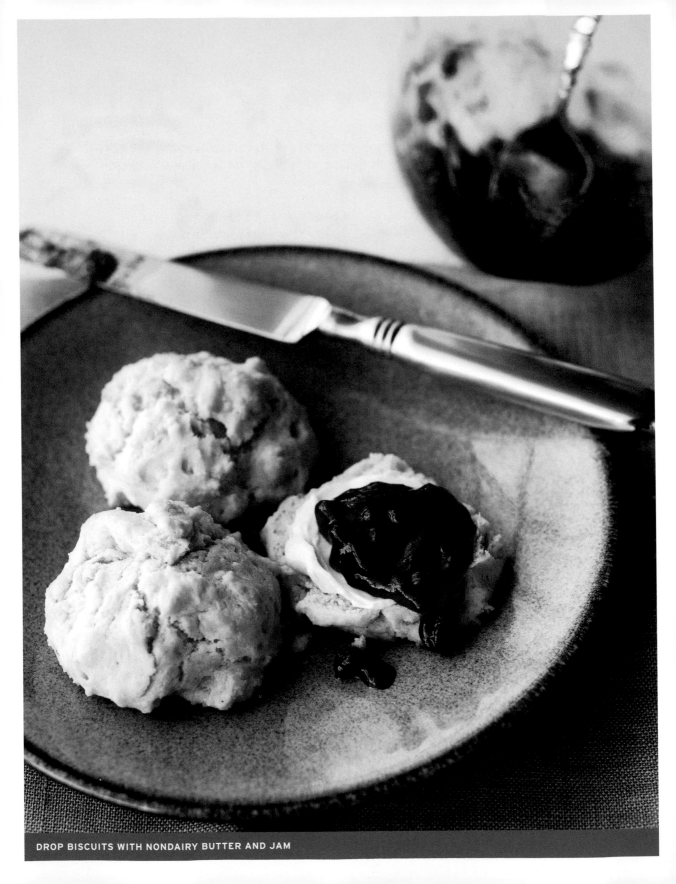

DROP BISCUITS WITH NONDAIRY BUTTER AND JAM

Drop Biscuits

YIELD: 12 BISCUITS

Perfect as the topping for fruit cobblers or as an accompaniment to soup, these biscuits are also delicious with gravy or doused with fruit compote. Alternatively, they are simply divine with some nondairy butter and fruit preserves. No need for a commercial biscuit mix; the preparation is 5 minutes.

$1^2/_3$ cups unbleached all-purpose flour
1 tablespoon baking powder
$1/_2$ teaspoon salt

$2/_3$ cup nondairy milk
$1/_3$ cup canola oil or melted
    nonhydrogenated, nondairy butter

Preheat the oven to 475 degrees. Lightly grease a baking or cookie sheet.

In a large bowl, mix together the flour, baking powder, and salt until combined. Add the milk and oil and stir just until the dry ingredients are moistened. It will be very sticky and thick, not smooth like cake batter. Scoop 2 tablespoons of batter onto the cookie sheet for each biscuit, spacing the biscuits about $1^1/_2$ inches apart.

Bake until the bottoms are golden brown, about 8 minutes. Serve hot.

Variations
Add any of the following for more flavorful biscuits:
- Melted nondairy butter instead of canola oil for a buttery flavor
- Sun-dried tomatoes: 5-6 tablespoons finely chopped
- Chives: $1/_4$ cup snipped fresh
- Rosemary: 1 teaspoon minced fresh or $1/_2$ teaspoon dried and crumbled
- Chili peppers: $1/_4$ to $1/_3$ cup drained canned diced chili pepper

DAY 26 Finding Harmony Living in a Mixed Household

In an early chapter preparing you for the 30-Day Vegan Challenge, I encouraged you to ask the people you live with to take the Challenge with you in order to make the experience more enjoyable. Even if they didn't join you, you may find that your partner, parent, or children are supportive of your changes, making the process a lot less challenging for you.

Not everyone has this experience, however, and new vegans are often surprised by how their own changes cause waves in an otherwise calm sea. Some non-vegan family members may be critical, resistant, or even hostile to your new way of eating. Understanding the reasons for their reaction will do wonders for your peace of mind and the ease of your journey.

CHALLENGE YOUR THINKING: Though we may have become awakened to our own compassion or had a revelation about our health, it doesn't mean everyone around us has had the same experience.

CHANGE YOUR BEHAVIOR: As much as we want our loved ones to be understanding and compassionate about our new lifestyle, we have to offer them the same understanding and compassion.

YOUR JOURNEY MAY NOT BE THEIR JOURNEY

You may have come to this Challenge because you have health issues you heard could be helped by a plant-based diet, you may have decided you didn't want to contribute to violence toward animals, or you may have become inspired by the desire to use fewer of the Earth's resources. By the time you arrived at this place, you most likely read, processed, and internalized a lot of information. When you picked up this book, you may already have decided to create some new habits. With conviction and zeal, you declared this to your family members and became disappointed by their less-than-stellar reaction.

We have to remember that even though we may have become awakened to our own compassion or had a revelation about our health, it doesn't mean everyone around us has had the same experience. Even though we may feel completely changed, we cannot forget to look at how our changes may affect our loved ones. As much as we want them to be understanding and compassionate, we have to offer to them the same compassion and understanding.

They may not have gone through the same process as you, read the same books, or watched the same videos. In fact, they may not be willing to. But demanding that they understand the transformation you've experienced or calling them closed-minded for not being supportive is ineffective and unfair. Just as you've taken the time to adjust to your new way of seeing the world, you have to honor the transition of the people with whom you share your life. That doesn't mean you should squelch your newfound enthusiasm; it just means you need to understand that not everyone around you may share it, at least right now.

Navigating these tricky waters requires a little patience, a dash of psychology, and a lot of really good food, no matter how old you are or what your living situation is.

VEGAN TWEENS AND TEENS LIVING WITH NON-VEGAN PARENTS

Part of becoming an adult means trying to see someone else's perspective, and I always encourage new teen vegans to put themselves in their parents' shoes in order to understand why they may react with panic when they learn their child wants to be vegan.

Frankly, no matter what your age, parents need time to adjust to your new lifestyle. Like all of us, they're creatures of habit and most likely have been cooking the same thing for you day after day, year after year. They've gone through your picky phases, they've cut the crusts off your bread, they've made special meals to accommodate your preferences. Now you tell them that's all going to change—and you wonder why they react so emotionally. Let them have their reaction, and remember that it has nothing to do with *you*.

On one hand, they're probably freaking out because they have no idea what to feed you. If they've been making your favorite meals for years, they're not exactly going to be enthusiastic about changing the repertoire.

On the other hand, though, I think one of the reasons parents take it so personally is because they've used food from the day we were born as a way to express their love for us, to nurture us, and to be close to us. When we reject the food they've chosen to feed us, it may feel like we're rejecting *them* and their affections. They may defensively ask, "What's wrong with the way I've raised you? You always loved what I fed you!" as if our decision to be vegan is a judgment of their parenting skills.

Tell them you understand how different this must be for them and how much you appreciate all the years they've spent feeding you and buying your favorite foods. Tell them this is not just another temporary fad; tell them why this means so much to you. Show them that you're serious. Be consistent. Tell them you need their support and that you're willing to help make it easier.

And then help make it easier.

It would be utterly unfair to expect Mom or Dad—or whoever does the cooking—to change instantly. You absolutely need to take responsibility for your decision and help cook. Not only will this take the burden off them and begin to hone your own cooking skills, but it will also show them how delicious and nutritious your new lifestyle is. I've never seen it fail. Even parents who were the most resistant in the beginning eventually come around and wind up being inspired and influenced, many becoming vegan themselves. I'm not saying that should be your expectation, but I've seen many parents change because their teenager changed first. Whatever the outcome, I can assure you they will respond differently given some time.

To help with the process:

- Sit down with your parents and write down all the dishes you all eat on a regular basis. Show them how you can veganize the family favorites.

- Look through cookbooks together and pick out recipes you'd like to try.

- Shop with them. Participate.

Beyond food, your parents are probably genuinely concerned that you're not going to get all the nutrients a growing person needs. Help alleviate their fears. Show them the chapters in this book on protein, calcium, iron, omega-3 fatty acids, and vitamin B_{12}. Read them the American Dietetic Association's position paper on vegetarianism; show them—by eating your vegetables—that you're not a junk-food vegan. You can't expect them to support you if all you eat is potato chips. Vegan? Yes. Healthful? No.

The goal is to find solutions together and not let it become a power struggle between vegan teenager and non-vegan parent.

VEGAN PARENTS OF NON-VEGAN CHILDREN

Teenagers aren't the only family members who bring veganism home. Often one or both parents make dietary changes that inevitably affect the entire family. Your children and teens may already be joining you in this Challenge, but they also might be resisting. The difference may have to do with how old they are.

There's no doubt that it's more difficult to change the food habits you instilled in your children, but that's not to say it can't be done. Communication, consistency, and confidence are essential ingredients.

I say "confidence" because I've often heard people criticize parents for raising their children vegan, accusing them of imposing their values on their children.

Balderdash! Parents impose their values on their children all the time. It's called parenting. So if transitioning your children from an animal-based diet to a plant-based one is what you feel is best for yourself and your family, be confident in your decision. There's nothing wrong with raising your children in such a way that reflects the values you've most likely taught them: compassion, kindness, empathy, and wellness.

I believe we come into this world fully compassionate, and the best gift we can give our children is to honor the compassion they have for animals by encouraging them to make choices that are aligned with these values. After all, we try to keep images of animal cruelty and suffering from children for a reason, so why would we go behind their backs and support the very thing they would (and we do) find anathema? Why should we pay other people to do to animals what we could never do and what children (and adults) are traumatized by when they do witness it?

CHALLENGE YOUR THINKING: Children raised to eat meat, dairy, and eggs are not given a choice. Parents raising vegan children are no different from parents raising non-vegan children in that they are instilling *their* values in their children. It's called parenting.

CHANGE YOUR BEHAVIOR: Honor the empathy children have for animals by encouraging them to make choices that are aligned with the values *you're* teaching them: compassion, kindness, and wellness.

Don't underestimate the compassion in your children. When they begin to understand that their new way of eating means animals will be helped, *they get it*. The actual transition process may be bumpy at first as they learn how to navigate in this new world, but as they internalize the lessons you're teaching them, it will become easier, and it will become their own.

In terms of health, I think the most compelling research coming out about what we eat and how well we live is that which indicates that not only do food habits instilled as children dictate how we eat as adults but that food choices made as children are strong predictors of disease later in life. In other words, what children eat during their formative years has a profound impact on their future health, and since American children eat so few whole plant sources, there is *much* room for improvement.

As you discuss with your children the benefits of eating their veggies—for everyone involved—you can start changing their meals, and this is where vegan versions of their familiar foods will be helpful.

- Instead of animal-based hot dogs and hamburgers, give them veggie dogs and veggie burgers.

- If they're accustomed to cow's milk in their cereal, gradually reduce it by a quarter, then half, until you're using 100 percent plant-based milk. Do the same if they eat yogurt, ice cream, sour cream, or cream cheese.

- Make or buy other vegan versions of their favorite foods, but don't make a big to-do about the new food. They may turn their nose up at it just because it's new. Over time, you can casually tell them they're eating the cruelty-free versions.

VEGAN, LIVING WITH A DIE-HARD MEAT-EATER

I've heard from a lot of vegan women over the years who lament that their husbands, riddled with health issues that could very well be improved or solved by eating a plant-based diet, fight tooth and nail when it comes to making any changes. This tends to cause understandable friction—the wife pleading with her husband to change, the husband insisting that he's just fine the way he is. Nobody wins, and everyone is miserable.

Keep in mind that some people may not want information about eating differently *because* it comes from you. I think family members can be the hardest to reach because of all the other underlying dynamics that are already built in. Sometimes it's much easier to receive information from strangers.

CHALLENGE YOUR THINKING: Sometimes family members may not want information about veganism *because* it comes from you. Sometimes it's easier for them to receive information from strangers.

CHANGE YOUR BEHAVIOR: Guide loved ones to resources, but try to remain detached from the outcome. Know that you have planted seeds, whose germination is not your business.

Certainly there's nothing wrong with directing them to resources (such as *The 30-Day Vegan Challenge*), but it's important to do so and then remain unattached to the outcome. Note the difference between "You should read this" and "Some things you said recently indicated that you might be interested in this. I'll leave it here in case you want to read it."

Also, when you're concerned about someone's health, communicate openly from your heart. Telling your husband (or wife) that you're genuinely concerned, that you love him and are scared to lose him, will go much farther than nagging about how unhealthful his diet is. Be sure to tell him that you cannot condone what you perceive as harmful behavior but that you won't hassle him about it anymore. And then be true to your word.

Planting seeds is a much more effective way of inspiring people than knocking them over the head.

I also hear from a lot of newly vegan women—who are still the primary cooks in most families—who feel obligated to continue cooking for their husband all the animal products he insists on eating. Add fussy kids or teens to the mix, and she winds up making two or three different meals every night for dinner. When did home kitchens become restaurants?

I absolutely do not advocate that people make more than one meal for their meat-, dairy-, and egg-eating family members. If you're the cook in the family and the expectation has always been that the rest of the family eats what you create, then that applies in this situation, too. If your family members feel they need to eat meat at every meal, then they can cook it themselves. If they eat outside the home for lunch, then they can get whatever they want at that time. But at dinner, if you're in charge of the meals, then *you* decide what's on the menu, and this also includes vegan variations of their favorite meals. If you live in a home that has meat in the house, and family members want to cook it themselves, then that's a compromise you'll have to decide on, but the point is not to become a short-order cook in your own kitchen.

After all, the surest way to inspire people to *eat* delicious plant-based food is to *make* delicious plant-based food. "If it tastes good, they will eat it" is my motto. If people eat food they find satisfying, filling, familiar, and tasty, they won't care if it has no animals in it.

The bottom line is that the joy you feel making compassionate, healthful choices will be a magnet to those around you. Your enthusiasm will be contagious and will arouse curiosity and interest, and the food will seal the deal.

Family gatherings, children's birthday parties, and school events tend to revolve around food, and vegan parents naturally want to make sure their children aren't left out. With a little forethought and preparation, this need not be a problem at all.

PREPARING FOR PARTIES

Depending on the event, you can always prepare something special for your child, or just ask the host if you can bring something to share with everyone. If your kids had a food allergy, you'd have no problem doing this, so why should it be any different when it comes to your family's vegan food choices?

Also, my vegan friends who have kids teach them that it's okay for them not to have what everyone else is having all the time. Even though it won't always be "equal" for them in terms of food options, they emphasize that they don't always have to have some sugary dessert in order to celebrate someone's birthday.

VEGAN KIDS IN THE CLASSROOM

I know some brilliant vegan parents who prepare at the beginning of the school year, first by making sure the teacher knows their children are vegan, and next by packing a bag of nonperishable treats that are kept in the classroom, replenishing the supply as needed. Whenever another student brings in non-vegan cupcakes or treats, the teacher gifts my friends' children with their own special treats from their vegan goodie bag. These kids have yet to feel awkward or left out when these sorts of celebrations happen at school.

The other option—depending on how much time you want to invest—is to whip up a batch of vegan cupcakes to have your child bring to the school when you know there is a birthday being celebrated.

Though it may seem daunting at first, I assure you that in time it gets easier. Family and friends ultimately want to make sure your children are included in celebrations and will often make sure there is something vegan for them to eat. Just give them time to come around, while being clear and consistent about your family's dietary choices.

DAY 27 Dealing with Changes

With the 30 days almost up, you're no doubt experiencing some changes, be they physical, mental, emotional, or spiritual. You may be noticing that this is a very gratifying and powerful way to live—choosing health and compassion over convenience and habit. I have witnessed thousands of people go through this transition and know that even as they feel more grounded, more energetic, and more joyful, they are often quite overwhelmed by how profound these transformations are. Some changes people experience are purely physiological, both the changes that take place in terms of cholesterol, blood pressure, and blood glucose—and also changes you can feel and see. Other changes people experience are less tangible.

Let's talk about some specific changes you might be experiencing and what to do about them, if anything at all. Simply getting validation that the changes are real and that you're not alone may be helpful enough.

PHYSICAL CHANGES

Consuming All That Fiber

Because there is no fiber in meat, dairy, eggs, or any animal product, many people are eating a very low-fiber diet. When you initially increase your intake of plant foods—and thus fiber—you may experience some discomfort. However, once your body adjusts, it's not really a problem for most people. In the beginning, if you feel you need to take in fewer high-fiber foods, you can still do so without adding animal products back into your diet. There are lower-fiber plant foods you can try, such as white rice instead of brown, bagels, pastas, crackers, tofu, nondairy yogurt, tomato sauce, pizza, fruit juices (with no pulp), applesauce, and bananas. As you get more comfortable—and you will—you can continue adding more fiber-rich foods into your diet, such as those in "Day 22: Keeping Things Moving with Fiber."

The Power of Fiber

Unlike the soluble fiber that helps to reduce cholesterol and stabilize blood sugar, insoluble fiber is the plant roughage that stays intact and helps push everything through and out of our bodies, manifesting in more trips to the bathroom. Some people get nervous about this, but I assure you it's not only normal, it's optimal. The average non-vegan has suboptimal fiber intakes, which contributes to less frequent bowel movements and constipation, marked by hard, dry, hard-to-pass stool. So, even though you may be surprised by the new sensations in your colon or by the change in your stool from hard pellets to a softer final product, you can celebrate the fact that this is contributing to a reduced risk of colon disease and cancer.

Discomforting Beans

It's the sugar molecules—called oligosaccharides—in beans that people have a hard time digesting, resulting in gas, cramping, or bloating. Rather than avoiding eating these incredibly healthful legumes, there are a number of things you can do if beans are giving you trouble.

- Gradually increase your intake of beans. Counterintuitive though it may seem, the more your body becomes adjusted to these oligosaccharides, the easier it is for it to digest them. Throw a few on a salad or into a soup, and slowly begin to eat more concentrated bean dishes.

- Eat more canned beans than beans made from scratch. In canned beans, the sugars have been aggressively cooked out, and the beans have been rinsed really well, making these oligosaccharides less prevalent.

- If you cook beans from scratch, do not cook the beans in the same water you soaked them in. Also, try adding a piece of kombu seaweed in with the beans while they're cooking, or add a little white vinegar to the beans just after they're cooked.

- People tend to do better with lentils than with the larger beans. Give that a try and see if it helps.

- Some species of a particular mold produce an anti-oligosaccharide enzyme, which facilitates digestion of oligosaccharides in the small intestine. This enzyme is currently sold in the United States under the brand name Beano. By taking this enzyme at the same time you begin to eat the beans, there's a very good chance that you won't experience the gas and bloating. However, the only problem with Beano is that it uses gelatin to make its capsule. Fret not. A vegan version called Bean-zyme is available in health food stores, large natural grocery stores, and online.

Reduced Premenstrual Symptoms

Hormones thrive on fat, so when you reduce your consumption of dietary fat—which happens naturally when you eliminate meat, dairy, and eggs—you may find that you have a shorter menstrual period, less bleeding, less cramping, and a more regular cycle. Women going through menopause may also experience fewer symptoms, and postmenopausal women may find they no longer need synthetic hormones (check with your doctor). To be sure, these are all positive changes, but they're worth mentioning here in case you've noticed these changes and were wondering if they were normal.

Cravings

When we eliminate animal flesh and secretions from our diet and experience what we call physical cravings, we are most likely craving fat and salt. Just as with any substance we have been habitually putting in our bodies, we will no doubt go through some withdrawal when it's removed. After some time has passed—30 days is often enough—your body and palate will have altered enough that you stop craving the heavy, fat- and salt-laden foods you once ate with abandon. Emotionally, you may be craving familiarity; don't underestimate its power. See "Day 12: Discovering That There *Is* Life After Cheese" for how to fulfill the true desire through healthy, compassionate means.

The Vegan Glow

When you eat a large amount of beta-carotene-rich foods, you may notice your skin begin to take on an orange glow. There is nothing wrong with this. However, if you want to tone down the tint, you can still eat carotenoid-rich foods that aren't orange. (To put it in perspective, 1 medium carrot contains 330 percent of your Daily Value of vitamin A; 1 cup of raw spinach contains 75 percent.)

There is another glow I've seen in many vegans, which is the light that emanates from within. Many talk about a sense of peace and calm that comes from aligning their values with their behavior, and it shines through their skin and their eyes. This is obviously not a problem to solve. Embrace it.

EMOTIONAL CHANGES

Anger

The stereotype of the "angry vegan" is well known, and though it is indeed a stereotype, there is no doubt that people feel anger once they learn about the heinous abuses committed against animals. And whereas many people feel a sense of peace at no longer participating in and paying for these abuses to take place, the awareness of so much cruelty and suffering can also have a devastating effect on our psyches, and the result is sometimes anger. And why shouldn't people be angry? Human greed and the desire for convenience and pleasure drive the socially sanctioned use and abuse of billions of nonhuman animals. We live in a world where it's considered normal to champion this and radical to oppose it.

Whenever we meet someone who's vegan, it seems to be a natural response to ask them *why* they're vegan—whether it's for health or ethical reasons—and I think we react differently depending on the answer. If we're told it's for health reasons, I think we tacitly applaud the person for doing something beneficial for themselves, but if we're told it's for ethical reasons, I think it makes us feel threatened or judged because a mirror is held up that forces us to look at our own ethics and choices.

Frankly, I think most vegans will tell you that though there may have been one thing that sparked their desire to be vegan, they remain so for a number of reasons.

I think one of the most pervasive myths that shapes people's perception about being vegan—and which I hope I've debunked by this point in the Challenge—is that it's about limitation and restriction. And yet, ironically, many people freely embrace a willingness to *limit* knowledge and *restrict* their awareness when they resist learning about how animals are bred, kept, and killed for human consumption. "Don't tell me about how the animals are treated," they say. "I don't want to know. I don't want to see. I don't want to look."

Personally, I don't believe that people who avoid looking are insensitive to animal suffering; I believe they're *so* sensitive to it that it makes them close their eyes and subsequently their hearts. The very idea that animals suffer is so anathema to them, so difficult to confront—particularly if they're still eating them—that it's easier not to go there at all.

And yet, on a very personal level, every time we say, "Don't tell me. I don't want to know," we limit the potential for growth, for change, for making possible everything we want to be and everything we want this world to be. So we walk around with blinders on, complacent in our comfort zones because we're afraid to look, afraid to know, afraid to change. To me, *that's* limiting. *That's* restrictive. On the contrary, being vegan is about being willing to know, willing to explore, willing to experience what is painful but true. Being vegan is about evolving, participating, and taking responsibility.

Animal suffering is methodically and purposefully hidden from view in our society, because the animal exploitation industries know that the public is outraged and offended whenever they see the truth about what the animals endure. The worst thing we can do to the perpetrators and the best thing we can do for the animals is to bear witness to the abuses. Awareness is the greatest weapon against violence. Of course looking at the truth can be painful, but it's what many of us need to knock ourselves into consciousness and become part of the solution.

If you feel that watching something will hinder you rather than energize you, then be true to yourself. Learn where your line is and be honest, but don't be so afraid of feeling sad that you avoid what is also a very human emotion. Being human, after all, is about embracing joy as well as sadness and anger.

Please visit "Resources and Recommendations" at the back of this book for a list of my favorite books and videos for further reading and viewing.

Of course people are angry. But *anger* is not a dirty word. It is a very real response whose roots go deep. It's what we do with anger that will make or break us.

I think it's very helpful to know that the root of the word *anger* means "sorrow" or "anguish." The earliest roots of the word *anger* referred to something being "painfully constricted," a "strangling, narrowing, squeezing, throttling." And it's anguish that we feel when we learn what happens to animals. If we reframe anger so we see it in its proper context, we can recognize that there isn't a contradiction between the peace that comes with eating nonviolently and the anger we feel in the face of so much cruelty. The key is transforming anger into action. It's easy to become cynical, disheartened, and hopeless, but that doesn't do anyone any good. The key is in becoming active and staying hopeful.

Change Is Change
Even when it's incredibly positive, change is still change, and many people find it very difficult to deal with. There's a reason we're so habit-oriented. We feel comforted by our habitual routines and choices. They add order and familiarity to our lives, which is why some people resist change—even when it can save their lives. In fact, our society is set up to *discourage* change. Instead of being taught to change poor habits, we're given Band-Aids to simply cover them up; we romanticize, ritualize, and justify harmful behavior just so we don't have to do anything about it.

I hope that once you realize that change is not so scary, you will feel empowered to continue. You start exercising muscles you never knew you had, and you begin to know yourself a little better. That alone is a reward, even though there is so much more.

DAY 28 Achieving and Sustaining Weight Loss

Among the changes people experience when they become vegan (see "Day 27: Dealing with Changes"), weight loss tends to be one of them. Although this isn't a guarantee, many people effortlessly lose weight because plants are much less calorie-dense than animal flesh and secretions. The research bears this out, indicating that people who eat a plant-based diet have a lower percentage of body fat and are less likely to be overweight or obese than people who eat animals.

The main reason for this is fat. Remember the basics behind macronutrients and calories? There are:

- 4 calories in 1 gram of protein
- 4 calories in 1 gram of carbohydrates
- 9 calories in 1 gram of fat

Most non-vegans' fat consumption comes from animal products—meat, dairy, and eggs—and though there is indeed fat in plant foods, there is generally much less than in animal products. As a result, on a plant-based diet, you tend to consume fewer calories without much effort. And everyone knows that eating fewer calories leads to weight loss.

When you burn more calories than you consume, you experience weight loss, so if you want to lose weight, you need to do one of two things: take in fewer calories or burn more calories. (Or do both at the same time.) If weight loss is your goal, it is a simple numbers game. Weight loss is all about decreasing your energy intake and increasing your calorie output so that you end up with a calorie deficit at the end of the day. Here's how it works.

One pound of body fat is equivalent to 3,500 calories. Let's say your goal is to lose 10 pounds in 10 weeks (70 days). You must *burn* 35,000 more calories than you consume during that period. Breaking it down, that amounts to an average daily deficit of 500 calories (35,000 calories divided by 70 days). You can do that either by eating 500 fewer calories a day or by burning 500 additional calories a day. (Or eating 250 fewer and burning 250 more.) If you want to speed up the weight loss, you can eat 500 fewer calories *and* burn 500 additional calories for a daily deficit of 1,000 calories, dropping the 10 pounds in 5 weeks instead of 10. You can have a lot of fun just deciding how you want to achieve this deficit. (Yes, I just said weight loss can be fun.)

CALORIE REDUCTION

Let's talk first about reducing the number of calories taken in. As I said, this may happen very naturally for you within these 30 days, but what I hope you realize is that *eating fewer calories does not necessarily mean eating less food*. We are talking not about a diet here but rather about a mathematical principle. Essentially, you can eat more and weigh less because a plant-based diet enables you to eat *more* food in terms of volume yet take in fewer calories.

It's true that there are fewer calories in plant foods because there is less fat in plant foods, but if weight loss is your goal, you'll want to have a smaller ratio of higher-fat plant foods such as avocados, nuts, and seeds. You'll also want to limit or eliminate deep-fried foods and empty-calorie snack foods, which is a good thing, because instead you'll be filling your body with high-nutrient plant foods.

THE COST OF CALORIES

In fact, what if we learned to reduce the calories we take in so we could experience weight loss in a joyful, empowering way? Think of it this way. There are inherent costs associated with what we eat: monetary costs, environmental costs, health costs, the costs to our values, the cost to the animals, and so on. There is also the cost of calories. Each time we eat, we either make an investment in or a withdrawal from our health and well-being.

The idea is this: choose the number of calories you want to spend (that is, take in) throughout each day, but choose to spend them as effectively as possible, spending calories that are nutrient-dense rather than empty. (We get empty calories from foods that are calorie-rich but nutrient-poor.) The goal is to make sure that every calorie we spend (i.e., *take in*) goes toward giving us the best bang for our calorie buck. We want the calories we take in to give us the most amount of energy, provide us with an abundance of healthful nutrients, contribute to short- and long-term health, and also give us pleasure.

We *can* have it all.

Just as when you do your financial budget you determine how much money you have and then figure out how you want to spend it, I suggest you do the same for your calorie budget. You can spend it however you like each day. You don't even have to deprive yourself of your favorite cookie or eggless mayonnaise on your sandwich. *You* can decide how to spend your calories, but like all good budgeters, you learn to spend them wisely.

And just as credit really isn't the best way to make purchases with your dollars, because you're spending money you don't have, you also learn that if you spend calories, you have to *pay* for them! So if you really want that piece of chocolate—let's say it's 200 calories, then you just have to realize that you need to pay for it by burning those 200 calories (or spending 200 fewer elsewhere).

HOW MANY CALORIES TO SPEND EACH DAY?

Since healthful weight loss is a matter of having a calorie *deficit,* the number of calories you consume each day matters less than the fact that you consume fewer calories than you burn (or burn more calories than you take in). For example, if you're aiming to lose 1 pound a week, then you'll want to have a calorie deficit of 500 calories a day (or 3,500 calories a week—the equivalent of 1 pound). So if you take in 1,500 calories in one day, and your goal is to have a deficit of 500 calories that day, then you need to burn a total of 2,000 calories, which you will do through normal activities as well as through intentional cardiovascular movement.

Your weight loss can be slow or fast depending on the deficit you choose, though most experts would recommend losing no more than 2 pounds a week.

WISELY SPENDING 500 CALORIES

Let's look at some ways to wisely spend 500 calories.

Breakfast

- One 6-ounce container of soy milk yogurt is between 160 and 170 calories. Add to that 2 tablespoons of walnuts (100 calories) and 1 tablespoon of ground flaxseeds (50 calories), and you've got plenty of calories to spend on fruit: 110 calories or so for a medium banana; about 40 calories for ½ cup of blueberries; 20 calories for ½ cup of whole strawberries.

- One-half cup of cooked oatmeal is about 150 calories. Add to that 1 tablespoon of brown sugar or maple syrup (about 50 calories) or whatever sweetener you like (they're all around the same calorie-wise), plus 1 apple, chopped (70 calories), 1 tablespoon of walnuts (50 calories), and 1 tablespoon of ground flaxseeds (50 calories). You still have calories to spare—add more fruit or oats.

- Fruit smoothies can be calorie-dense or calorie-light, depending on your goal. Calculate 1 banana (110), ½ cup of blueberries (40), 1 tablespoon of peanut butter (80), 1 tablespoon of ground flaxseeds (50 calories), and 1 cup of nondairy milk (90 calories). Make it less calorie-dense by using a reduced-calorie soy milk or halving the milk and adding cold filtered water. The options abound!

- If you want to spend 500 calories on a heartier breakfast, there are 150 calories in an average-size pancake (see page 82). People usually have 3 or more, so that's about 450 calories. Adding 1 teaspoon of Earth Balance will add 33.3 calories, and 2 tablespoons of maple syrup will add 100 more.

- When choosing cereals, I recommend the ones that are the least processed, such as Grape-Nuts (200 calories for ½ cup) or Shredded Wheat (183 calories for 1 cup for bite-sized Shredded Wheat). Although they're a little more processed, All-Bran (81 calories for ½ cup) and bran flakes (95 calories for ¾ cup) are also options. Add to your cereal bowl some nondairy milk (all of them average about 90 calories for 8 fluid ounces), and of course 1 banana (110) and ½ cup of berries (40), and you're good to go.

- You're not going to get a lot of nutritional bang for your calorie buck if you just have a bagel (about 350 calories) and peanut butter (190 calories for 2 tablespoons), but you can still choose that option, picking whole-grain versions. The question to ask is, "Is that how I want to spend my precious calories?" The answer is up to you.

Lunch/Dinner

- Five Tofurky slices (100 calories) on 2 slices of whole-wheat bread (200 calories) or whole-wheat pita bread (170 calories), with 1 tablespoon of vegan mayonnaise (80 calories) or mustard (15 calories per tablespoon), allows you to pile on the lettuce and tomato. Make a bunch of Kale Chips to go with that sandwich (see page 232). One whole bunch of kale is only 50 calories, and only 1 teaspoon of oil (40 calories) is needed to make the whole bunch of chips. That still leaves room for 2 or 3 carrots, cut up.

- Two Wildwood Southwest Tofu Burgers are 336 calories; two Dr. Praeger's California Burgers are 220 calories; two Amy's California Veggie Burgers are 140 calories. Add a whole-grain bun (or not), a side of sautéed veggies or a salad, and you're good to go.

- One cup of whole-wheat penne pasta; ¼ cup of canned white beans, rinsed and drained; 1½ cups of cherry tomatoes, halved; 1 tablespoon of olive oil; 1 tablespoon of balsamic vinegar; ½ cup of fresh basil, chopped; and 2 minced garlic cloves come in at around 500 calories.

- Green salads are the best way to spend your calories wisely. Use any lettuce, or finely chop kale or chard. The amount of greens needed for an entire salad provides about 50 calories—but with loads of nutrients. Top with beans (a can of rinsed and drained beans averages 330 calories, so use half a can if you want to spend more calories on raw veggies) or 3 ounces of extra-firm tofu (around 90 calories). Pile on the veggies: 1 tomato is 15 calories; 1 medium raw carrot is 35 calories; 1 cup of cauliflower is 25 calories. There are lots of low-cal dressings, though my favorite is just seasoned rice vinegar mixed with minced garlic and miso. Another favorite is a little balsamic vinegar (only 20 calories a tablespoon) mixed with a smidge of oil (1 tablespoon of olive oil is 120 calories).

Snacks
- The best way to spend calories for weight loss and nutrition is on raw veggies and fruit. Cut them up so you can savor each bite, and choose according to what's in season. Raw carrots, bell peppers, and cauliflower florets are wonderful snacks. Dip them in a little hummus or peanut butter.

- One cup of air-popped popcorn is 30 calories (though I never eat just a cup). Toss it with a few mists of spray-on olive oil, nutritional yeast, and salt.

- Vegan ice creams vary, but 1 cup of ice cream is anywhere from 250 to 400 calories, depending on the brand and flavor. My favorite "ice cream" is just frozen bananas thrown in the blender, along with some almond milk, vanilla extract, and cinnamon. Try varying the flavor by adding some frozen strawberries, mango, pineapple, or other favorite frozen fruit. Add a few walnuts and a little maple syrup and vanilla for maple-walnut ice cream!

Beverages
Beverages can be a part of your total calories for the day, but they can really add a lot of calories very quickly. If that's where you want to spend your calories, that's up to you, but consider:

- A 4-ounce glass of red table wine is about 100 calories; a dry white is between 80 and 100.

- A 12-ounce bottle of beer is typically 150 calories.

- Nondairy milk is about 90 calories for 8 ounces.

- Orange juice is 110 calories for 8 ounces.

- Exotic coffee drinks vary. Ask the vendor.

When you realize *you* have the power to spend calories the way you want to, then you can allow yourself to have more indulgent food for a special occasion or dinner at a special restaurant. You can have the birthday cake, but you just have to cough up the calories, just as you have to cough up the dough if you buy a new pair of fabulous leather-free shoes. There are no free rides.

A Few Tips
- Set a goal.

- Keep temptations out of the house.

- Write down your calorie intake for the first 30 days, after which time you'll have a better idea of the calorie content of your favorite foods.

CALORIE BURN

We are creatures who are built to *move*. We aren't designed to lead the sedentary lives we currently live. We need to move—and we need to give our bones a reason to live.

In terms of intentional calorie burn, we have a million options. When I say "intentional calorie burn," I mean the kind that's in the form of cardiovascular exercise versus the calories we burn just breathing and being alive. The best form of exercise for you is whatever makes you most excited and gets you most motivated.

The number of calories you burn during cardiovascular exercise depends on your weight, but on average, you burn about:

- 140 calories for a 2-mile walk
- 320 calories in a 3-mile run
- 350 calories for a 1-hour light bicycle ride
- 500 calories for 1 hour of swimming laps

Basically, the more muscle groups involved in your activities, the more calories you are likely to burn.

There are so many additional ways to get moving. Take your pick: join a gym, jump rope, dance, lift weights, join a sports team, practice yoga, play tennis, bowl, skate, Rollerblade, ski, golf, take an aerobics class, buy a workout video. Though they all vary in terms of calories burned, the point is to get moving.

Mini-Exercising

A lot of people ask about splitting up your cardio exercise throughout the day; that's fine (and certainly better than nothing), but one of the benefits of sustained cardiovascular exercise is the afterburn, which refers to your elevated metabolism after a workout. Afterburn can last anywhere from fifteen minutes to twenty-four hours, depending on the intensity and duration of your workout, and increases the number of calories you burn.

However, since you're trying to burn calories, there are some modifications you can make in your daily habits that can get you moving more in addition to an intentional cardio routine. These suggestions aren't meant to replace a cardio routine. They're meant to burn additional calories throughout your normal day.

- Take the stairs instead of the elevator (down *and* up).

- Go for a walk with a friend at lunch instead of sitting in a restaurant.

- When you walk, instead of strolling, pick up the pace.

- Get up from your desk several times a day to stretch or take a brief walk. Or if you work from home, get up from your desk and do 3 minutes of jumping jacks, running in place, or rope jumping (you don't need a rope to mimic the motion) every 30 or 45 minutes. Download—for free—a computer program called Time Out, which inspires you to get up from your computer every ten minutes or so.

- For your daily commute, walk or bicycle to work or to the bus stop.

- When you send your kids outside to play, run around with them!

- Walk your dog twice a day instead of once.

- Do jumping jacks or jump rope during TV commercials. Jumping rope requires a little extra space and minimal skill to effectively burn calories and build cardiovascular endurance. In just 10 minutes, a 160-pound person can burn 120 calories. It may be challenging to keep up that pace for a full 30 to 60 minutes, but it's a great way to expend 120 calories in 10 minutes!

- Go on an after-dinner walk with your partner, friend, or family. Ask neighbors to join you.

You might be asking how to calculate calories burned throughout the day to better keep track of your weight loss. You have a couple of options.

1. **ESTIMATE.** Once you have an idea of how many calories you burn in a cardio interval (let's say 500 for a 5-mile run), that's a start. I know a lot of machines in gyms have read-outs telling you how many calories you burned, but they're not always *that* accurate. Frankly, I'd knock 100 calories off whatever it tells you, especially if you are using a machine that doesn't ask you to enter your weight and other information. There are a number of calculators online, such as at healthstatus.com, that enable you to calculate various activities.

2. **USE A MONITOR.** There are a number of monitors available to track your calorie burn throughout the day. The best and most heavily studied device is an armband sold as GoWear Fit by BodyMedia and as the Bodybugg by 24 Hour Fitness. You plug the device into your computer, and you basically upload the information to your online account every day or however often you want to see the results. You can also purchase the Display Device, which is essentially a watch that gives you the read-out of calories burned at any given moment.

So get moving—even if weight loss isn't your goal. Lack of physical activity is associated with several diseases, including cardiovascular disease, high blood pressure, diabetes, osteoporosis, and depression, and it's a leading cause of obesity. On the positive side, cardiovascular exercise has numerous physiological, psychological, emotional, and even social benefits, especially if we use it as an opportunity to connect with friends.

Compassionate Fashion: It's Cool to Be Kind

As you wrap up your 30 days, reaping the many benefits of a compassionate, plant-fueled diet, you may be more keenly aware not only of the animals you once put in your mouth but also of the animals you may be wearing on your body in the form of leather shoes, leather purses, wool suits and dresses, silk ties, pashmina scarves, and cashmere sweaters. You may suddenly realize there's goose down in your winter coat, duck feathers in your pillows and comforter, and fur lining your gloves.

As our awareness expands, so does our desire to be consistent in our values, which is why many people extend their compassionate ethic beyond their diet to their wardrobe and home goods. But just as we have been conditioned to believe that meat, dairy, and eggs are healthful, so, too, have animal skin, fur, and hair been touted as "natural," "humane," and even "eco-friendly," leading many compassionate people to unknowingly support practices they really are opposed to. Below is a brief overview of leather, wool, feathers and down, silk, and fur, with many recommendations for choosing compassionate versions.

LEATHER

When I was about 17 years old, there was a leather store in the mall near where I lived that sold everything from coats, belts, and jackets to purses, wallets, and shoes—all made out of leather. I was obsessed with a particular black leather skirt they carried, and I saved up my money to buy it. Around the same time, I had a brown leather bomber jacket that I wore with affection, as well as a pair of brown leather cowboy boots. I absolutely loved all of these things, and I had no idea what I was contributing to. I was already someone who cared about animals, and yet I had successfully compartmentalized my compassion and my understanding, and I was blissfully ignorant of the impact I was having. In fact, I continued to wear leather shoes even after I had stopped eating land animals—I simply did not make the connection.

Denial is deep and vast, and it tends to manifest itself in the excuses we tell ourselves in order to justify our behavior—not only to feel *better* about what we're doing but also to feel *good* about it. When it comes to leather, we often declare that it is just a by-product of the meat industry and say we feel good knowing they're at least doing something with the leftover parts of the animals instead of having them go to waste. As much as we like to believe that the leather industry is motivated by waste-conscious altruism, it is not the case. The U.S. leather industry is a $1.5 billion business tanning over 100 million animal skins every year; worldwide, it's even bigger, representing $46 billion, ranking among the most important internationally traded commodities.

What most people don't understand is that the meat industry is *not* sustainable on its own. It *relies* on skin sales to remain profitable. Let me put this another way: one of the reasons meat is so cheap (aside from the subsidies it receives from the government) is because they can sell so much of the animal's other body parts, such as the skin and fat, for a profit. According to the U.S. Department of Agriculture, the skin represents the most economically important by-product of the meatpacking industry, accounting for 55 to 60 percent of the by-product value of cattle. In other words, the leather industry essentially subsidizes the meat industry.

Most leather is from cattle—bulls, steers, cows, and calves—though not all. Buckskin comes from deer; suede is made from lambs, goats, pigs, calves, and deer; pigskin is from pigs and often used to make riding saddles; horses' skin tends to be used for baseballs; and a shearling garment is created from the skin of young lambs, which is tanned with the wool still on. And even though the slaughter industry relies on the leather industry to be profitable, that doesn't mean wild animals are safe. Some animals in the United States, such as deer, sharks, and alligators, are killed only for their skins, and animals killed outside the United States include zebras, bison, water buffaloes, kangaroos, elephants, eels, dolphins, seals, walruses, frogs, crocodiles, and lizards. Australia exports approximately 3 million kangaroo skins every year, and though you won't see "kangaroo" on the label, you will see "K leather" or "RKT."

Much of the leather sold in the United States comes from overseas, especially from India. That may surprise people who thought cattle were considered sacred in that country. Not everyone in India follows Hindu principles, so the law dictates that cattle can be killed in certain provinces. In fact, they can be raised in one province but killed in another, which often means the cattle are forced to travel hundreds of miles on foot, in the hot sun, with their noses tied together. China is also another of the world's leading exporters of leather. In addition to using cattle and sheep, an estimated 2 million cats and dogs in China are killed for their hides each year.

From an environmental and health perspective, the tanning process is incredibly energy-intensive and pollution-producing. In fact, tanneries are listed as top polluters on the Environmental Protection Agency's Superfund list, which identifies the most critical industrial sites in need of environmental cleanup. Because of their high levels of toxins, many old tannery sites can't even be used for agriculture, built on, or even sold. Tanning is bad for the workers, bad for people who live near these tanneries, bad for the rivers that ultimately collect these toxins (formaldehyde, coal tar derivatives, oils, dyes, and cyanide-based compounds), and bad for the animals and ecosystems affected by these toxins in the environment.

ALTERNATIVES TO LEATHER

What's a compassionate fashionista to do? Well, once you've decided not to contribute to the leather and meat industries, you have plenty of options, and they're everywhere you look!

The main thing to look for on the label when you're buying synthetic leather is "man-made materials." (Note that you might see "man-made materials" for the main part of the shoe but "leather uppers," so just look at the label.) You can find man-made shoes in virtually every store from Macy's and Saks Fifth Avenue to Birkenstock and Payless. Even high-end lines, including Chinese Laundry, Kenneth Cole, Nine West, and Kate Spade, feature synthetic footwear and accessories.

As a runner, I have to make sure I have the best running sneakers in terms of comfort and safety, and I never have a problem finding what I need. New Balance is my go-to brand for running sneakers—though there are many other brands featuring leather-free sneakers, too—and Merrell makes great walking and hiking shoes. Whenever I visit a shoe store, I just ask them to tell me which ones are leather-free, and they're always happy to assist; or on websites, I just search for "synthetic" or "vegan."

There are also many online and brick-and-mortar stores dedicated only to vegan shoes, and the options continue to expand. MooShoes (mooshoes.com) has a beautiful shoe store in New York City as well as their entire inventory online. In addition to selling vegan shoes, the store's suppliers are fair-trade, ensuring that workers get fair pay and safe working conditions, and none of the materials (down to the glues) is tested on animals. They go to great lengths to get high-quality, ethical shoes that are fashionable.

Alternative Outfitters (alternativeoutfitters.com) is another fabulous fashion-conscious vegan-owned store, and they carry super-cute shoes, bags, wallets, and accessories. They also carry the vegan ethic to all aspects of their business and ensure that the products made outside of the United States and Canada are made under fair-trade conditions and are not manufactured with child labor or under sweatshop conditions.

Outside of the United States, there are the pioneers: Vegetarian Shoes and Bags (vegetarianshoesandbags.com). A vegan-owned shoe store based in England, they have been around since 1990. They're also concerned with human rights as well as animal rights and work to make sure they are buying from companies that don't exploit humans. But there are so many other online retailers, including zappos.com (search for "vegan"), over stock.com (search for "faux"), veganchic.com, veganessentials.com, and veganstore.com.

Many of these companies also carry nonleather wallets, guitar straps, briefcases, gloves, purses, and belts for men and women, including those from Truth Belts (vegetarianbelts .com) and Matt and Nat (mattandnat.com), and Cynthia King (cynthiakingdance.com) makes leather-free ballet slippers. Of course, there are also other wonderful alternatives to leather, such as microsuede, microfiber, a whole range of other synthetics, cotton, linen, rubber, ramie, canvas, bamboo. None of these materials produce the same toxins as the leather tanning industry, but when you can choose and afford organic versions, it's always a good idea to do so.

FEATHERS AND DOWN

Sometimes our attachment to certain comfort items can be so strong that we genuinely believe that no one is harmed in their production; what's more, we give more credence to the people selling the goods than we give to our own consciences, economic realities, and sheer common sense. Ask people how they think feathers and down are acquired, and many will insist they just fall off the birds and are then collected by opportunists. Some even think the feathers are massaged off, while the birds live a pampered life. Unfortunately, this is not the case.

Geese and ducks are the primary victims of the feather and down industries (chickens and turkeys don't produce down), but ostriches are also exploited for their beautiful plumes. A very lucrative multimillion-dollar industry, most of it is situated in China, Hungary, and Poland, though more than twenty-five countries are involved in the production of feathers and down, taken either from live geese (referred to by the industry as "live plucking" or "ripping") or dead ones. Feathers from live animals are considered better quality and thus have a higher value. The geese are plucked three to four times a year before they're finally killed. Many are often used to produce foie gras before they meet their end. Overfed to engorge their livers, birds suffer a great deal for this "luxury" product.

ALTERNATIVES TO FEATHER AND DOWN

Feather- and down-free blankets, coats, and sleeping bags are widely available. The Company Store (www.thecompanystore.com) sells down-free comforters in every color and size. Look for "down alternatives" or Primaloft on their website. Many other companies market their own down-free versions, called Micromax, Nature's Touch, Sensuelle, and Thinsulate.

Consider another advantage of synthetic down: when wet, animal-based down loses virtually all of its insulating properties, making it a much worse insulator than equally wet synthetic fills. To make up for this, sleeping bags insulated with down also require the use of a sleeping pad to provide insulation from warmth that would otherwise be conducted into the ground. So, essentially, the down is useless. And that goes for coats, too. Coats made with down are not waterproof, whereas if you get a down-free jacket with a waterproof material such as Gore-Tex, you have the advantage of good insulation.

In fact, many outdoor clothing stores and brands (REI, Patagonia, North Face) carry puffy, warm, down-free jackets and vests, using synthetic Primaloft and recycled Thermogreen materials. Many options abound, and they're less expensive than the animal versions. Just visit sporting goods stores and ask the salespeople which coats are down-free, or search for "synthetic down" on their websites.

WOOL

Wool is not unlike leather in that you can't support the hide/wool industry without supporting the meat industry, and all sheep raised for their wool are eventually killed for their flesh. Australia and China dominate the wool industry, with Iran, New Zealand, and Turkey following close behind.

Sheep are sheared at an incredible pace (shearers who are hired are paid by volume, not by the hour), a rough process that stresses out these already sensitive prey animals and often results in cuts and wounds that are left untreated. Just as with dairy cows, when it's no longer considered economically viable to provide veterinary care for sheep, they are culled from the herd, usually at 4 or 5 years old (their life expectancy is 15 to 20 years) and sold to slaughter. With so many "excess animals," the live animal export industry cropped up, annually shipping around 6.5 million sheep from Australia to the Middle East and North Africa.

Livestock ships can carry up to 100,000 animals for voyages that last up to three weeks, a painful, arduous journey during which time many sheep die. Once the sheep arrive at their destination, unloading them at the ports takes its own toll, and the sheep are sent straight to backyard butchers or dirty slaughterhouses where anti-cruelty laws are nonexistent. I'll spare you the gruesome details, though you can view undercover footage online.

In addition to being used for their milk and meat, goats are also bred and killed for their hair, which goes by several names: mohair, fleece, goat wool, angora, cashmere, or pashmina, depending on the breed being used for the desired purpose. (Angora goats produce the fiber known as mohair.) Their end is the same as for all other animals used only for what we can get out of them.

ALTERNATIVES TO WOOL

Wool-free materials have been around forever, mostly due to the fact that so many people are allergic to wool clothing and blankets. Check labels and look for cotton, cotton flannel, polyester fleece, synthetic shearling, and other cruelty-free fibers such as Tencel (breathable, durable, and biodegradable) and Polartec Wind Pro (made primarily from recycled plastic soda bottles). Olefin—also known as polypropylene, polyethylene, or polyolefin—is a synthetic fiber used to make clothing, rugs, upholstery, wallpaper, and car interiors.

During the winter months, it's true that many stores tout their wool and cashmere clothing lines, but many less expensive brands make beautiful sweaters, pants, suits, and coats using acrylic, nylon, and polyester. And for those of you who are avid knitters, wool-free yarn is available; just search for it online.

Aside from countless mainstream retailers selling clothing made from synthetic fibers, there are a growing number of fashion designers dedicated to creating vegan and often eco-friendly clothing, shoes, and accessories, especially Leanne Mai-ly Hilgart of Vaute Couture (vautecouture.com), Stella McCartney (stellamccartney.com), and Steve Madden (stevemadden.com). Nonwool tuxedos can be found at etuxedo.com and cheaptux.com. As far as area rugs, many options are available and are less expensive than those made with animal hair. Check out www.rugsusa.com or your favorite home goods store and look for synthetic versions.

There are also a number of online bloggers dedicated to vegan fashion for both men and women, but the three go-to experts I recommend are Girlie Girl Army (girliegirlarmy.com), the Discerning Brute (thediscerningbrute.com), and the Ethical Man (theethicalman.com).

SILK

Many people may have a hard time including worms in their circle of compassion, but if our intention is to foster kindness rather than harm, it's a no-brainer, especially once you know that silk is obtained from silkworms by submerging them in boiling water just before the adult moths emerge.

ALTERNATIVES TO SILK

Artificial silk, namely rayon, has the same beautiful sheen and texture as silk made by worms, and nylon has been used as an alternative to silk since the 1930s. Many clothing items for both men and women, including scarves, blouses, and dresses, are made from these materials. For men's suits and neckties, bow ties, and ascots, check out Jaan J. (jaanj.com) or places such as Men's Warehouse.

FUR

Despite losing popularity in the 1990s due to successful anti-fur campaigns by animal activists, fur has returned on runways across the globe, in large part due to efforts of the fur industry to reach out to designers. Worldwide, more than 30 million animals are killed each year on fur farms. In the United States alone, 3 million animals die on farms and another 4 million are trapped. Half of the fur sold in the United States is from China, where domestic dogs and cats are brutally killed for their fur. Whether they are raised in confinement or trapped in the wild, the gruesomeness of this industry is something we would all rather put out of our minds.

ALTERNATIVES TO FUR

Fur can be found as trim on parkas, sweaters, boots, and gloves or as the basis for an entire coat, and though synthetic fur is most definitely available, investigations revealed that because of a loophole in the labeling law, real fur was often mislabeled as faux fur. Because of the dedication of the Humane Society of the United States, a bill was recently signed into law that has closed this loophole. If you're unsure that a faux fur garment is indeed synthetic, you can check yourself by spreading apart the hairs to reveal the material at their base. If you see threadwork stitching from which the "hairs" emerge, it's synthetic. If you're still not certain, perhaps pass on the item.

All of the items at Fabulous Furs (fabulousfurs.com) are made of faux fur, and other designers and manufacturers are specializing in faux furs as well, including Charly Calder, Faux, Purrfect Fur, and Sweet Herb. Wearing faux fur is one of those tricky decisions that each person has to make on his or her own. On one hand, it's great for the public to see that they can be compassionate as well as trendy, but if people just assume you're wearing authentic animal fur, then you might be inadvertently promoting the fur industry.

If you have old furs you want to get rid of, check out Coats for Cubs (coatsforcubs.com), an organization that collects fur and fur-trimmed garments for donation to wildlife rehabilitators, who use the furs to provide warmth and comfort for the injured or orphaned animals under their care.

DAY 30   Keeping It in Perspective: Intention, Not Perfection

Perhaps in these last 30 days, you've received questions from people all around you—strangers, friends, coworkers, family members—and, unfortunately, some of them may be antagonistic. Some may try to undermine your decision, some may challenge the entire concept of being vegan, some may try to find fault with your choices. Because many people mistakenly believe that being vegan is about being perfect, they often accuse vegans of being hypocrites and sometimes don't hesitate to point out all the areas where they're imperfect.

This pressure might not even come from others; it might come from *you*. Perhaps over these last few weeks, while striving to do your best, you've accidentally eaten something that wasn't vegan and feel bad for doing so.

Because you are looking at the world through this new lens, you notice animal products in things you never even thought of before. You feel guilty, you feel overwhelmed, and you feel judged by everyone around you for "not doing it right" or for "not being perfect." You just wait for the vegan police to come knocking on your door to take away your vegan status.

> **CHALLENGE YOUR THINKING:**
> There is no such thing as a certified vegan. If perfection and purity are what you're trying to attain in this imperfect world, you will be gravely disappointed. Being vegan is a means to an end—not an end in itself.

Let me assuage your fears: there is no such thing as a certified vegan, and if perfection and purity are what you're trying to attain in a world that is by its nature imperfect, then I'm afraid you'll be gravely disappointed. As I said in the very first chapter, being vegan is not an end in itself; it's a *means* to an end, and if we forget this, then we're missing the entire point of what it means to be vegan, whether we're doing it from a health perspective or an ethical one.

Unfortunately, I think this expectation of perfection is what stops many people from even giving veganism a try. They're afraid they're going to be expected to change everything in one fell swoop, and their fear is justified when they proudly declare to someone that they're vegan but are met with a smug reminder that the shoes they're wearing are made of leather. "Ha!" the other person seems to say, deriving pleasure in catching you at not being perfect after all.

Whenever I've been in the situation where it seems someone's trying to catch me, I'm aware of what a great privilege and responsibility it is to help change the perception of what it means to be vegan. Unabashedly, I admit that I'm far from perfect, that I'm doing the best I can, and that I'm trying to make a difference where I'm able.

I remind them that not to do anything because we can't do everything makes absolutely no sense. Don't do nothing because you can't do everything, say I. Do something. Anything.

Some new vegans simply can't stand the thought of wearing any of the animal products that once gave them so much pleasure, and so they slowly replace them with the array of beautiful skin-free products available. Most people can't afford to do this all at once, and so they do it over time. That's *fine*. You do what you can as you're able, and you feel confident that you're doing the best you can.

Whenever you're faced with this dilemma, the question to ask is: "How does keeping this leather couch, for instance, contribute to animal cruelty?" Or flip it around: "How does getting rid of it *help* animals?" As it becomes difficult to even have the couch in your home, then sell it and save for a new one. Or sell it and donate the money to an animal organization.

The most counterproductive response is to beat yourself up for once having purchased these things. All we can do is the best we can with the information we have at the time; as we grow and learn, we can strive to make the most compassionate, healthful decisions possible. Keep in mind that being vegan is about intention, not perfection.

ACCIDENTS HAPPEN

Though vegans try to avoid all animal products, it can be difficult to shun every hidden animal-derived ingredient. Keeping in mind your goals—whether you're trying to avoid contributing to violence toward animals, to eat only life-enhancing foods rather than life-taking ones, to reduce the use of the Earth's resources, or all of these things—will help keep things in perspective when you accidentally eat something that has gelatin or

CHALLENGE YOUR THINKING: Being vegan is about reflecting our compassion and desire for health in our actions. It doesn't mean we're going to succeed all the time, but just having the intention means we will manifest these values more often than not.

CHANGE YOUR BEHAVIOR: Don't do nothing because you can't do everything. Do something. Anything.

IS HONEY VEGAN?

A great debate rages over whether honey is vegan or not, and I confess, I don't understand.

I believe that one of the reasons we're in such a sorry state in terms of our relationship with animals is because we view them as here for us to do with as we please. We see their flesh, skin, bones, reproductive outputs (milk and eggs), and hair as here for us to use and consume. Of course there are natural cycles we all benefit from (bees pollinating trees enabling us to eat nuts and fruit, for instance), but that need not include taking everything animals produce and making commodities of them.

Some people feel that honey is the deal breaker for people—that many who would try to be vegan would just change their minds upon realizing they'd have to give up honey, too. Honestly, I don't think that's what keeps people from becoming vegan. If it weren't honey, it would be something else. I just don't believe that people are *this* close to being vegan but then say, "Oh—it means I couldn't eat honey, either? Well, just forget the whole thing."

I think the other aspect of the honey issue is that there is still debate as to whether keeping bees constitutes cruelty or whether bees really are harmed when their food is taken. As a result, some people argue that including honey in the fold of products that vegans avoid makes veganism seem difficult, unreasonable, rigid, or impossible. I just don't agree. If someone is already resistant to being vegan, then he or she will make that same argument about other animal products, too.

To me, the bottom line is that honey is not made for me; the bees make it for themselves as a source of food, and it's just not something I eat.

And besides, honey fills no nutritional need; it's just one of many liquid sweeteners. The people who sell honey and its by-product royal jelly (secreted from the heads of bees to feed their new queen) will tell you it's a "wonder" food, which is ridiculous. We have no more need to consume the regurgitated food of bees than we do to consume the colostrum of cows, which is also sold in health food stores with promises of optimal health.

Agave nectar is a wonderful plant-based liquid sweetener that has the viscosity and flavor of honey. It comes from a cactuslike plant, and if you've ever had tequila, you've had agave. For baking, you can use it for such desserts as baklava, or use it to sweeten tea. Of course, other liquid sweeteners include maple syrup, rice syrup, molasses, sorghum syrup, and barley malt, but we don't have any nutritional need for any of them, either. Although many of them are touted as health food, just keep in mind that they're all sweeteners. But when we want them as a treat, at least we have many choices in the plant kingdom and can live without the *one* in the animal kingdom.

eggs. Here's how I handle that situation: I write it off as an accident, and I move on. Every vegan I know has bitten into a sandwich that contained some non-vegan ingredient. Even in vegan-friendly restaurants, I've witnessed vegan friends chew on what they thought was tofu but turned out to be chicken. I myself have eaten what I realized was pork after I swallowed—in both Mexican and Asian restaurants.

Although it's not pleasant, and it can be emotionally upsetting, accidents happen. I certainly recommend talking to the server and explaining the mistake, and competent management will rectify the situation. But in terms of dwelling on it, there's no point. Take whatever lessons can be gleaned from the experience and utilize them for the future.

DRAWING THE LINE

Living with integrity in a world that seems to value convenience and pleasure over ethics can be challenging at best, and since we can't be perfect, we do have to draw the line somewhere. After all, the rubber in my car tires has the remnants of animals in it; I kill insects every time I walk on the ground or drive my car; many municipal water systems use animal bones as filtering agents; and white sugar is sometimes refined through activated charcoal, most of which comes from animal bones. Clearly, we have to find a line to draw, or we'll drive ourselves crazy.

Some people draw that line at white sugar (choosing unrefined cane sugar, raw sugar, turbinado sugar, beet sugar, Sucanat, or white sugar clearly labeled "vegan," as in Whole Foods' 365 brand). Some people draw it at honey. (See sidebar on page 290.)

KEEPING IT IN PERSPECTIVE

I was once asked by someone if I'm a "hard-core" vegan. I asked her what she meant. She said, "Do you ever cheat? Do you ever sneak a piece of cheese, or are you hard-core?" I told her that if by "hard-core" she meant "consistent," then by that definition, yes, I suppose I'm hard-core.

For me, being vegan is about expansiveness and openness. Not restriction. Not limitation. Not rules. Not doctrine. I'm not *forbidden* to eat animals or their secretions. I don't *want* to eat animals and their secretions.

For me, being vegan is about living my life with integrity and compassion, knowing that every decision I make is done with the intention of not contributing to the suffering and exploitation of human and nonhuman animals. And there is freedom and serenity in that choice.

Beyond the 30 Days: Being a Joyful Vegan in a Non-Vegan World

My intention in creating the 30-Day Vegan Challenge was to provide you with the tools and resources you need to do it for 30 days while I held your hand, answered your most pressing questions, debunked prevailing myths, and helped create a strong foundation on which to stand should you want to continue.

Giving you what you need to eat delicious food and live as healthfully as possible is the easy part, and my hope is that this book will continue to serve as a resource and recipe guide for you long after you finish the 30 days. But there is still much to say about the social, ethical, and spiritual aspects of living in a world that seeks to encourage empathy, kindness, and compassion in children but seems suspicious of these same values in adults. We live in a world where human privilege and the desire for convenience and pleasure drive the socially sanctioned use and abuse of billions and billions of nonhuman animals. We live in a world where it's considered normal to champion this and radical to oppose it.

The excuses we humans come up with to justify tradition and habit can range from the absurd to the offensive, and new vegans are often caught off guard by the defensiveness that seems to be directed toward what to them is simply a healthful, kind way for them to live. Even when the reaction isn't hostile, vegans are often asked to defend how and why they eat the way they do. Although non-vegans are never asked to explain why they eat meat, dairy, and eggs, the most common question meat-eaters ask those who don't is "Why are you vegan?"

This can be difficult for some people to reconcile; not all of us want to have to answer for our food choices every time we sit down to eat. And I understand that. Not everyone who is vegan is necessarily an activist. But the truth is whether we like it or not, if we're the vegan someone meets, if we're the vegan someone comes to, we represent *all vegans*. I realize that puts a lot of pressure on vegans, but with so many myths perpetuated about and against veganism, if we brush off people's questions or answer without patience and understanding, then we may be squandering an opportunity to show how positive and healthful this way of living really is.

We certainly don't have to become experts in nutrition, anthropology, animal husbandry, or the culinary arts, but I do believe we have an obligation to speak our truth when someone asks us why we're vegan—not only for ourselves (and for the animals, if that's part of your story) but also for the benefit of the person asking. When someone asks me why I'm vegan, I don't spout off all the statistics and studies that support the benefits of a vegan diet—and there are plenty. When someone asks me why I'm vegan, I simply tell *my* truth, *my* story, *my* reason for being vegan, which is—in short—*to not contribute to suffering and violence where I have the power to do so.* Nobody can take away *my* story. Nobody can say "That's wrong" or "That's not true." All I can do is speak the truth and trust that the truth will inspire others to act on their own values. And if they don't, that's not mine to worry about.

Whenever I speak to anyone about the joys and benefits of being vegan, I make sure I'm clear about my intention, and my intention is never to change someone else's mind. It's not my role to *make* anyone do anything. That's why I abhor the word *convert*. I prefer *inspire* or *empower*. I never set out to convert anyone.

When I speak on behalf of animals, on behalf of a healthful, compassionate life, in my mind, I make sure I'm clear about my goal, and my goal is this:

- To raise awareness about the joys and benefits of living compassionately
- To be a voice for animals
- To speak my truth

I believe we're here to be teachers for one another, and I'm grateful for my role as a conduit, but that's all any of us is. I believe intention is everything, and when our intention is simply to plant seeds and remain unattached to the outcome, we can't but succeed in having a pleasant and effective dialogue with people who inquire about our lifestyle (and they will inquire).

Having a clear intention about your goal and making that goal about *truth* rather than *outcome* will make you a successful, effective spokesperson 100 percent of the time. Don't feel so much pressure to have all the answers or speak so eloquently on behalf of a vegan lifestyle that you wind up not speaking at all. In your truth lies your eloquence. In *your* story lies someone else's. But in order to tell your story, you first have to remember it.

REMEMBERING OUR STORIES

In an earlier chapter, I talk about the phenomenon of non-vegans feeling threatened in the presence of a vegan because a mirror is held up to them that forces them to look at their own behavior. I call this being the "vegan in the room." But just as non-vegans need to confront this reflection and choose to either accept or reject what comes up for them, so, too, do vegans need to look in the mirror when we meet someone who is still eating animal meat, milk, and eggs and look squarely at what comes up for us. Is it impatience? Judgment? Self-righteousness? Arrogance? All of the above?

These reactions are understandable. When you stop eating animals, you become keenly aware of how often people are eating this stuff, and it can be very upsetting. You're now looking at the world through an entirely different lens, and you want to shake everyone and make them see what you see. But I can tell you that you will neither make nor keep many friends if that's your approach. You will neither inspire people nor do yourself any good. If we're pushy, hostile, angry, passive-aggressive, self-righteous, or arrogant, we *will* turn people away. *That* I can guarantee.

We absolutely have to remember that we were once unaware, that we once ate animals, that we once may have made excuses for eating them and perhaps even made fun of "those crazy vegans." In forgetting our own stories and our own process, we lose our humility and the ability to be effective, compassionate spokespeople for this wonderful lifestyle.

Remember your story, and tell your story. Connect with other vegans, either online or in person, and ask them to tell their story. Creating a community of like-minded people is vital to staying a joyful vegan, but finding common ground with people who aren't where you're at yet is also essential.

> **CHANGE YOUR BEHAVIOR:** Remember your story, and connect with like-minded people. Ask them to tell their story.

LOOKING FORWARD, NOT BACKWARD

When animals were first herded and domesticated for human use and consumption about ten thousand years ago, they became the alternatives to the plant foods that were then the foundation of the human diet. While humans ate mostly small animals and little of them, plant foods played the larger role. Thousands of years later, entrenched in an archaic animal-based agricultural system controlled by those who benefit financially, we find that the roles have reversed. Animal-based products are dominant in most people's diets, while plant foods are regarded as side dishes or garnish.

With a determination that belies an irrational attachment to animal flesh and fluids, otherwise sensible and sensitive people spend time and energy extolling the human history of eating and domesticating animals. Using lyrical and exalted language, they wax poetic about the virtues of animal husbandry and glorify the prehistoric hunter-gatherer, who anthropologists now assert was more likely a gatherer-hunter. Still, the argument goes something like this: since early humans ate animals, we're justified in continuing to eat them now.

Some contemporary food writers even charge vegetarians and vegans with turning their backs on their "evolutionary heritage," strangely perceiving Darwinian evolution as a moral system by which we should justify our actions. By eschewing meat, they say unabashedly, we're "sacrificing a part of our identity." It seems to me that we have the ability and responsibility to make moral and rational decisions—not abdicate our ethics to an amoral process. Surely our identities are defined by more than our paleontological past. And yet, determined to dwell perpetually on this past, these same people even romanticize the life of cavemen in order to rationalize our contemporary consumption of animals. Certainly there are lessons to learn from our human predecessors, but do we really want to use Neanderthals as the model for our ethics? Can't we do better than that?

We often say that we want to do better than we did a generation ago, two generations ago. I presume we want to do better than we did tens of thousands of years ago. That's the point of being human, isn't it? To learn from our past and make better, more healthful, more compassionate choices once we know better, especially once we have the ability and opportunity to do so?

TAKING THE LONG VIEW

Having coined the word *vegan*, founded the first vegan organization, and dedicated his life to inspiring a compassionate world, Donald Watson was asked in an interview a few years before he died if he had any message for the millions of people who are now vegan.

His answer was this: "Take the broad view of what veganism stands for—something beyond finding a new alternative to scrambled eggs on toast or a new recipe for Christmas cake. Realize that you're on to something really big and something which is meeting every reasonable criticism that anyone can level against it. And this doesn't involve weeks or months of studying diet charts or reading books by so-called experts; it means grasping a few simple facts and applying them.

"We don't know the spiritual advancements that long-term veganism—over generations—would have for human life. It would be certainly a different civilization, and the first one in the whole of our history that would truly deserve the title of being a civilization."

May you realize you are indeed on to something really big. It's up to each one of us to reflect our deepest values in our daily choices and in doing so create the healthful, compassionate world we all imagine. If not you, then who? If not now, then when?

Weekly Menu Ideas for Breakfast, Lunch, and Dinner

In the spirit of helping you to choose at a glance from the many options you have for every day of the 30-Day Vegan Challenge—and beyond—I've crafted these weekly menu ideas, within which you'll find new quick recipes, simple suggestions, or references to the recipes included throughout this book. Mix and match, repeat again and again, use your own ideas, or just treat this as a helpful reference guide.

Although weekday and weekend lunches tend to be pretty similar (sandwiches, salads, soups), you most likely make different choices during the workweek than you do on the weekends when it comes to breakfast and dinner, so I've organized these suggestions with that in mind.

WEEK ONE BREAKFAST IDEAS (WEEKDAYS)

As you're just starting off the Challenge this week, let's keep things as simple and familiar as possible. Although you will be stocking your kitchen with some new staples, you will most likely have some items in your cupboards and refrigerator that you can use for your meals this week.

Oatmeal: Quick-cooking oats can be used to make a hearty and healthful bowl of oatmeal. Add any or all of the following: fresh fruit, dried fruit, nuts, seeds, 1 tablespoon of ground flaxseeds, and your favorite sweetener with some cinnamon. Once the oats have soaked up the water and you've stirred in your goodies, top it with some of your favorite nondairy milk.

Cereal: Enjoy your favorite cereal (best is a high-fiber, low-sugar choice) with nondairy milk and a sliced banana. Stir in 1 tablespoon of ground flaxseeds, too.

Fruit Smoothie: A variety of options are available on page 83. Though the recipes I provide create a pretty substantial amount, if that's not filling enough for you, supplement it with some whole-grain toast with nondairy butter and jam or peanut butter.

Nondairy Yogurt: Serve with fresh fruit, granola, nuts, seeds, and ground flaxseeds.

Toasted Whole-Grain Bread or Bagel with Fresh Fruit: Keep it simple, but be sure to add some fresh fruit. For instance, spread a couple of pieces of toast with peanut or almond butter, then top with sliced bananas.

WEEK ONE BREAKFAST IDEAS (WEEKEND)

Blueberry Pancakes: See page 82 for a quick and simple recipe for fluffy pancakes. Top with fresh fruit or preserves. Serve with Tempeh Bacon (recipe on page 77).

Banana Chocolate Chip Muffins: Also super-fast and utterly delicious, these are a great excuse for using up your ripe bananas. Serve with fresh fruit. Recipe is on page 175.

WEEK ONE LUNCH IDEAS (WEEKEND AND WEEKDAYS)

Our lunch choices tend to remain the same whether it's during the week or on the weekend, depending, of course, on how much time you want to spend. I've made a point to focus on simple, familiar fare: salads, sandwiches, and soup. Though I'm including seven options here, one for each day of the week, realistically you'll most likely go out to eat one or two of these days or bring leftovers from dinner the night before.

Better-Than-Tuna Salad Sandwich: With eggless mayonnaise on your shopping list, now is the time to try this delicious recipe (see page 162) loved by kids and adults alike.

Green Salad: Despite the stereotype, salads are *not* the only things vegans eat, but they're certainly the most healthful. If you're in a rush, visit the salad bar at your local supermarket, and pile on the veggies.

Soup: If you haven't made your own soup from scratch, you can bring canned soup to heat up at the office. (See pages 34–35 for favorite brands.) Serve with a salad or sandwich.

Peanut Butter and Jelly Sandwiches: I don't care what anyone says—these are great when you're a kid and even better when you're an adult!

Veggie Grain or Pasta Salad: Consult the 10 One-Dish Salads on pages 92–93 and the Mix-and-Match Grain Salads on page 100 to prepare a large salad that you can take to work with you.

Tomato Sandwich: A super-easy and delicious sandwich that transports well: whole-grain bread (my preference is to toast it first), sliced tomatoes, whole basil leaves, lettuce, and eggless mayonnaise. Add Tempeh Bacon (page 77) for added deliciousness.

Veggie Lunch Meat/Veggie Sandwich: You can use the Sloppy Col recipe on page 109 as a guide, but feel free to add some veggie lunch meats to this sandwich filled to the brim with raw veggies.

WEEK ONE DINNER IDEAS (WEEKDAYS)

No doubt we want it quick and easy during the week, but we may be willing to spend a little more time on the weekends; hence the structure below. Serve each with a side salad.

Pasta with Marinara Sauce: Serve with a green salad.

Quick (No-Queso) Quesadillas: A favorite of my cookbook readers and cooking class students, these are loved by people of all ages. See page 130 for recipe.

Vegetable Fajitas: Sauté some bell peppers, onions, and mushrooms (or grill them), flavor with a packet of fajita spices, and serve on warmed tortillas with nondairy sour cream.

Easy Asian Menu: Thai Salad with Orange-Ginger Vinaigrette (page 215), miso soup (follow instructions on miso container), edamame salad (boil frozen shelled edamame for just a few minutes, then drain, rinse, cool, and toss with sesame oil, tamari soy sauce, and toasted sesame seeds).

Veggie Burgers with French Fries: See page 43 for recommended veggie burgers and frozen fries or potato puffs.

WEEK ONE DINNER IDEAS (WEEKEND)

Bean Chili: See the easy recipe on page 158 that utilizes convenient and nutritious canned beans.

Marinated Portobello Mushroom Steaks: See recipe on page 99, and serve with mashed potatoes (use nondairy milk and nondairy butter) or Herbed Scalloped Potatoes (page 138). Serve with grilled asparagus or Brussels sprouts and a green salad.

WEEK TWO BREAKFAST IDEAS (WEEKDAYS)

By week two, you'll most likely be rotating some menu items from week one, and that's fine. But here are even more ideas for the purposes of variety, again divvying up breakfasts between the workweek and the weekend.

Sliced Apple with Nut Butter: A quick, nutritious breakfast. Add a glass of orange juice, and you're good to go.

Fruit Salad: Serve in a pretty parfait glass to make it fancy. Top with some nondairy yogurt and chopped nuts.

Breakfast Quinoa: Use the grain-cooking chart on page 52 to cook this nutritious grain, and serve as you would oatmeal—with some brown sugar or maple syrup, raisins, nuts, and chopped apple.

Peanut Butter and Jam Sandwiches with Banana Slices: This healthful sandwich need not be confined to lunch. If it's too weird to eat a sandwich for breakfast, just toast up some whole-grain bread or waffles (check the frozen section of your grocery store for vegan options), and slather on the peanut butter and preserves.

Muesli with Nondairy Milk: Add fresh fruit and a handful of nuts.

WEEK TWO BREAKFAST IDEAS (WEEKEND)

French Toast: See recipe on page 79; serve with vegan breakfast sausages, such as Gimme Lean or Yves.

Vegetable Sauté: Sauté sliced peppers, onions, zucchini, mushrooms, and tomatoes. Flavor with a little salt and red pepper flakes. Serve with buttered toast. Simple and delicious.

WEEK TWO LUNCH IDEAS (WEEKDAYS AND WEEKEND)

Sandwiches and salads are so easy to prepare and transport. Here are seven for the week.

Potato Salad: Just make it the way you always have, using eggless mayonnaise.

Sloppy Joe Sandwich: See recipe on page 100. Delicious and filling, it's best on a hearty bun.

Sloppy Col Sandwich: A fresh, healthful version of a Sloppy Joe; see page 103 for the actual recipe.

Cannellini Bean Salad with Fresh Herbs: See page 107 for recipe. Bring along a small green salad as well.

Hummus Wrap: Along the lines of the Sloppy Col Sandwich, this wrap is so easy to whip up before leaving the house for the day. Spread hummus on tortillas or lavash, then add roasted red peppers or even beans or any favorite raw veggies. Roll up burrito-style.

Caesar Salad with Croutons: Add sautéed tofu or Tempeh Bacon (page 77) to the recipe on page 133 for a heartier meal. Pair with your favorite canned or homemade soup.

Sesame Soba Noodles with Shredded Vegetables: Make the night before from the recipe on page 104, and let marinate in the fridge. Serve with salted edamame and miso soup.

WEEK TWO DINNER IDEAS (WEEKDAYS)

Another week of ideas to help guide you.

Simple Bean Burritos: So easy and transportable. Check out the recipe on page 166.

Polenta Squares: Prepare in fifteen minutes in the morning, and let it set up during the day. All you need to do when you come home from work is to fry it up (or bake it). Serve with marinara sauce and a large green salad. Recipe on page 228.

Split Pea Soup: Prepare the night before so all you have to do is heat it up. See recipe on page 233. Serve with salad and Drop Biscuits (page 259).

Chickpea Burgers with Tahini Sauce: Page 164. Serve with salad, french fries, or Kale Chips (recipe on page 232).

BBQ Tofu and Cannellini Bean Salad: Marinate extra-firm tofu (preferably frozen and thawed—see "Day 21: Demystifying Tofu") in your favorite bottled BBQ sauce, and bake in a 350-degree oven until the tofu is heated through and the sauce is cooked into it. Serve with a green salad and Cannellini Bean Salad with Fresh Herbs on page 107.

WEEK TWO DINNER IDEAS (WEEKEND)

Garlic and Greens Soup: One of my staple recipes (page 231), this soup is incredibly healthful and a perfect meal served with a crusty bread or the Drop Biscuits on page 259.

Creamy Macaroni and Cheese with Field Roast Sausages: See page 43 for more about Field Roast and page 134 for mac and cheese recipe. Serve with a large green salad.

WEEK THREE BREAKFAST IDEAS (WEEKDAYS)

Overwhelmed by the variety yet? Here are seven more weekday and weekend ideas.

Frozen Waffles with Maple Syrup and Fresh Fruit: Many brands now make vegan waffles; you'll have the best chance of finding them in a large natural foods store.

Fruit Smoothie: My favorite breakfast in the warmer months. Check out the variations on page 83.

English Muffin: See page 44 for a vegan version. Spread on preserves and your favorite nut butter.

Breakfast Polenta: Using the grain chart on page 52, whip up some creamy polenta. Flavor and top with nuts, dried fruit, and your favorite sweetener.

Nondairy Yogurt and Fruit: Try another brand or another flavor.

WEEK THREE BREAKFAST IDEAS (WEEKEND)

Mushroom Scramble: Chop up your favorite mushrooms and sauté them in some non-dairy butter or oil. Add some chard or spinach, and serve on top of toast and alongside a fresh fruit salad and/or roasted tomatoes.

Cinnamon Coffee Cake: Though this could easily be made during the week since it takes virtually no time at all to prepare, it is definitely a special breakfast to wake up to on a Sunday morn with the cinnamon aroma filling the air. Recipe on page 176.

WEEK THREE LUNCH IDEAS (WEEKDAYS AND WEEKEND)

Aside from leftovers from dinner, here are some more ideas for both weekday and weekend lunches.

Better-Than-Egg Salad: Make the easy recipe on page 97, and bring with you to work or on a picnic as a salad or as a sandwich on a roll or in a pita pocket.

Taco Salad: Add a can of pinto beans (or any bean you prefer) to a pot with ¼ cup water, add some corn kernels and kale leaves, and stir in some chili powder, cumin, and salt. Cook for about 10 minutes until it starts to thicken, adding more water, if necessary. Eat right away, or transfer to a container to take with you on the road. Serve with tortilla chips or taco shells and salsa.

English Muffin Pizzas: Toast some Rudi's English Muffins, then add pizza sauce, some shredded veggies, and/or some shredded vegan cheese. Bake until the cheese melts, and either serve right away or wrap up to take on the road.

Tempeh Bacon, Lettuce, and Tomato Sandwich: Prepare the Tempeh Bacon on page 77, and build a sandwich with lettuce, eggless mayonnaise, and tomato slices.

Grain Salad: Using the chart on page 52, build your own grain salad using grains, veggies, and dressings from each column.

Green Salad: Green salads should be in your daily rotation, which is why it bears repeating here. For variety, use chard or kale as your base or at least dispersed throughout the other greens. Make it hearty with lots of raw veggies, beans, and even croutons.

Veggie Sub Sandwich: Build a veggie sandwich on a hearty sub roll; add veggie lunch meats, if desired. Add shredded lettuce, mustard, oil, and vinegar, and prepare to be stuffed. Serve with Kale Chips recipe on page 232.

WEEK THREE DINNER IDEAS (WEEKDAYS)

Realistically, on at least one weeknight, you'll be eating leftovers, calling the pizza guy and ordering a custom-made vegan pizza (no cheese, lots of veggies and fresh herbs), or eating some meals in a restaurant or at a friend's house. Still, here are some suggestions to provide a little extra inspiration.

Vegetable Stir-Fry: Slice some veggies, cube some tofu, and sauté them with a bottled stir-fry sauce (ginger, peanut, sesame). Serve with brown rice or quinoa.

Frozen Pizza with a Green Salad: Tofutti, Amy's, and Tofurky make great vegan pizzas that can be heated up in no time. Make sure you eat a big green salad first.

Baked Potato: A favorite in many homes, choose yellow varieties, such as Yukon Gold, or just poke some holes in a sweet potato, and throw in a 350-degree oven until crispy on the outside and tender on the inside. Serve with nondairy butter, or pile on sautéed or roasted veggies or even salsa. A green salad is always an essential accompaniment.

Ensalada de Frijoles: With the addition of some brown rice (which you've made in advance), this salad couldn't be easier to prepare. Open a can of black beans and rinse. In a large bowl, toss together the rice, beans, corn kernels (thawed if using frozen), 1 chopped bell pepper, 1 chopped tomato, and your favorite salsa. Serve over a bed of greens or with tortillas.

Pasta and Pesto: Cook your favorite pasta, and toss with Basil Pesto (page 131). Add chopped tomatoes for added nutrition.

WEEK THREE DINNER IDEAS (WEEKEND)

African Sweet Potato and Peanut Stew: Serve over quinoa, couscous, or your favorite rice. See recipe on page 161.

Butternut Squash Risotto with Toasted Sage: Risotto is so much easier to make than most people think, but I still thought it would be more appropriate for the weekend. See recipe on page 249.

WEEK FOUR BREAKFAST IDEAS (WEEKDAYS)

Fruit Smoothie: Choose from the three on page 83.

Bagel with Nondairy Cream Cheese: Tofutti and Follow Your Heart brands are widely available. Or use nondairy butter and your favorite nut butter.

Barley Porridge: While the barley is cooking (see page 52 for grain-cooking chart), stir in some brown sugar, raisins, and cinnamon. When thick, pour into bowls, add some nondairy milk, and top with walnuts and ground flaxseeds.

Sliced Banana with Nut Butter: One of my favorite simple breakfasts. You can use peanut butter or almond butter—and throw in a sliced apple or pear for good measure.

Baked Apples: Slice up an apple or two (don't peel), and add to a pot with ¼ cup nondairy milk. Add brown sugar, cinnamon, and a touch of nutmeg. Cook for 10 minutes until the apples soften a bit, and serve topped with toasted nuts, granola, and raisins. Add a bit more nondairy milk if desired.

WEEK FOUR BREAKFAST IDEAS (WEEKEND)

Drop Biscuits with Jam or Gravy: Make the Drop Biscuits on page 259, and serve with your favorite preserves or—in the spirit of an old southern standby—with Mushroom Gravy (page 252).

Breakfast Burrito with Home Fries: Either make it bean-based just like a typical lunch-time burrito, or roll up your Tofu Scramble (page 80) in a flour or corn tortilla along with salsa, chopped avocado, and lettuce.

WEEK FOUR LUNCH IDEAS (WEEKDAYS AND WEEKEND)

Better-Than-Chicken Sandwich: See recipe on page 97.

Corn and Tomato Salad: Use thawed frozen or fresh corn. Toss with a diced tomato, fresh herbs, chopped red onion, some balsamic vinegar, salt and pepper, and a touch of olive oil.

Rolled Collard Leaves: Spread peanut or almond butter on raw (rinsed and patted dry) collard leaves, and roll up. Alternatively, you can use hummus, add a thin layer of roasted red peppers and alfalfa sprouts, and roll up.

Macaroni Salad: Cook up some elbow macaroni, and toss with eggless mayonnaise, chopped carrots, chopped bell pepper, and chopped celery. Add salt and pepper to taste.

Avocado and Tomato Sandwich: Add whole basil leaves, lettuce, and Muhammara (see page 227).

BBQ Tempeh Sandwich: Steam up some tempeh slices, transfer to a glass dish, and cover with BBQ sauce. Bake for 30 minutes at 350 degrees to allow the tempeh to absorb the sauce. Serve on a hearty bun.

Kale Salad: My favorite kale salads are made with curly kale and Lacinato (dinosaur). Pull leaves from stem, rinse, and pat dry. Transfer to a large bowl and massage for about 5 minutes to tenderize the kale. Add some cauliflower slices, shredded carrots, and any of your favorite vegetables, thinly sliced. Toss with some orange juice, seasoned rice vinegar or apple cider vinegar, and agave nectar. Sprinkle with salt.

WEEK FOUR DINNER IDEAS (WEEKDAYS)

Roasted Vegetables: One of my favorite meals is just a huge plate of roasted veggies. Take ten minutes before you leave for work to chop all the veggies you want to roast—potatoes, cauliflower (yes, cauliflower), Brussels sprouts, asparagus—and store them in the fridge until you get home. (Chopped potatoes should be stored in water.) When you come home, before you take your coat off, preheat the oven to 450 degrees. Toss the veggies with just enough olive oil to coat them, sprinkle on some salt and pepper, and place them on a baking sheet. Transfer to the hot oven and cook until the veggies are crisp on the outside and tender on the inside. Serve with a big salad or a main dish such as tofu, tempeh, seitan, or mushrooms.

Veggie Dogs and Potato Puffs: Make tonight's dinner quick and dirty. Serve hot dogs in buns with relish, ketchup, onions, and mustard, and heat up some frozen potato puffs or "tater tots," or whatever they're called in your area. Cascadian Farms makes my favorite.

Stuffed Shells: Make the tofu ricotta from the Hearty Lasagna on page 137, and stuff into pasta shells. Cover with tomato sauce and bake. Serve with garlic bread and a large salad.

Mediterranean Meal: Make Muhammara on page 227, slice up a baguette, and cut up some carrots, celery, and a bell pepper. Open a can of white beans (cannellini, great northern, etc.) and rinse and drain. Add to a pot with ¼ cup water, and add salt and ¼ to ½ teaspoon rubbed sage. Cook until the beans thicken, mashing them as they cook. Spread some Muhammara on the baguette and top with the white beans. Serve with olives and raw veggies.

Carrot-Ginger Soup: This is one of my go-to recipes; it's been a staple in my home for years. It's silky smooth and takes very little time to prepare. If you're following my suggestions for prepping in advance, then you will already have your carrots, onions, garlic, and potatoes prepared, so you can just throw it all together when you get home. Recipe is on page 226.

WEEK FOUR DINNER IDEAS (WEEKEND)

Thai Curry with Vegetables: Make green, red, yellow, or Massaman curry with the curry pastes and coconut milks you've stocked your cupboards with. Use a variety of favorite vegetables, extra-firm tofu, and even canned bamboo shoots. Garnish with some Thai basil and serve over brown rice.

Harvest-Stuffed Acorn Squash: Perfect for the autumnal months or for a Thanksgiving dinner, this is a beautiful centerpiece and delicious main dish. See recipe on page 254.

WINTER HOLIDAY MENU IDEAS

Check out "Day 25: Celebrating the Holidays" for some menu ideas for such autumnal holidays as Thanksgiving. In addition, consider using the following recipes for fall and winter feasts:

- Caesar Salad (page 133)
- Garlic and Greens Soup (page 231)
- Carrot-Ginger Soup (page 226)
- African Sweet Potato and Peanut Stew (page 161)
- Butternut Squash Risotto with Toasted Sage (page 249)
- Harvest-Stuffed Acorn Squash (page 254)
- Polenta Squares (page 228)
- Hearty Lasagna (page 137)
- Marinated Portobello Mushroom Steaks (page 99)
- Drop Biscuits (page 259)
- Mushroom Gravy (page 252)
- Herbed Scalloped Potatoes (page 138)
- Roasted Brussels Sprouts with Caramelized Onions and Toasted Pistachios (page 255)
- Oatmeal Raisin Cookies (page 180)
- Apple Cobbler (page 256)
- Pecan Balls (page 173)

Resources and Recommendations

Here are a number of resources for your edification and enjoyment, organized by the chapters in *The 30-Day Vegan Challenge*. Feel free to visit my store at www.compassionate cooks.com to purchase my favorite books, kitchen tools, and videos and find many more recommendations and resources.

WELCOME TO POSITIVE CHANGE

These experts specialize in the fields of research and treatment of preventable diseases. Many of them have several seminal books, which you can find on their websites.

Caldwell Esselstyn, M.D., heartattackproof.com
Dr. T. Colin Campbell, tcolincampbell.org
John Robbins, johnrobbins.info
Jack Norris, R.D., veganhealth.org
Vesanto Melina, R.D., nutrispeak.com
John McDougall, M.D., drmcdougall.com
Michael Greger, M.D., drgreger.org
Michael Klaper, M.D., vegsource.com/klaper
Dr. Joel Fuhrman, drfuhrman.com
Dr. Pam Popper, wellnessforum.com
Physicians Committee for Responsible Medicine, pcrm.org
World Peace Diet, worldpeacediet.com
Rip Esselstyn, engine2diet.com
Brenda Davis, R.D., brendadavisrd.com
Becoming Vegan by Brenda Davis and Vesanto Melina is *the* bible of vegan nutrition, and their new book, *Becoming Raw,* will demystify the questions around raw diets.

KNOW YOUR NUMBERS

In addition to the blood and urine panel you'll get from your doctor, visit b12.com for the most accurate testing of your vitamin B_{12} levels.

The Vitamin D Council has partnered with ZRT Labs to make a discounted take-home vitamin D test kit that you can order at zrtlab.com/vitamindcouncil.

STOCKING A VEGAN KITCHEN

Earth Balance butter, earthbalancenatural.com

Whole Soy & Co. yogurt, wholesoyco.com

Turtle Mountain/So Delicious yogurt, ice cream, and coconut milk beverage, turtle mountain.com

Ricera yogurt, ricerafoods.com

Wildwood Organics yogurt, milk, tofu, tempeh, and tofu burgers, pulmuonewildwood .com

Amande almond-milk yogurt, cascadefresh.com

Follow Your Heart eggless mayonnaise (Vegenaise), cream cheese, and Vegan Gourmet cheese, followyourheart.com

Nasoya tofu and eggless mayonnaise (Nayonaise), nasoya.com

Tofurky deli slices, sausages, franks, pizza, tempeh bacon, jerky, and Tofurky roast, tofurky.com

Field Roast deli slices, sausages, cutlets, and meat loaf, fieldroast.com

Gardein meatless meals and meats, gardein.com

Yves deli slices, franks, and sausages, yvesveggie.com

Match Meat sausages and ground meatless meats, matchmeats.com

Rudi's Organic Bakery sliced breads, rudisbakery.com

Chicago Soydairy Temptations ice cream and Dandies vegan marshmallows, chicago soydairy.com

Sweet and Sara vegan marshmallows, sweetandsara.com

Soyatoo whipped cream (soy and rice versions), soyatoo.com

Visit peta.org/accidentallyVegan for more standard brands whose products happen to be vegan.

BREAKFAST IDEAS

Rudi's Organic Bakery bread, English muffins, buns, rolls, and bagels, rudisbakery .com

Tofutti cream cheese and sour cream, tofutti.com

Lightlife Gimme Lean sausage, Smart Bacon, and Smart Sausages, lightlife.com

LIFE AFTER CHEESE

Dr. Cow's Tree Nut Cheese, dr-cow.com

Sheese by Bute Island Foods, buteisland.com

Sunergia Soy Foods, sunergiasoyfoods.com

Parma in the Raw, eatintheraw.com
Galaxy Nutritional Foods, galaxyfoods.com
Daiya, daiyafoods.com
Chicago Soydairy (Tecse), chicagosoydairy.com
Redwood Foods (Cheezly), redwoodfoods.es
Follow Your Heart, followyourheart.com

PLANT-BASED MILKS

There are almost too many brands to name, but here are a few.

Soymilks: Wildwood (pulmuonewildwood.com), Earth Balance (earthbalancenatural
.com), Eden Soy (edenfoods.com), Soy Dream (imaginefoods.com), Vitasoy (vitasoy
.com), Whole Foods 365 (wholefoods.com)
Almond milks: Almond Breeze (bluediamond.com), Pacific Foods (pacificfoods.com), Al-
mond Dream (tastethedream.com), Whole Foods 365
Rice milks: Rice Dream (imaginefoods.com), Pacific Foods
Hemp milks: Tempt Living Harvest (livingharvest.com), Hemp Bliss by Manitoba Harvest (manitobaharvest.com), Pacific Foods
Coconut milk (beverage and creamer): So Delicious by Turtle Mountain (turtlemountain
.com)
Coffee creamers: MimicCreme (mimiccreme.com), Silk Creamers (silksoymilk.com),
Wildwood, Trader Joe's
Vegan dry milk powders: Better Than Milk Vegan Beverage Mix, Soy (Original, Vanilla,
and Light) and Better Than Milk Vegan Beverage Mix, Rice (Original and Light)—buy
at veganessentials.com

ATHLETES

Protein powders: Nutiva hemp-based (nutiva.com), Nutribiotic rice-based (nutribiotic
.com), Vega pea protein (myvega.com)
Resources and community for vegan athletes: Organic Athlete (organicathlete.org),
Brendan Brazier (brendanbrazier.com), Vegan Body Building (veganbodybuilding
.com)

VEGAN DOG FOOD AND TREATS

V-Dog, vdog.com
Evolution Diet, petfoodshop.com
Natural Life Pet Products, nlpp.com
Natural Balance, naturalbalanceinc.com
Nature's Recipe, naturesrecipe.com

Pet Guard, petguard.com
Wow Bow Distributors, wow-bow.com
Boston Baked Bonz, bostonbakedbonz.com
Vegan Cats (for supplements, info, and dog food), vegancats.com

SUPPLEMENTS

Dr. Fuhrman, drfuhrman.com, for multivitamin, vitamin D, DHA Purity, and other supplements for various stages of life (also sold through compassionatecooks.com)
O-Mega Zen3 and other supplements sold by NuTru, nutru.com
DEVA Omega-3 DHA, devanutrition.com
VegLife sold in various online stores

FINDING HARMONY IN A MIXED HOUSEHOLD

vegfamily.com
vegetarianbaby.com
vegetarianteen.com
The Teen's Vegetarian Cookbook by Judy Krizmanic
Help! My Child Has Stopped Eating Meat! by Carol Adams

BOOKS FOR VEGAN CHILDREN

A Turkey for Thanksgiving by Eve Bunting
Herb the Vegetarian Dragon by Jules Bass and Debbie Harter
'Twas the Night Before Thanksgiving by Dav Pilkey
Victor's Picnic and *Victor, the Vegetarian* by Radha Vignola
Benji Bean Sprout Doesn't Eat Meat by Sarah Rudy
This Is Why We Don't Eat Animals by Ruby Roth
Our Farm: By the Animals of Farm Sanctuary by Maya Gottfried

BEARING WITNESS—RECOMMENDED READING

More and more books continue to be published about the plights of animals bred and killed for food and the system that makes it possible. Here are a few of my favorites.

Diet for a New America: How Your Food Choices Affect Your Health, Happiness and the Future of Life on Earth by John Robbins
An Unnatural Order: Roots of Our Destruction of Nature by Jim Mason
Animal Liberation by Peter Singer
Slaughterhouse: The Shocking Story of Greed, Neglect, and Inhumane Treatment Inside the U.S. Meat Industry by Gail Eisnitz

Mad Cowboy: Plain Truth from the Cattle Rancher Who Won't Eat Meat by Howard Lyman

Dominion: The Power of Man, the Suffering of Animals, and the Call to Mercy by Matthew Scully

For the Prevention of Cruelty: The History and Legacy of Animal Rights Activism in the United States by Diane Beers

Food Politics: How the Food Industry Influences Nutrition and Health by Marion Nestle

Vegan Outreach and their pamphlets, *Why Vegan, Even if You Like Meat,* and *Guide to Cruelty-free Eating*

Why We Love Dogs, Eat Pigs, and Wear Cows: An Introduction to Carnism by Melanie Joy, Ph.D.

RECOMMENDED VIEWING

The people who work undercover to get footage of the plights of animals are unsung heroes, and the best way we can honor their work is to view what they have documented via video, audio, and still photos. Many animal organizations have videos of undercover investigations available to view on their websites. Please visit hsus.org, farmsanctuary.org, mercyforanimals.org, cok.net, and peta.org.

Earthlings by Shaun Monson of Nation Earth. Narrated by Joaquin Phoenix, *Earthlings* is an award-winning documentary film about the suffering of animals for food, fashion, pets, entertainment and medical research. Considered the most persuasive documentary ever made, *Earthlings* features 95 minutes of sensitive footage shot at animal shelters, pet stores, puppy mills, factory farms, slaughterhouses, the leather and fur trades, sporting events, circuses, and research labs. Available for free download (low-res) or in a high-resolution DVD for purchase in ten languages at earthlings .com.

Meet Your Meat by PETA. Though this short video contains footage I admit is difficult to watch, I think it is essential viewing for anyone who does or has eaten meat, dairy, and eggs. View at meetyourmeat.com.

The Witness by Tribe of Heart. In this award-winning documentary, Eddie Lama explains how he feared and avoided animals for most of his life, until the love of a kitten opened his heart, inspiring him to rescue abandoned animals, become a vegetarian, and ultimately to bring his message of compassion to the streets of New York. Purchase at tribeofheart.org.

Vegucated by kindgreenplanet.org.

EPILOGUE: BEYOND THE THIRTY DAYS

There are many ways to find like-minded folks in your area. Visit meetup.com and search for vegan and vegetarian groups near your city, or do a search online for vegetarian/vegan organizations, associations, and social events such as "vegan drinks" in your area.

AUTHOR'S WEBSITES

colleenpatrickyoudream.com (*main website*)

30dayveganchallenge.com (*30-Day Vegan Challenge*)

vegetarianfoodforthought.com (podcast)

joyofveganbaking.com (*Joy of Vegan Baking* cookbook)

vegantable.com (*Vegan Table* cookbook)

colormevegan.com (*Color Me Vegan* cookbook)

vegansdailycompanion.com (*Vegan's Daily Companion* book)

joyfulvegan.wordpress.com (*Joyful Vegan* blog)

Acknowledgments

The making of a book starts with a seed that grows with the help of many hands, and I'm incredibly thankful for everyone who helped my idea for this book germinate, take root, and blossom.

First and foremost, thank you to my husband, David Goudreau, my beautiful partner in life, love, laughter, compassion, and dance! Every day with you is better than the one before.

Thanks to my friend Patti Breitman, whose own abundant workload turned into a blessing for me when she introduced me to Carole Bidnick, the best agent a girl could dream of. Carole's enthusiasm for this book was immediate, and she expertly guided it from inception to birth with unwavering zeal and seasoned expertise. Looking for an advocate for my book, I also gained a friend in Carole, and for that I am grateful.

My top-notch editor, Marnie Cochran, never missed a beat from the moment she laid eyes on the proposal. I can't imagine a more skilled, passionate, or diligent editor. Her regard for my vision made the process truly collaborative and resulted in the gorgeous book we envisioned from the start. In short, everyone I've worked with at Ballantine Books has been a dream.

Thanks also to Carole for recommending Sara Remington, the most delightful, professional, talented photographer of people, food, and animals! Her crack team of stylists and assistants made our cover shoot and food shoot unforgettably delightful—from food stylist Katie Christ and food stylist assistant Lillian Kang to prop stylist Nissa Quanstrom, camera assistants Kass Medeiros and Annie Martin to people stylist Tietjen Fischer and my much-adored and perpetual laugh stylist Michael Scribner.

When it comes to gathering the most accurate, up-to-date, unbiased nutrition information, it doesn't get better than Brenda Davis, R.D., who is tirelessly committed to empowering people to live compassionately and healthfully. The time, energy, generosity, and thoughtfulness Brenda brought to this book are beyond measure, as she scrupulously and expertly ensured that every word, every detail, every fact lived up to the high standards we both seek to reflect in our work. I revere her as a colleague and adore her as a friend.

Many beloved colleagues and friends generously gave (and continue to give!) their precious time and input, including Michael Greger, Melanie Joy, Robin Brande, Chris Marco, Amanda Mitchell, and Michael Scribner. I value their perspective, intuition, and expertise so very much, and I've quite come to rely on their advice and support. I hope I am able to give them back all that they give me. Thanks also to Lauren Ornelas, Lisa Shapiro, and John and Mary McDougall for all their help making connections.

I'm blessed to be surrounded by so many loving friends (including those named above) and supportive family members, especially Diane Miller, Cadry Nelson, David Busch, Kenda Swartz, Kristin Schwarz, Shad Clark, Abby Kaster, Cheri and Mark Arellano, John Keathley, Randy Lind, Cathleen Young, Stephanie Arthur, Deborah Underwood, Rae Sikora, Pam Webb, Ryan Thibodaux, Poppy Nguyen, mom Arlene, dad John, and parents-by-marriage, Mary Jane and Paul.

I'm kept sane and productive by a number of people who lovingly donate their time and skills to help me accomplish my mission, particularly Amanda Mitchell, Tami Hiltz, Jennifer Stadtmiller, Juliet Lynn, Aaron Weinstein, Stephen and Danielle Tschirhart, Brett Renville, and Blake Wiers.

I am so incredibly grateful to have the honor and privilege of hearing from so many remarkable people whose eyes and hearts have been opened and who let me be part of their journey. Thank you to anyone who has ever listened to my podcast, read my books, used my recipes, watched my videos, attended my talks, or shared with me your story. You are the reason I awaken with hope every day. Thank you to each and every person who uses his or her voice to speak for those who have no voice. Whether you do it formally as part of a larger organization or on your own as a grassroots activist, every seed you plant contributes to the compassionate world we all envision.

What a blessing it is to live in the company of cats, who bring me immense joy every moment of every day. I cherish every second I get to spend with Schuster, our magical feline boy of eighteen years, and Charlie, our little two-year-young monkey cat. Simon and Cassandra continue to live in our hearts.

My greatest inspirations are the nonhuman animals of the world, and I dedicate my work to them. My hope is that we can navigate through this world and our lives with the grace and integrity of those who most need our protection. May we have the sense of humor and liveliness of the goats; may we have the maternal instincts and protective nature of the hens and the sassiness of the roosters. May we have the gentleness and strength of the cattle, and the wisdom, humility, and serenity of the donkeys. May we appreciate the need for community as do the sheep and choose our companions as carefully as do the rabbits. May we have the faithfulness and commitment to family of the geese, the adaptability and affability of the ducks. May we have the intelligence, loyalty, and affection of the pigs and the inquisitiveness, sensitivity, and playfulness of the turkeys.

My hope is that we can learn from the animals what we need to become better people.

Index

protein bars/shakes, 167
protein powders, 156

quesadillas, 130
quinoa, 41, 185

rabbits, 187
raw foods, 221-22
reading labels, 53-56
recipes, 6, 28
    African Sweet Potato and
      Peanut Stew, 160-61
    Apple Cobbler, 256
    Banana Chocolate Chip
      Muffins, 174-75
    Basil Pesto, 131
    Bean Chili, 158
    Better-Than-Chicken Salad,
      90, 97
    Better-Than-Egg Salad, 90,
      97, 211
    Better-Than-Tuna Salad, 90,
      162-63
    Blueberry Pancakes, 82
    Butternut Squash Risotto with
      Toasted Sage, 249
    Caesar Salad, 132-33, 213
    Cannellini Bean Salad with
      Fresh Herbs, 92, 106-7
    Carrot-Ginger Soup, 226
    Cashew Cheese, 127
    Charoset, 245, 257
    Chickpea Burgers with Tahini
      Sauce, 164-65
    Chocolate Cake, 48, 178-79
    Chocolate Frosting, 182
    Chocolate Mousse, 216-17
    Cinnamon Coffee Cake, 176-77
    Creamy Macaroni and Cheese,
      134-35
    Drop Biscuits, 48, 243, 258-59
    French Toast, 78-79
    Fresh Strawberry Pie with
      Chocolate Chunks, 234
    Fruit Smoothie Trio, 83-84
    Garlic and Greens Soup, 49,
      230-31
    Harvest-Stuffed Acorn Squash,
      254
    Hearty Lasagna, 136-37, 212
    Herbed Scalloped Potatoes,
      138-39
    Homemade Hummus, 159
    Kale Chips, 232, 275

    Marinated Portobello
      Mushroom Steaks, 91,
      98-99
    Muhammara, 49, 227
    Mushroom Gravy, 243, 252-53
    Oatmeal Raisin Cookies,
      180-81
    Orange-Ginger Vinaigrette,
      215
    Pecan Balls, 173
    Polenta Squares, 228-29
    Quick (No-Queso) Quesadillas,
      130
    Roasted Brussels Sprouts with
      Caramelized Onions and
      Toasted Pistachios, 49, 255
    Sesame Soba Noodles with
      Shredded Vegetables,
      104-5
    Simple Bean Burritos, 166
    Sloppy Col Sandwich, 102-3
    Sloppy Joes, 100-101
    Split Pea Soup, 233
    Tempeh Bacon, 77, 91, 120
    Tempeh Pâté, 250-51
    Thai Salad, 214-15
    Tofu Scramble, 80-81, 211
red food, 224-25, 227, 234, 246
rennet/rennin, 56, 207-9
resources, 306-12
restaurant meals, 47, 85-89
    communicating your desires,
      87-89
    international foods, 85-86
rice, 41, 157
    milk, 151
    risotto, 249
    stuffing, 254

salads/salad dressings, 35, 86,
    213
    Better-Than salads, 90, 93, 97,
      162-63
    Caesar, 132-33, 213
    cannellini salad, 92, 106-7
    green salad, 93, 277
    low-cal dressings, 277
    noodle salad, 93, 104-5
    one-dish salads, 92-94, 104-7
    orange-ginger vinaigrette, 215
    pasta salad, 92
    potato salad, 93
    taco salad, 93
    Thai, 214-15

Salley, John, 167
salmon, 188
salmonella, 4
salsa, 35
salt, 120, 125
salt coagulants, 209
sandwiches/wraps, 86, 90-92
    nut butters, 90-91
    recipes, 97-103
    spreads, 92
saturated fats, 4
sauces, 35
    barbecue sauce, 38
    pesto, 126, 131
    tahini, 38, 164
    tamari soy sauce, 38, 120, 219
scalloped potatoes, 138-39
schedules, 71, 108-9
Schweitzer, Albert, viii
scrambles, 74, 80-81, 91, 211
Seder plates, 245-46, 257
seeds, 95
    butters, 38
    egg substitutes, 169
    fiber, 222
    iron, 185
    omega-3 fatty acids, 189-91,
      200
    protein, 157
seitan, 119
selenium, 201-3
Shakespeare, William, 61
shea butter, 10
shearling, 282
sherbet, 44, 86
shiitake mushrooms, 120
shoes, 281-84
shopping
    grocery store layouts, 57-59
    label information, 53-56
    lists, 50
    See also costs; staples
silk, 286
silken tofu, 58, 170, 209, 210-11
skin health, 5
skipping meals, 75-76
slicing/spreading cheeses, 127
sloppy-joe style sandwiches, 91,
    100-103
smartphone apps, 115
smoked peppers, 120
smoothies, 72, 83-84, 96, 110,
    275
snacks, 94-96, 277

ABOUT THE AUTHOR

Raised on a typical American diet of meat, dairy, and eggs, Colleen Patrick-Goudreau was moved to change when she read *Diet for a New America* at nineteen. No longer able to justify eating animals and their "products," Colleen began a journey of discovery that continues to this day.

For over eleven years, Colleen Patrick-Goudreau has guided people to becoming and staying vegan through sold-out cooking classes, bestselling books, inspiring lectures, engaging videos, and her immensely popular audio podcast, "Vegetarian Food for Thought." Using her unique blend of passion, humor, and common sense, she empowers and inspires people to live according to their own values of compassion and wellness.

With a master's degree in English literature and a command of traditional and new media, Colleen is an exhilarating speaker, a powerful writer, a talented chef, and a persuasive advocate, whose success can be measured by the thousands of people whose lives have been changed by her compassionate message.

The award-winning author of five books, including the bestselling *The Joy of Vegan Baking, The Vegan Table, Color Me Vegan,* and *Vegan's Daily Companion,* Colleen also contributes to National Public Radio and *The Christian Science Monitor* and has appeared on the Food Network and PBS.

She lives with her husband and feline boys in the San Francisco Bay area. Visit her at colleenpatrickgoudreau.com.

Colleen Patrick-Goudreau is available for select readings and lectures. To inquire about a possible appearance, please contact the Random House Speakers Bureau at rhspeakers@randomhouse.com.